Life Before Birth

Life Before Birth

The Moral and Legal Status of Embryos and Fetuses

SECOND EDITION ■

BONNIE STEINBOCK

OXFORD
UNIVERSITY PRESS

5/20/15
WW
$41.95

OXFORD
UNIVERSITY PRESS

Published in the United States of America by Oxford University Press, Inc.,
198 Madison Avenue, New York, NY, 10016
United States of America

Oxford University Press, Inc., publishes works that further Oxford University's
objective of excellence in research, scholarship, and education

Oxford is a registered trade mark of Oxford University Press
in the UK and in certain other countries

© Oxford University Press, Inc. 2011, 1992

First Edition published in 1992

Library of Congress Cataloging-in-Publication Data

Steinbock, Bonnie, author.
   Life before birth : the moral and legal status of embryos and fetuses / Bonnie Steinbock. — Second Edition.
      p. ; cm.
   Includes bibliographical references and index.
   ISBN 978-0-19-534162-1 (alk. paper)
1. Fetus—Legal status, laws, etc. 2. Abortion—Law and legislation.
3. Abortion—Moral and ethical aspects. 4. Fetus—Research—Moral and ethical aspects.
5. Prenatal care—Moral and ethical aspects. 6. Prenatal care—Law and legislation. I. Title.
[DNLM: 1. Fetus. 2. Abortion, Induced. 3. Embryo, Mammalian. 4. Legislation as Topic.
5. Morals. 6. Reproductive Techniques, Assisted. WQ 210]
K642.S74 2011   179.7'6—dc22

Typeset in Minion Pro Font
Printed on acid-free paper
Printed in the United States of America

For Sue and Ron
—my posse

CONTENTS

ACKNOWLEDGMENTS

As I said in the Acknowledgments in the first edition, I have been influenced by more people than I can name here. A second thank-you is due to those who improved the first edition. There are many more people whose work has influenced the second edition; many of them are given credit in the footnotes. I am especially grateful to David Boonin, David DeGrazia, and Jeff McMahan. Their writings on abortion have influenced my own thinking, and they have improved Chapter 2.

I thank David Shoemaker, who read all of Chapter 2 and made invaluable suggestions. I asked my son, Nick, to go through Chapter 3, to make sure I was accurate on the law. He did that, but much more. Like the former law review editor he is, he painstakingly tracked down every footnote, correcting errors and letting me know when my paraphrases were too close to the original wording. I cannot thank him enough. Although not a blood relative, Sean Philpott agreed to read Chapter 6. I am very grateful for his amazing editorial skills, including gently pointing out several places where there was a "flow" problem; that is, my arguments were opaque. Sean also prevented me from making several blunders on the science of stem cell research. (Any remaining mistakes are all his fault.)

The Hastings Center remains my professional "home away from home," and it has always been a source of inspiration for me. In particular, the project on Prenatal Testing for Disability gave me a much deeper understanding of the disability critique, which has informed my views on the nonidentity problem and procreative responsibility, and helped shape Chapter 5. Thanks to Erik Parens and Adrienne Asch for including me in the group, and to all of the group's members for animated conversations and abiding friendship.

I am especially indebted to the Rockefeller Foundation for giving me a scholarly residency at its Bellagio Center on Lake Como, Italy, in September and October 2008. The 4 weeks I spent there writing a draft of Chapter 6 were among the happiest and most productive of my life. To all of my Bellagio buddies, thank you for your inspiration, your friendship, and your support.

I thank my colleagues in the Department of Philosophy for providing such a collegial atmosphere. In particular, I thank Rachel Cohon and Ron McClamrock for helpful discussions over the years.

I thank my graduate students, especially Wes McMichael and Susan Parrillo, who engaged me and challenged me in an independent study in fall 2007 on the interest view. I am also grateful to the students in my Philosophy and Public Policy seminar in fall 2009, especially Leah Pelish, who really pressed me on my view that a pregnant woman could have obligations to her future child, while not having any obligations to the fetus per se. Those discussions found their way into and, I hope, improved Chapter 2.

The research necessary for this edition to be written could not have been done, or done so easily, without the terrific library supported provided by the University at Albany. The amount of material available at hand is truly amazing, and when it was necessary to use either the electronic delivery service or interlibrary loan, I received the material very quickly. Hats off to the superb UAlbany librarians!

I am also grateful to Paul Menzel for providing intellectual stimulation, being understanding when I was totally focused on writing, and for providing a wonderful atmosphere on Whidbey Island in which to work during the summers of 2009 and 2010.

Credit for the idea of writing a second edition goes to the editor of the first edition, Jeffrey House, while Peter Ohlin deserves credit for actually shepherding the project to completion. Antonio Orrantia, the production editor at Oxford University Press, and Viswanath Prasanna, the project manager assisting Mr. Orrantia, were professional, efficient, and very patient. I am very grateful to them, and to the entire production team.

As I noted in the Acknowledgments to the first edition, the book's impetus and theoretical framework were provided by the work of Joel Feinberg. His death in 2004 was a tremendous loss to philosophy, to the profession, and to me personally. I owe him more than I can say. I have also been influenced, as has virtually everyone writing on abortion, by Mary Anne Warren, and mourn her untimely death on August 9, 2010.

The idea to do a new edition of this book came from my editor, Jeff House. At first reluctant (on a "been there, done that" basis), I eventually came to the conclusion that such a project was well worth doing. A great deal has happened since 1992, when the first edition of this book was published. Some of the issues covered in the first edition, such as abortion and maternal–fetal conflict, are still sources of controversy. Assisted reproduction, which I addressed in combination with embryo research in the first edition, now has a chapter to itself, while stem cell research, not in existence when the first edition was written, has a new chapter all to itself. In addition to doing updates on the factual material, I have considered the philosophical literature that has amassed in the last 15 years, on topics ranging from abortion to the nonidentity problem.

Issues like abortion, maternal–fetal conflict, and embryonic stem cell research raise the question of the moral status of the unborn: Are embryos and fetuses part of the pregnant woman or are they persons? Are they sources of tissue, research tools, or "preborn children"? They also have legal implications. The U.S. Supreme Court's legalization of abortion in 1973 was based in part on the unborn's never having been recognized in law as a full legal person. At the same time, fetuses have been considered as persons for the purposes of insurance coverage, wrongful-death suits, and vehicular homicide statutes. The legal status of the unborn thus appears to vary from jurisdiction to jurisdiction, from context to context, according to our purposes.

Medical and technological advances have compounded confusion over the status of the unborn. The threshold of viability—the point at which the fetus can survive outside the womb—has been pushed back into the second trimester of pregnancy. The same fetus might be a candidate for legal abortion and aggressive life-saving intervention. The emergence of perinatology and fetal surgery has made the fetus a patient in its own right. While such surgery is regarded as miraculous by couples whose unborn babies would otherwise certainly die, it is also troubling, because it creates the potential for conflict with the pregnant woman. A few courts have authorized compulsory cesarean sections, where this was deemed necessary to preserve the life or health of the fetus. Some commentators have suggested that, as in utero surgery becomes standard treatment, it could be legally imposed on pregnant women for the sake of the unborn, even though women currently have the right to choose abortion up until viability, between 24 and 28 weeks gestation. (This too is under attack. For example, Nebraska has a law banning abortion after 20 weeks, in clear contradiction to *Roe v. Wade*.)

In short, there seem to be inconsistencies, both in morality and the law, in our attitudes toward and treatment of the unborn. Some consider this evidence of confusion, or even hypocrisy. A politician once dismissed an antismoking campaign that emphasized the effects of cigarette smoking on fetuses. With heavy sarcasm, he said, "Yet the anti-smoking lobby doesn't oppose abortion, which I suppose is also detrimental to fetal health."

This book is an attempt to show that at least some of these alleged inconsistencies and contradictions can be dispelled. The key is a theory of moral status—that is, a theory about which kinds of beings can be the object of moral concern. The question of moral status is fundamental to all of the aforementioned issues. None of them can be resolved, or even adequately understood, without a plausible account of moral status. Consider, for example, an issue that often comes up during the abortion debate—namely, religion. Those who defend the right to abortion often argue that the state has no right to impose the religious views of one group on all citizens. This presupposes the fetus's lack of moral standing, and so it will be regarded as question-begging by those who believe that abortion violates the unborn's right to life.

In Chapter 1, I present a theory of moral status, "the interest view." In subsequent chapters, I apply this theory to problems involving embryos and fetuses. However, I do not restrict myself to the status of the unborn in the first chapter, because I want to present a general theory of moral status. The reason for giving a general theory is to avoid "cooking the evidence." That is, the theory should not be driven by the purposes to which it is put. It should be independently plausible. For this reason, I consider the implications of the interest view for animals, dead people, permanently unconscious people, and future generations, as well as for the unborn.

The basic idea of the interest view is that all and only beings who have interests have moral status. Chapter 1 explains and defends this thesis, and it gives an account of interests as conceptually connected with sentience (the ability to experience pain and pleasure) or conscious awareness. Mere things—rocks, planets, automobiles—are not conscious or sentient and so do not have interests. Nor do plants, although, unlike mere things, they are alive. Plants have their own natural growth and development, independent of human designs and purposes. However, plants lack interests because it does not matter to plants what is done to them. It is this notion of *mattering* that is key to moral status. Beings that have moral status must be capable of caring about what is done to them. They must be capable of being made, if only in a rudimentary sense, happy or miserable, comfortable or distressed. Whatever reasons we may have for preserving or protecting nonsentient beings, these reasons do not refer to their own interests. For without conscious awareness, beings cannot have interests. Without interests, they cannot have a welfare of their own. Without a welfare of their own, nothing can be done for their sake. Hence, they lack moral standing or status.

The exposition of the interest view in Chapter 1 is aimed primarily at philosophers. It not only presents the interest view but defends it against possible objections. This takes us into such rarified areas as the theory of belief and problems of identity. These issues are important to a thorough defense of the interest view, but they are unlikely to be of great interest to nonphilosophers, who can get a good enough idea of the interest view by reading the beginning of Chapter 1, stopping at the section titled "Is Consciousness Necessary for Interests?" and then skipping to the last section, "Potential People: Embryos and Fetuses." Some readers may be more inter-ested in the specific practical problems I discuss than in the underlying theory. This book should be of value to these readers as well. They are advised to skip Chapter 1 and go directly to the chapters where these problems are discussed. They will find enough of the interest view incorporated in the subsequent chapters to make the general approach clear.

My primary concern, however, is to develop a view that can help dispel some of the apparent inconsistencies in our attitudes toward the unborn. I think that the interest view is useful in this respect. For example, it explains why the right of recov-ery for prenatally inflicted injuries does not conflict with a right to abortion. If an abortion is performed before the fetus becomes sentient (probably toward the end of the second trimester), the fetus is killed, but not harmed, paradoxical as this may sound. For to be harmed is to have one's interests set back or thwarted. Without thoughts or feelings or awareness of any kind, the embryo or fetus has no interests. Without interests, it cannot be harmed. It has the potential to develop into the kind of being that will have interests, but, as I argue in Chapter 2, this potential does not give it the actual interests necessary for moral standing. We may choose to respect embryos and preconscious fetuses as powerful symbols of human life, but we cannot protect them for their own sake. Without interests, beings do not have a welfare of their own.

The idea that the unborn do not have legally protectable interests has a long history in Anglo-American law. Chapter 3 reviews the legal status of the unborn in areas outside abortion, considering such issues as prenatal torts and wrongful-death actions, the fetus as homicide victim, and wrongful-life suits. I believe that the inter-est view can help us develop a consistent, coherent legal conception of the unborn. This avoids a completely ad hoc approach that is intellectually unsatisfying, likely to generate cynicism, and incapable of offering guidance as new questions arise.

An important distinction, only relatively recently acknowledged by the courts, is between the fetus per se and the not-yet-born child. That is, although fetuses do not have legally protected interests, born children do. One of their important interests is an interest in healthy, unimpaired existence. Children who are born maimed may be condemned to a lifetime of suffering and limitation. Prenatal injury clearly harms such children. If the injury is due to negligent or intentional wrongdoing, they deserve to be compensated. Recognizing this, and allowing surviving children to recover damages for prenatal torts, poses no conflict with permitting abortion.

Along the same lines, we can reconcile abortion and maternal obligations to the unborn. The interests of preconscious fetuses do not have to be considered in the decision to abort, since preconscious fetuses do not have interests. However, if a woman decides not to abort, but to carry the fetus to term, she is morally required to think about the effects of her actions on the baby who will be born. Drinking heavily, smoking cigarettes, using crack cocaine—all of these can harm the child she bears, and therefore I claim in Chapter 4 that there is a prima facie moral obligation not to engage in these dangerous behaviors. Whether a woman should be blamed for the harm she causes her unborn child depends on the choices she had and the extent to which her behavior was free. Whether we should allow children to sue their moth-ers, whether we should jail pregnant drug users, or impose additional criminal pen-alties for drug use during pregnancy—these are far more complicated matters. They go beyond the interest principle, raising both philosophical and pragmatic questions.

How much intervention into people's lives should be tolerated? How successful are coercive measures likely to be in the protection of the "not-yet-born"?

Chapter 5, "Assisted Reproductive Technology," is almost entirely new. In this chapter, I outline the developments in assisted reproduction, as well as the challenges they pose. In particular, what obligations do prospective parents owe the children they bring into the world? What makes procreation responsible or irresponsible? What limits, if any, should society impose on attempts to procreate? My view, which I call "procreative responsibility," builds on the procreative liberty framework developed by John Robertson.

Chapter 6 is entirely new, as human embryonic stem cell research did not exist when I wrote the first edition of this book. The chapter addresses both adult and embryonic stem cell research, since one of the arguments against embryonic stem cell research is that it is unnecessary because adult stem cells (and induced pluripotent stem cells) provide an ethically acceptable alternative to destroying human embryos. The chapter also includes a discussion of cloning, since cloned human embryos might one day be a source of stem cells, and in the farther future, a huge advance in regenerative medicine. I discuss the possibility of reproductive cloning as well, since one of the arguments against "therapeutic" cloning is that it could lead to reproductive cloning.

It will by now be clear that while the interest view plays a fundamental role in finding answers to the dilemmas posed in this book, it is not the only factor. Matters like abortion, maternal–fetal conflict, assisted reproductive technologies, and stem cell research raise a host of issues, such as the function of the state and the proper province of law; the importance of privacy and the need for communal values; the role of women in society and the importance of the traditional family; and respect for human life and the deeply held moral or religious views of others. I will discuss these issues as they arise, but I will not do so on the basis of an overarching moral or political theory. Some philosophers may find this unsatisfactory, but I am not convinced that a basic moral theory is necessary for doing applied ethics. In this I am relieved to find myself aligned with Joel Feinberg, who freely confesses to the absence of a "deep structure" theory in his important work *Harm to Others*. "Progress on the penultimate questions," Feinberg notes, "need not wait for solutions to the ultimate ones."[1]

This book is not intended to give a startlingly original conception of the status of the unborn. Instead, it attempts to elicit a view that is implicit in our legal traditions and ordinary moral thinking. Some philosophers may find this disappointing. They would prefer a novel theory, however counterintuitive. I believe, however, that a view that is espoused by many different people who have all thought long and hard about a topic is more likely to be true, or at least plausible. I have found variations on the interest view in philosophical works, law review articles, and judicial opinions, and I have cited these where appropriate. In this book I hope to give the view a firmer grounding and to make it more plausible to those who remain unconvinced. My aim is to provide a theoretical basis for some of our intuitive judgments and convictions, which can also help us to reach answers to new problems in bioethics in a coherent and consistent way.

---

1. Joel Feinberg. 1984. *Harm to Others*. New York: Oxford University Press, p. 18.

The Interest View

Moral problems typically involve conflicts between parties. These conflicts often arise because the interests of the individuals clash or cannot be mutually satisfied. For example, smokers' interest in smoking where they please conflicts with non-smokers' interest in not being subjected to smoke. One factor relevant to a moral resolution of such conflicts is the relative importance of interests. Which is a more pressing claim: health or liberty? Equally important is the *moral standing* of the claimants. A being has moral standing if it counts, morally speaking; if its claims must be considered in moral deliberations, or from "the moral point of view."[1]

In the first edition of this book, I used the term "moral status" to refer to a being's having moral claims on us. However, I have become persuaded that there are two distinct aspects of moral considerability. A being is morally considerable if it has claims on our moral attention, if its interests must be considered from the moral point of view. We can refer to this aspect of moral considerability as having *moral standing*. A separate question is whether all beings that have moral standing count equally in moral deliberations. That is, given interests of equal seriousness or weight, do different characteristics of the being make its interests more important? We can refer to this aspect of moral considerability as *moral status*. That a being has moral standing tells us that its interests count; its moral status tells us how much those interests count. It may be that the right account accords all beings with moral standing equal moral status, or it may be that the right account accords beings with moral standing differential moral status. The distinction between moral standing and moral status enables us to address that substantive meta-ethical question.[2]

I believe that the correct account of moral standing is provided by "the interest view." The interest view maintains that the possession of interests is both necessary and sufficient for moral standing. In a sense, this is trivially true. To have moral standing is to be the sort of being whose interests must be considered from the moral point of view. Obviously, only beings with interests can have their interests considered. But the point is not trivial. The focus on interests requires us to consider the being itself—what is important to it—rather than what makes it valuable or

1. See Kurt Baier. 1965. *The Moral Point of View*. New York: Random House, especially Chapter Five.

2. I owe the distinction between moral standing and moral status to Allen Buchanan. 2009. "Moral Status and Human Enhancement," *Philosophy & Public Affairs* 37 (4): 346–381.

significant to others. Gold, for example, is valuable, but that fact does not endow gold with moral standing.

As many readers no doubt realize, the interest view is based on Joel Feinberg's "interest principle,"[3] which Feinberg proposed as an answer to the question "What kinds of beings can have rights?" However, my concern is not with the logic of rights ascription, but with the more basic question of moral standing. The question of who counts morally is more basic in that it is an issue for all moral views, even those that reject rights. Feinberg's central insight—that interests are essential to rights—can be applied to moral standing as well. Interests are the content of rights; without interests, there would be nothing for rights to protect. Equally, if a being has no interests, it can have no claims against others, nothing that they are required to consider from a moral perspective. The possession of interests is therefore a minimal condition for both rights and moral standing. All beings that have moral rights have moral standing, because to say that someone has a moral right to something is to say that he or she has a moral claim against others that they act (or refrain from acting) in certain ways. And to say that someone has a moral claim to the attention or concern of others is just another way of asserting moral standing.

All moral theories agree that *people* have moral standing, that their claims must be considered from the moral point of view. Indeed, the willingness to consider, impartially and dispassionately, the claims of other people is definitive of taking the moral point of view. There is also considerable, though not unanimous, consensus that mere things—pencils, rocks, and refrigerators—lack moral standing. In between people and rocks, there are lots of what have come to be known as "marginal cases," including animals, embryos, fetuses, and permanently unconscious individuals. How these marginal cases are handled depends on the justification for assigning moral standing to entities. For example, the Judeo-Christian tradition and Anglo-American law hold that moral standing is primarily, if not exclusively, held by *human beings*. In both law and commonsense morality, it is primarily humans who count and whose interests must be considered. While there has been considerable debate about when a human life begins and when it ends, the significance of humanity to the possession of moral standing is not disputed in commonsense morality. The importance of being human is simply taken for granted by most people.

In recent years a number of philosophers have challenged this commonsense view, in two ways. First, they maintain that it is unjustified to base moral standing on anything as arbitrary as membership in a particular species. Second, they view the widespread acceptance of human beings as having a moral status that is superior to that of nonhuman animals as due partly to the religious belief that God created human beings in his own image, and partly to human arrogance and complacence. Whatever its cause, "speciesism" is alleged to be as unjustified as racism or sexism.[4]

In the next chapter, I will argue that the special moral status of human beings can be justified. For now, I want to point out that, even within commonsense morality, human beings are not the only ones who count or matter morally. It is not

3. Joel Feinberg. 1974. "The Rights of Animals and Unborn Generations," in William T. Blackstone, ed., *Philosophy & Environmental Crisis*. Athens: University of Georgia Press, pp. 43–68.

4. Peter Singer. 1975. *Animal Liberation*. New York: Avon Books.

permissible morally to do anything one likes to animals, for example. Cruelty to animals has long been considered to be morally wrong, and in many places it is legally prohibited, although typically such prohibitions are limited to animals connected in some way to human beings. For example, in 1999, New York passed "Buster's Law," which makes it a felony intentionally to kill or cause serious physical injury, with aggravated cruelty, to a companion animal. The reference to "companion animal" was deliberate. The statute makes it clear that it cannot be construed to prohibit or interfere in any way with anyone lawfully engaged in hunting, fishing, or trapping. In other words, cruelty toward wild animals is not prohibited by Buster's Law, nor does this law restrict inhumane farming practices. It applies only to pets. Nevertheless, most people recognize the wrongness of cruelty—understood as the unnecessary infliction of severe pain—to animals, even those who are not companion animals. While it has been suggested that the basis for this moral and sometimes legal prohibition is the avoidance of cruelty to human beings,[5] or the offense to human sensibilities,[6] a more plausible explanation concerns the direct effect of such cruelty on the animals themselves. Certain treatment *hurts* animals: that is what makes it wrong. So animals do count; they have moral standing. Whether they count as much as human beings—whether, that is, they have equal moral *status*—is a topic to which I will return in the next chapter. But animals do count, and any plausible account of moral standing must reflect this.

A far more inclusive principle for determining moral standing is suggested by Albert Schweitzer's ethics of reverence for life.[7] Schweitzer holds that life is sacred. It is good to cherish and maintain life; it is evil to destroy and check life. Admittedly, expressed this way, no claim about moral standing necessarily follows. Life might be seen simply as a value to be promoted, like beauty or truth, without any suggestion that living things are entitled to our moral concern. However, Schweitzer's characterization of life as a "will-to-live" and his claim that ethics consists in "the necessity of practicing the same reverence for life toward a will-to-live, as toward my own" suggests a kind of golden-rule approach toward all living beings. Because we want to live, we should respect the claim of others to live. Animals and plants may not "want" to live, in the sense of having conscious desires, but they still strive to exist and that is why we ought to respect their lives. All living beings count, in Schweitzer's view. He says:

> A man is really ethical only when he obeys the constraint laid on him to help all life which he is able to succour, and when he goes out of his way to avoid injuring anything living. He does not ask how far this or that life deserves sympathy as valuable in itself, nor how far it is capable of feeling. To him life as such is sacred. He shatters no ice crystal that sparkles in the sun, tears no leaf from its tree, breaks off no flower, and is careful not to crush any insect as he walks. If he

5. Immanuel Kant, "Duties to Animals," in Tom Regan/Peter Singer, eds. 1976. *Animal Rights and Human Obligations*. Englewood Cliffs, NJ: Prentice-Hall, pp. 122–123.

6. Louis B. Schwartz, 1963. "Moral Offenses and the Model Penal Code." *Columbia Law Review* 63, p. 669.

7. Albert Schweitzer, "The Ethics of Reverence for Life," in Regan/Singer, *Animal Rights and Human Obligations* (see note 5).

works by lamplight on a summer evening, he prefers to keep the window shut and to breathe stifling air, rather than to see insect after insect fall on his table with singed and sinking wings.[8]

Every living being, no matter how seemingly insignificant, thus has a claim to our moral attention and concern. Of course, we cannot completely avoid killing, if we are to survive. But we can avoid killing and inflicting suffering unnecessarily. Interestingly, Schweitzer does not oppose the use of animals in laboratory experiments, as do many of today's animal liberationists. He simply requires scientists "to ponder in every separate case whether it is really and truly necessary thus to sacrifice an animal for humanity."[9] The willingness to sacrifice animals for humanity, when truly necessary, but not, presumably, human beings for animals, even if equally necessary, indicates acceptance of a moral-status scale that ranks human life as more valuable than other forms of life. Thus, Schweitzer's ethic is closer to commonsense morality than it may appear at first sight. Its main departure from ordinary morality lies in its insistence that people should be willing to make significant sacrifices of comfort and convenience to avoid killing living things.

How plausible is the ethic of the reverence for life? It seems to me a well-intentioned confusion of distinct moral principles. For example, reluctance to break off an ice crystal might express appreciation for natural beauty or a feeling that human beings should leave the natural environment undisturbed, as far as possible, in recognition of the delicate balance of ecosystems. It cannot exemplify reverence for life, since ice crystals are not alive. Similarly, Schweitzer's condemnation of the unnecessary use of animals in scientific experimentation is better explained by a principle that it is wrong to cause needless suffering than by reverence for life. The use of live cells that are discarded and destroyed after the experiment is over does not provoke moral outrage, nor does Schweitzer suggest that it should.

If the ethic of reverence for life implies that it is seriously wrong to destroy any living thing, it is implausible. After all, all sorts of things are alive, including bacteria and viruses. I doubt that anyone seriously believes that we should have moral qualms about using antibiotics. Bacteria are not the kind of beings that can have moral claims against us. But why is this? The interest view provides an answer. Only beings with interests can have claims against moral agents. Biological life alone does not endow a being with interests because interests are compounded out of beliefs, aims, goals, and concerns. Therefore, nonsentient, nonconscious beings do not have interests. Without interests, they cannot have moral standing.

Admittedly, most of us feel that there is something wrong with the wanton destruction of some nonsentient life-forms, such as trees and flowers. We might stop a child from peeling the bark off a birch tree, saying, "Don't do that; it will kill the tree." When vandals lopped the heads off hundreds of tulips, days before the annual Tulip Festival in Albany, New York, many people were morally outraged, and not just by the destruction of property. Perhaps this can be explained by a moral principle that condemns vandalism in general, and particularly the wanton destruction of beautiful things that give many people pleasure. However, it might be argued that the

8. Ibid., p. 134.

9. Ibid., p. 137.

killing of living flowers is worse than vandalism directed at nonliving things. Perhaps the fact that a thing is alive gives it a value that no nonliving thing has. (I am not sure that this is true. After all, one can always plant more tulips. If a work of art is destroyed, it is usually nonreplaceable.) But even if living things do have a special value, the mere fact that something is alive does not endow it with moral standing. If that were so, then weeds as well as tulips would have a claim to our moral attention and concern. The ethic of reverence for life is simply too broad. It does not provide a reasonable account of moral standing. The interest view, which is broader than the Judeo-Christian tradition but narrower than the ethic of reverence for life, is a much more plausible candidate.

In the first section, I argue first that the capacity for conscious awareness is a necessary condition for the possession of interests. This rules out both functional objects and organic beings, such as plants, bodily organs, and presentient fetuses. Next, I argue that conscious awareness is also a sufficient condition for having interests, opposing those philosophers who maintain that possession of language is essential to the having of interests. I believe that nonlinguistic beings, like animals and babies, can have interests, and so, moral standing. In the second section, I apply the interest view to the postconscious and the never-conscious. Postconscious beings include the dead and those in permanent vegetative state (PVS). I argue that while the dead and those in PVS no longer have occurrent interests, the interests they once had can exert a claim on us even after they are no longer alive or conscious. The never-conscious include anencephalic infants. Their moral and legal status has practical significance because of the possibility that they could be used as organ donors. The interest view seems to imply that this is morally permissible; however, the matter is complicated both by factual disagreements and the symbolic status of even the most radically impaired infants as family members.

The third section considers future people. At first glance, their situation seems to be exactly the reverse of that of dead people: the interests they will have can have a claim on us even before they come to exist. However, this is complicated by what has come to be known as the Nonidentity Problem, or the Parfit Problem. Sometimes choices made in the present do not merely affect people in the future, especially in the farther future, but actually affect their identity, that is, affect who gets born. The possibility of what Parfit terms "Different People Choices"—that is, choices that affect the identity of the people who come into existence—creates a problem with maintaining that future people can be harmed. This issue will be discussed under the rubric of wrongful life suits in Chapter 3 and revisited in a discussion of the morality of certain procreative decisions in Chapter 5. The fourth section considers the moral standing of potential people: embryos and fetuses.

CONSCIOUSNESS AND INTERESTS

The restriction of interests to beings capable of conscious awareness stems from a certain conception of what it is to have interests. Feinberg usefully analogizes having an interest in something to having a "stake" in it: "In general, a person has a stake in X . . . when he stands to gain or lose depending on the nature or condition of X."[10]

10. Joel Feinberg. 1984. *Harm to Others*. New York: Oxford University Press, p. 34.

I am better off if the things in which I have a stake, such as my health, my career, my assets, and my family, flourish or prosper. Their flourishing is in my interest.

> One's interests, then, taken as a miscellaneous collection, consist of all those things in which one has a stake, whereas one's interest in the singular, one's personal interest or self-interest, consists in the harmonious advancement of all one's interests in the plural. These interests . . . are distinguishable components of a person's well-being: he flourishes or languishes as they flourish or languish. What promotes them is to his advantage or *in his interest*; what thwarts them is to his detriment or *against his interest*.[11]

This way of thinking about interests connects them to what we care about or want, to our concerns and goals, to what is important or matters to us. How large a stake people have in the advancement of their careers, financial success, physical health, or spiritual development depends on how important these things are to them.

If we think of interests as stakes in things, and understand what we have a stake in as defined by our concerns, by what matters to us, then the connection between interests and the capacity for conscious awareness becomes clear. Without conscious awareness, beings cannot care about anything. Conscious awareness is a prerequisite to desires, preferences, hopes, aims, and goals. Nothing matters to nonsentient, nonconscious beings. Whether they are preserved or destroyed, cherished or neglected, is of no concern to them. Therefore, when we care for things, or do what is necessary to keep them in mint condition, we are not acting out of concern for *them*.

This point is underscored when we think of devices that are used to get us to think of inanimate objects as having a welfare of their own. For example, children's books and cartoons often portray inanimate objects such as locomotives, automobiles, toasters, radios, and vacuum cleaners as feeling pride, envy, loneliness, or despair. In such stories, the little train does mind when it rusts or is not used; the radio is terrified of having its tubes removed. We are meant to feel sorry for the neglected train and relief when the radio is saved. But such feelings are appropriate—or possible— on the assumption that the object has feelings and concerns of its own. If the object lacks feelings and concerns, we cannot be upset or aggrieved on its behalf. We cannot hope that it is restored and used, for its own sake. Mere things do not have a sake of their own, because what happens to them is of no concern to them at all.

Of course, the fact that it does not matter to "mere things" what is done to them does not mean that it does not matter at all. There are good reasons to preserve, protect, and maintain all sorts of things, from beautiful paintings to natural wildernesses. An obvious reason for preserving a beautiful painting is the interest of people in looking at it. However, the reasons for taking care of things need not stem only from the actual interests of people (and other interested beings). Perhaps there are things people ought to be interested in, although they are too ignorant or insensitive to realize this. Environmentalists attempt to awaken our interests in remote wildernesses and get us to appreciate the natural world, even though we may never observe parts of it or have any direct interest in its preservation. They may even maintain that preservation of the natural environment has *intrinsic value*. If this means that the natural environment is something that sensitive, intelligent people *ought* to

11. Ibid.

appreciate, a proponent of the interest view can agree. All the interest view denies is that the environment has a stake in its own preservation. The obligation to preserve wilderness areas is not one that we can owe *to* the wilderness. We can have obligations *regarding* mere things, but these obligations are not *to them*.[12] We have no obligations to them because it does not matter to them how we treat them. It is not *for their sake* that we take steps to preserve them, but for the sake of beings who have interests, such as existing people or animals, or future generations.

On the view I have been presenting, a being can have interests only if it can matter to the being what is done to it. Interested beings can be made happy or miserable; they can feel pleasure or pain. Of course, they do not always know what will make them happy or sad. They can often be wrong about what is in their interest. I am not claiming that if someone asserts that he does not care about X, then X is not in his interest. For X may be necessary for him to achieve Y, about which he does care, and he may be ignorant or willfully blind about the connection between X and Y. All I am claiming is that if nothing at all can possibly matter to a being, then that being has no interests. Its interests therefore cannot be considered, and so the being lacks moral standing.

Although the connection between consciousness and interests seems to be a natural and intuitive one, it is not universally accepted. The idea that all and only beings capable of conscious awareness have interests has been criticized as being too restrictive, and not restrictive enough. Those who regard it as too restrictive maintain that consciousness is not necessary for the possession of interests. Those who regard it as not restrictive enough believe that conscious awareness is not sufficient for the possession of interests. I discuss these objections in turn.

Is Consciousness Necessary for Having Interests?

REGAN'S ARGUMENT

Tom Regan denies that consciousness is necessary for the possession of interests.[13] He thinks that even mere things, like a violin or an automobile, can have interests. The failure to realize this, he alleges, stems from a failure to recognize an ambiguity in the word *interest*. One sense of interest (interest$_1$) refers to those things that are *in the interest* of a being—that is, those things that promote its welfare or good. Another sense of interest (interest$_2$) refers to the things individuals *take an interest in*—that is, the objects of their desires, preferences, aims, and goals. Regan agrees

12. See H.L.A. Hart. 1955. "Are There Any Natural Rights?" *Philosophical Review* 64 (2): 175–191. Hart argues that if X promises Y that he will look after Y's aged mother, then it is Y, and not Y's mother, to whom performance is owed. Y's mother is a person *concerning whom* X has an obligation and a person who will benefit by its performance, but the person *to whom* X has an obligation is Y. "It is important for the whole logic of rights that, while the person who stands to benefit by the performance of a duty is discovered by considering what will happen if the duty is not performed, the person who has a right (to whom performance is owed or due) is discovered by examining the transaction or antecedent situation or relations of the parties out of which the 'duty' arises" (p. 181).

13. Tom Regan. 1976. "Feinberg on What Sorts of Beings Can Have Rights," *Southern Journal of Philosophy* 14: 485–498.

that only conscious beings who have desires, preferences, and the rest can have interests$_2$. But it does not follow, and, in Regan's view, is not true, that only conscious beings can have interests. All that is necessary for having interests$_1$ is a good or sake of one's own. Whatever promotes or produces that good will be *in* the thing's interest. Feinberg's mistake, according to Regan, is thinking that there can be only one kind of good of one's own, "namely the kind of good that we tend to equate with the integrated satisfaction of our desires—i.e., happiness."[14] Mere things cannot be happy or unhappy, but they can nevertheless have a good of their own. Their good or welfare is promoted by those things that enable them to be good instances of their kind. This is reflected when we say, for example, that having the oil changed every 3,000 miles is good for a car. It's good for the car because it enables the car to run well. Similarly, excessive humidity is bad for oil paintings because it can damage them.

Feinberg acknowledges that we do often speak this way of what is good or bad for a thing, but he denies that this implies that the thing in question has interests *of its own*. Instead, the reference is to the interests of, for example, the car's owner, who wants a car that runs well, which in this context means something like "uses oil efficiently and doesn't need to be serviced too often." If running well were not something car owners had an interest in, this would not be a criterion of goodness in cars. In other words, to say that periodic oil changes are good for a car is an elliptical way of saying that periodic oil changes enable the car to perform in ways that advance the interests of people.

Regan thinks that this analysis confuses goodness and value. "That a car fulfills our purposes is not what makes it a good car; it is not even one of the good-making characteristics of a car."[15] Rather, a car fulfills our purposes because it is good; and it is good because it has good-making characteristics. To say that a car fulfills our purposes explains why we *value* or choose it; it does not explain what makes the car *good*.

Since human purposes do not explain what makes a car good, Regan thinks that the good-making characteristics of a thing must be independent of human interests and purposes. A good car would not cease to be good, he points out, just because people lost interest in driving cars. Regan concludes that talk of what is good for the car does not refer obliquely to what people want, but rather to the car's *own* good. Thus, he identifies what makes a car good (its good-making characteristics) with the car's good or welfare.

There are two errors in Regan's argument for ascribing to mere things a good of their own (and thus interests that advance that good). First, he confuses the application of good-making characteristics with their genesis. It is true that a good car would not cease to be good simply because people lost interest in driving cars. It would still be a good car insofar as it met the standards of goodness for cars. The reason for this is that standards, *once created*, can be applied independently of the actual interests and purposes of people. It does not follow that the standards themselves have an origin independent of human purposes. *People* determine the

14. Ibid., p. 490.

15. Ibid., pp. 492–493.

standards or criteria of goodness in functional objects, according to human interests and purposes.

Regan's second error is in confusing a thing's *being good* with its *having a good*. Functional objects can, of course, *be* good (or bad), depending on whether they meet (or fail to meet) the criteria for goodness. To say that they *have* a good, by contrast, is to suggest that they have a stake in fulfilling the good-making criteria. But mere things have no such stake. A car doesn't care whether it runs well or breaks down. If it cannot possibly matter to a being how it is treated, it is absurd to claim that we should give it such treatment *for its own sake*. And if we cannot treat it in certain ways for its own sake, then it makes no sense to ascribe to it a good or sake of its own.

The case is very different for beings with interests, beings to whom it can matter how they are treated. They can not only *be good* in the sense of meeting standards set by human beings, but they have a good or welfare of their own that is independent of human purposes. In fact, what is good for such beings, what is in their own true interests, may even conflict with the standards of goodness created by human beings. Consider the clipping of the ears of certain breeds of dogs. This is done because clipped ears are thought to have aesthetic value. An unclipped boxer will not win any prizes; such a dog will be considered "no good." But clipped ears have nothing directly to do with the *dog's* own welfare or well-being. Of course, a prize-winning dog may be treated better, and so indirectly benefit from having its ears clipped. However, not all dogs whose ears are clipped enter competitions, and not all who enter win. So most dogs are unlikely to benefit even indirectly by having their ears clipped. Clipping their ears does not promote their health or comfort; on the contrary.

Now compare clipping the dog's ears with having it vaccinated against distemper. It is in the owner's interest to have her animal vaccinated, since owners usually want healthy animals. But it is also in the dog's own interest, since a dog that gets distemper will experience considerable discomfort and will probably die. We might reasonably reproach an owner who neglected to have her dog vaccinated by saying, "It isn't fair to the dog. Even if you don't care if the dog dies, you should vaccinate the dog for its *own* sake."

This example shows us how standards of goodness can diverge from what is "good for" an animal. Such a divergence is impossible in the case of functional objects, because they have no good apart from the standards created by human interests and purposes. It is only when a being can have this kind of good that it makes sense to attribute to it a good or welfare or sake *of its own*. Feinberg does not, as Regan thinks, *confuse* interests$_1$ and interests$_2$. Rather, he correctly maintains that the ability to have interests$_2$ is necessary for the ability to have interests$_1$. It is only if treatment can matter to a being that it can be said to have a sake or welfare *of its own*.

THE NATURAL-FUNCTION VIEW

It is possible to accept the criticism presented above of Regan's argument criticism and still maintain that conscious awareness is not necessary for the possession of interests. That is, one might agree that mere things cannot have interests that advance their own good because things do not have a good or welfare of their own, independent of human interests and purposes. However, one might argue that living beings, unlike mere things, have natural functions that are not determined by human interests. Their good is achieved when they fulfill their natural function. Whatever enables them to achieve this function is in their interest. So living beings have interests$_1$, even though they may not have interests$_2$.

The natural-function view has a certain plausibility. We do not need to attribute imaginary mental states to hearts or livers, as we do to toasters and vacuum cleaners, to talk about doing things for *their* sake. For example, smoking is bad for the heart. Giving up cigarettes promotes cardiac health. Thus, we might tell someone to "Stop smoking—for your heart's sake." Why should we not say that certain things (such as not smoking, moderate exercise, and a low-cholesterol diet) are in one's heart's interest? This is true even if the individual in question does not care about, that is, has no interest$_2$ in, giving up smoking, exercising, or eating properly. The possibility of divergence in the case of conscious beings between interests$_1$ and interests$_2$ is one reason for developing an analysis of interests$_1$ based not on interests$_2$, but rather on natural functions.

Plants are another example of nonsentient beings that may be thought to have interests$_1$ and a welfare of their own. Unlike mere things, they are living beings with natural tendencies of growth and development. Plants can live or die, be healthy or sick. And what counts as healthy or thriving or flourishing is not determined solely by human interests and purposes, but stems from the plant's own biological nature. Human interests may even diverge from what is "good for" the plant with respect to its natural development and growth, as when a bonsai or espaliered tree is created.

Unlike mere things, then, both plants and bodily organs have what may be called "autonomous goodness"[16]—that is, a good that stems from their own nature, as opposed to the purposes imposed by people. Whatever promotes a being's autonomous goodness can be said to be in its interest, so long as we understand "interest" in this context as being merely teleological. That is, to say that something is good or bad for a plant is just to say that the thing in question promotes or thwarts its natural growth and flourishing. However, having autonomous goodness is importantly different from having "a welfare of one's own." The difference can be illustrated by thinking about when it does, and does not, make sense to act "for the sake of" a being. I suggested earlier that it is perfectly intelligible to admonish someone to stop smoking "for your heart's sake." By saying this, we are reminding the smoker that his habit damages his heart, and we are suggesting implicitly that it is in his interest to maintain cardiac health. But what if the smoker has incurable lung cancer and only months to live?[17] Smoking cigarettes cannot hurt him anymore, and indeed they may help to relax him. His decision to smoke need not be the result of ignorance, self-deception, or a weak will. It may be a perfectly rational attitude. If so, can we nevertheless recommend to him that he ought to stop anyway, "for his heart's sake"? Surely this would be absurd. The reason, I suggest, is that one's heart does not have a

16. Philippa Foot. 2003. *Natural Goodness.* Oxford: Oxford University Press. Although I use Mrs. Foot's term, "autonomous goodness," I do not think that she would have differentiated, as I do, between having autonomous goodness and having and a welfare of one's own, nor would she have approved of the phrase "merely teleological" with respect to interests.

17. This example comes from Peter Ubel, "When Bad Advice Is the Best Advice," *New York Times,* April 27, 2009. http://www.nytimes.com/2009/04/28/health/28case.html, accessed March 11, 2011.

sake of its own. The expression "Do it for your heart's sake" makes sense only in a context where proper cardiac functioning contributes to the well-being of its owner.

By contrast, a dog, for example, has a sake of its own. Because of this, we can tell its owner that she ought to have her dog vaccinated, for the dog's own sake. What explains this difference between dogs and hearts? Both are organic beings, and both have "autonomous goodness" in the sense that what is good for them does not depend on human interests and purposes. But dogs, unlike hearts, have a stake in their own well-being. When they are sick, they do not feel well, and they cannot do the things they enjoy doing. For this reason, it matters to the dog whether it is sick or healthy, and therefore it makes sense to suggest that steps be taken to preserve its health for its *own* sake.

What about plants? Plants are organic wholes, and not parts of organisms, like hearts and livers. Is this difference important for the possession of interests or moral standing? I cannot see why it should be. Whether something has a sake of its own depends on whether it has a stake in its own well-being. In this respect, plants are like bodily parts and mere things. They do not have nervous systems; they are not sentient. They are alive, but they do not experience anything. Without experiences, they cannot have interests$_2$—desires, plans, hopes, and goals. They cannot take an interest in anything, including their own health, lives, or well-being. Of course, plants can be healthy or sick, alive or dead, and so we can speak of their own well-being (a well-being that can be entirely independent of human wants and purposes), and we can identify the things that promote their own well-being, such as the right amount of water and sunshine, and the right kinds of nutrients in the soil. There is no harm in saying that these are in the plant's interest, or ascribing to plants interests in water, sun, and nutritional soil, so long as it is realized that the sense in which plants have interests is purely teleological. That is, these conditions must obtain if the plant is to live and thrive. However, whether these conditions obtain is not anything that matters to plants. Not being conscious or aware, plants cannot care whether they live or die, thrive or sicken. They are totally indifferent to treatment that furthers or hinders their well-being. By contrast, conscious, sentient beings do have a stake in their own well-being. It matters to sentient beings how you treat them. Morally, this is a crucial difference. Feinberg makes the point this way: "Having no conscious wants or goals of their own, trees cannot know satisfaction or frustration, pleasure or pain. Hence, there is no possibility of kind or cruel treatment of trees. In these morally crucial respects, trees differ from the higher species of animals."[18]

Defoliating a forest with Agent Orange may be *morally* wrong—that is, there may be moral reasons why people should not do this—but it is not a wrong *to* the trees. To preserve this difference between people and animals on the one hand, and plants on the other, I suggested earlier that we label the kind of well-being of which plants are capable "autonomous goodness." This captures the idea that the well-being of plants is independent of human purposes, while reserving the idea of "a welfare of one's own" for beings who have a stake in their own well-being. Whatever reasons we have to promote a plant's good, enabling it to flourish or thrive, these reasons do not derive from the plant's own concerns, aims, or goals. This does not, as I have tried to indicate, rule out an "environmental ethic," but it does mean that such

---

18. Feinberg, *Harm to Others* (see note 10), p. 491.

an ethic cannot be based on "golden-rule" or "fair-play" reasons. Such reasons require us to put ourselves in the other's place, to take the other's point of view. This is literally impossible in the case of plants, because plants do not have a point of view. While there may be moral reasons to preserve or protect plants, plants cannot have claims against us, nor are we morally obligated *to them* to protect them. The ascription of moral standing, by contrast, involves precisely these kinds of assertions, and that is why plants and trees, like bodily parts and mere things, do not have moral standing.[19]

Animals, on the other hand, can have interests. As Feinberg notes, "Many of the higher animals at least have appetites, conative urges, and rudimentary purposes, the integrated satisfaction of which constitutes their welfare or good."[20] Because they have a welfare of their own, we can not only preserve animals, as we can forests, but treat them humanely. Sentient beings can be given treatment that is good for them, for their own sake.

Is Consciousness Sufficient for Having Interests?

Some philosophers deny that animals have interests. R. G. Frey, for example, argues that animals lack the cognitive equipment necessary for interests—namely, wants and beliefs.[21] He acknowledges that animals can have *needs*—that is, whatever is necessary for them to survive or function well—but then, so can plants and even mere things. Needs are not the same as interests, and they are not sufficient for moral standing or rights.

Frey's argument is this: To want something is to have certain beliefs—in particular, the belief that one does not now have what one wants. Animals cannot have beliefs, according to Frey, because to have a belief is to believe that a certain sentence is true. Only creatures with linguistic ability can regard sentences as true. Since animals lack linguistic proficiency, they cannot have beliefs. Without beliefs, they cannot have wants; without wants, they cannot have interests. Without interests, they cannot have rights. Equally, they lack moral standing.

I think we must agree that the ability to have wants implies the ability to have beliefs. The question is whether only language users can have beliefs. An alternative model attributes beliefs to animals on the grounds that this is the best way to explain their behavior. This intuitive or commonsense belief-desire model arises out of our attempt to explain human behavior. In countless examples, the only remotely plausible explanation we can offer is in terms of the subject's beliefs and desires. The situation is quite parallel for at least higher animals. As Stephen Stich says:

> . . . it would be remarkable indeed if a theory could be produced which explains the behavior of higher animals without appeal to beliefs and desires, and if

19. Christopher Stone (1996) maintains that trees can have legal standing in *Should Trees Have Standing?* (New York: Oceana Publications), but rather than providing a conceptual analysis of legal standing, Stone is providing a legal basis for an environmental ethic that allows for the intrinsic value of plants.

20. Feinberg, *Harm to Others* (see note 10), p. 491.

21. R. G. Frey. 1980. *Interests and Rights: The Case Against Animals.* Oxford: Clarendon Press.

this theory could not be adapted to explain human behavior as well. In light of the evolutionary links and behavioral similarities between humans and higher animals, it is hard to believe that belief-desire psychology could explain human behavior, but not animal behavior. If humans have beliefs, so do animals.[22]

However, a problem arises when we attempt to specify just *what* a non–language user believes. If we cannot say what the animal believes, how can we use the belief to explain its behavior? Donald Davidson makes the point this way:

> We identify thoughts, distinguish between them, describe them for what they are, only as they can be located within a dense network of related beliefs. If we really can intelligibly ascribe single beliefs to a dog, we must be able to imagine how we would decide whether the dog has many other beliefs of the kind necessary for making sense of the first. It seems to me that no matter where we start, we very soon come to beliefs such that we have no idea at all how to tell whether a dog has them, and yet such that, without them, our confident first attribution looks shaky.[23]

We are presented, then, with a dilemma. On the one hand, it seems as reasonable to think that a belief-desire psychology can explain the behavior of higher animals as it is to think that such a theory can explain the behavior of people. On the other hand, we seem quite unable to say what it is that an animal believes, and thus we are unable to explain its behavior in terms of its beliefs and desires. Stich suggests that the dilemma of animal belief arises because we have two very different conceptions of belief. On the one hand, we take beliefs to be functional states that interact with desires to produce action. Viewed this way, we attribute beliefs to creatures whose behavior is amenable to explanation on the belief-desire model. On the other hand, beliefs are states with content; they are propositional attitudes. If a state is a belief, it must be a belief *that* something or other; we expect there to be some way of expressing its content.

The problem, according to Stich, is not that we lack information about animal behavior and reactions, and thus animal concepts. Even with complete information, we still would not be able to specify precisely what the animal *believes*. The reason is that we are not clear about the nature of belief. How central to our concept of belief is the having of specifiable content? "Is a belief-like state which lacks a specifiable content simply a somewhat peculiar belief, or is it, in virtue of lacking content, no belief at all?"[24] Stich provides the case for concluding they are not beliefs: "But what are we to say of a belief whose content we cannot specify? Under what condition is it true or false? There is, it seems, no obvious account of truth for such beliefs. In depriving beliefs of expressible content we have also deprived them of

22. Stephen Stich. 1979. "Do Animals Have Beliefs?" *Australasian Journal of Philosophy* 57 (1): 15–28, p. 18.

23. Donald Davidson. 1982. "Rational Animals," *Dialectica* 36 (4): 317–327, pp. 320–321.

24. Stich, "Do Animals Have Beliefs?" (see note 22), p. 27.

truth values."[25] To paraphrase a song from *Showboat*, beliefs without truth values ain't no beliefs at all.

The problem of truth is a difficult one. But I do not think that the solution is this extremely restrictive theory of belief. It rules out not only animals but also prelinguistic children, to whom we unhesitatingly ascribe all sorts of wants and preferences.[26] Admittedly, we are often uncertain *why* a child wants something—that is, what it is about the object that makes it appealing. However, it seems perverse to maintain that a child who is crying and reaching for an object does not want *anything* because we are not capable of specifying precisely what he wants.

Even if one accepts the restrictive Davidsonian account of belief, I do not think that Frey's conclusion that animals do not have interests (or rights or moral standing) follows. Whether propositional content is necessary for full-fledged beliefs, it is not necessary for interests$_2$. "Belief-like states" will do. So long as animals experience their treatment as painful or pleasant, it matters to them how they are treated. Sentient beings thus have at least one interest$_2$ an interest in not experiencing pain. This is sufficient to make them candidates for moral concern.

Once we demonstrate that animals can have interests, and so can meaningfully be ascribed moral standing, the next question is whether they *do* have moral standing, whether they are *entitled to* moral concern. To put the point another way, given that we *can* treat sentient creatures kindly and humanely, why are we *required* to do so? The only answer, it seems to me, is that pain is objectively bad. This answer is given by both utilitarians, such as Jeremy Bentham and Peter Singer, and Kantians, like Thomas Nagel. In *The Possibility of Altruism*,[27] Nagel points out that we tend to regard our own pain as objectively bad—that is, as giving others and not just ourselves reasons for action. If we then shift our perspective and see things from another's point of view, we will regard ourselves as having reasons provided by the other's pain. It is our ability to do this that makes us susceptible to arguments of the form "You wouldn't like it if someone did that to you." The success of such arguments does not depend on our thinking that the other *will* do whatever it is to us. The argument is not a prudential one. Rather, its success depends on our acknowledgment of objective reasons for action.

If the pain of other people provides us with at least some reason for doing certain things, it would seem that the pain experienced by nonhumans would also yield objective reasons for action.[28] Pain is pain, no matter who feels it. So long as a being

25. Ibid., p. 26.

26. In fact, as Stich points out, Davidson's view seems to restrict beliefs not only to language users, but to language users who share a significant number of our background beliefs. For, according to Davidson, we can say what someone believes only if there is a shared fund of background beliefs. This means that people from radically different cultures, or very distant eras, could not be said to have beliefs. Stich comments, "But surely all of this is perverse and amounts to no more than a reduction of the principle that beliefs must have a specifiable content." "Do Animals Have Beliefs?" (see note 22), p. 25.

27. Thomas Nagel. 1970. *The Possibility of Altruism*. Oxford: Clarendon Press.

28. Kant notoriously denied that animals were entitled to humane treatment for their own sake, and therefore he would not regard their pain as objectively bad. Rather, he explained our duty to treat animals humanely as a duty that concerns animals but is really a duty to people: "If he is

is sentient—that is, capable of experiencing pleasure and pain—it has an interest in not feeling pain, and its interest provides moral agents with prima facie reasons for acting. Sentience, then, is sufficient to give a being moral standing.[29]

I should stress that the interest view gives only a minimal condition for having moral standing—namely, the possession of interests. It does not locate beings on a scale of moral importance. In particular, it is silent as to whether all beings who have moral standing have it equally, that is, whether all have the same moral status. Perhaps such features as species membership, rationality, and potentiality are relevant to moral status, providing principled reasons for counting the interests of some beings more heavily than others. I will return to this issue in the next chapter.

So far I have argued that mere things and nonconscious living things fall below the moral-standing line; animals and people lie above it. It is now time to turn to more problematic cases: individuals who used to be, but will never again be, conscious, those who will never attain consciousness, and those who have the potential for conscious awareness.

THE INTERESTS OF NONCONSCIOUS INDIVIDUALS

Can the dead have interests? Or people in permanent vegetative states? These questions may seem remote from the topic of this book: the moral and legal status of embryos and fetuses. However, the topics are importantly connected. By understanding how the dead can have interests, we also come to understand how not-yet-born and even not-yet-conceived individuals can have interests, and thus a claim to our moral concern.

Dead People

Dead bodies—corpses—do not have interests. A corpse is a piece of decaying organic matter, without feelings, thoughts, or experiences of any kind. Without feelings and thoughts, it is impossible to have a stake or interest in anything. At the same time, most people have desires about what is to happen to their bodies, their property, their family and friends, or their own reputations after they are dead. They take an interest in what happens in the world even after they are no longer around to know about it. Thus, it seems that dead people both do and do not have interests.

---

not to stifle his human feelings, he must practice kindness towards animals, for he who is cruel to animals becomes hard also in his dealings with men" (Kant, *Lectures on Ethics*, translated and edited by P. Heath and J. B. Schneewind, Cambridge: Cambridge University Press, 1997, p. 240). This seems totally implausible, and few Kantians today would accept this explanation of the wrongness of cruelty to animals.

29. Among the philosophers who emphasize the importance of sentience to moral standing are L. W. Sumner. 1981. *Abortion and Moral Theory* (Princeton, NJ: Princeton University Press) and Mary Anne Warren. 2000. *Moral Status: Obligations to Persons and Other Living Things* (New York: Oxford University Press). Peter Singer argues that not only must the interests of all sentient beings be considered, but the comparable interests of all sentient beings must count equally. *Animal Liberation* (see note 4), pp. 8–9 and 23–34.

How are we to resolve this apparent inconsistency? Feinberg says, "I would like to suggest that we can think of some of a person's interests as surviving his death, just as some of the debts and claims of his estate do, and that in virtue of the defeat of these interests, either by death itself or by subsequent events, we can think of the person who was, as harmed."[30] The interests that survive are not the interests of the decaying corpse (that, as Feinberg says, would be absurd), but rather of the once-living person who is no longer with us. Feinberg refers to the once-living person as the "antemortem person" and the dead body as the "postmortem person." It is ante-mortem persons who have surviving interests, and who can be harmed and wronged.[31]

But how, it may be asked, can interests, which are derived from and linked to wants, continue to exist after the person who has those wants is dead? Are interests the kinds of things that can somehow survive independent of the individual whose interests they are? To explain this, Feinberg uses W. D. Ross's distinction between want-fulfillment and want-satisfaction.[32] The fulfillment of a want is the coming into existence of that which is desired. The satisfaction of a want is the pleasant feeling of gratification that normally occurs in the mind of the desirer when she believes that her desire has been fulfilled. Want-fulfillment and want-satisfaction are logically distinct. The fulfillment of wants does not always bring satisfaction. As George Bernard Shaw put it in *Man and Superman*, "There are two tragedies in life. One is to lose your heart's desire. The other is to gain it." Nor does a feeling of satisfaction imply that one's wants have actually been fulfilled, since the feeling may result from being deceived.

Dead people, as the Rolling Stones might say, can't get no want-satisfaction. But that does not mean that they cannot have their wants fulfilled after they have died. Their wants are fulfilled just in case events happen after their death as they wanted or planned while they were alive. The fulfillment of these wants is as much a part of their good as the fulfillment of wants while they are alive.

Admittedly, dead people cannot know that their wishes were carried out, their families provided for, their reputations intact. Nor can they know whether their wills are violated, their families impoverished, their reputations destroyed. But why should their mere lack of knowledge of these events imply that they have not been harmed? This does not seem to be true of living people who are unknowingly victimized. If ignorance does not prevent the living from being harmed, neither can it prevent the dead from being harmed.

A more troubling aspect of Feinberg's account has to do with the appearance of retroactivity. The antemortem person is harmed and wronged after her death by betrayals, broken promises, defamatory lies, and the like. But how, it may be asked, can an event that occurs after a person's death harm the living person she was before she died? How can an event that occurs at one time cause harm to someone living at an earlier time? Feinberg's answer is that posthumous harms do not entail backward

---

30. Feinberg, *Harm to Others* (see note 10), p. 83.

31. Ibid., p. 90 (borrowing these categories from George Pitcher). 1984. "The Misfortunes of the Dead," *American Philosophical Quarterly* 21 (2): 183–188, p. 184.

32. W. D. Ross. 1939. *Foundations of Ethics*. Oxford: Clarendon Press, p. 300. Cited in Feinberg, *Harm to Others* (see note 10), p. 84.

causation because they do not entail physical causation at all.[33] The occurrence of the harmful posthumous event *makes it true* that the antemortem person is harmed; it does not retroactively cause her to be harmed. Feinberg maintains that the subject of posthumous harm has been harmed all along, or at least at the point when she acquired the interest that would be defeated. It is just that until the harmful event actually occurs, no one could know of her harmed condition.

The claim that the antemortem person is harmed all along, by virtue of the future defeating of her interests, seems very counterintuitive.[34] It does not appear to square with our judgments about living people. We do not ordinarily think that someone who will fall off her bicycle or break her ankle in 6 weeks is *now* in a harmed condition in virtue of that future harm. Why, then, should we maintain that antemortem persons are now in a harmed condition, due to events after their death?

Feinberg's account can be made more plausible if we distinguish between propositions that ascribe properties timelessly and propositions that ascribe properties in the present. Whatever harms will befall me are timelessly true of me. That is, supposing that I will break my ankle in 6 weeks' time, then it is true of me now that I break my ankle on such and such a date (6 weeks from today). This does not imply that I am harmed *now*, 6 weeks before the accident. I am not harmed "all along." Rather, I have "all along" the property of being harmed at a particular time. This does not involve a belief in predestination, since the claim is not that breaking my ankle is something that will or must occur, but only that if it does occur, then the statement of its occurrence is timelessly true.[35]

Though the puzzles raised by posthumous harming are admittedly difficult, I do not think they are insurmountable. The common saying that the dead are beyond harming refers, I think, to the fact that the dead cannot be hurt, angered, or distressed. But their surviving interests, that is, the interests people have in events that will occur after their deaths, can be defeated. When someone's interests are set back or defeated, the individual is harmed. The subject of posthumous harm is the antemortem person, for it is the antemortem person who cared about what would happen after he died. If, after my death, the cause to which I have devoted my life fails, if the security I have worked to provide for my children is destroyed, if my own reputation is blackened, the interests I have now in these things are defeated, and I am harmed.[36]

33. Feinberg, *Harm to Others* (see note 10), p. 91.

34. Several critics have found this paradoxical. See, for example, Joan Callahan. 1987. "On Harming the Dead," *Ethics* 97 (2): 341–352, Nancy K. Rhoden. 1988. "Litigating Life and Death," *Harvard Law Review* 102 (2): 375–446, and Judith Thomson. 1986. "Feinberg on Harm, Offense, and the Criminal Law: A Review Essay," *Philosophy & Public Affairs* 15 (4): 381–395.

35. I owe this way of explaining postmortem harm to my colleague, Dr. Robert Meyers.

36. It goes without saying that not all interests are—or should be—protected by law. For example, under Anglo-American law, one cannot libel the dead; that is, the estate of a dead person cannot recover damages for libel. The rationale for this is a societal interest in free speech that might be hampered if authors and publishers had to be concerned about lawsuits. The dead no longer can suffer from a loss of reputation; they do not have to worry about losing their jobs or their friends. Therefore, their interest in maintaining a good reputation, real as it is, can be

Permanently Unconscious People

According to an article published in 2005, there may be as many as 15,000 patients in the United States in PVS.[37] The American Academy of Neurology places the number higher: between 10,000 and 25,000 adults and 6,000 to 10,000 children in the United States are diagnosed as being in PVS.[38] Some maintain that withholding or withdrawing any treatment necessary to sustain life is murder. Others would allow some forms of treatment to be stopped (e.g., respirators), but they oppose the removal of nasogastric feeding tubes. Still others argue that we should regard PVS patients as already dead. I will argue that this involves too great a conceptual shift. Nevertheless, the interest view supports the conviction that we are not required to sustain the lives of those who will never again be conscious.

First, some relevant facts and terminological distinctions. Patients who suffer acute brain damage may become comatose. Thanks to ever-improving intensive care medicine, they typically begin to awaken and recover consciousness within days or weeks, or they may enter a vegetative state (VS). The American Academy of Neurology defines the vegetative state as "a clinical condition of complete unawareness of the self and the environment accompanied by sleep-wake cycles with either complete or partial preservation of hypothalamic and brainstem autonomic functions."[39] Patients in this state have suffered severe neurological destruction of the cerebral hemispheres, which contain the function of consciousness or awareness, as well as voluntary action. Vegetative state may be "a transitional state on the route to further recovery or . . . progress to a long-standing, sometimes irreversible condition."[40] A vegetative state that persists for 4 weeks is considered to be a PVS. In common usage, the term "persistent vegetative state" is sometimes used interchangeably with "permanent vegetative state," but neurologists caution that the two terms should be distinguished " . . . because some persistent vegetative state patients, especially those with traumatic head injuries, may gradually improve to higher levels of cognitive and motor functions in the first few months."[41]

outweighed by the interest society has in the unrestricted flow of ideas. Nevertheless, someone who maliciously and knowingly sets out to defame a dead person not only acts wrongly; he wrongs and harms the once-living person who is now dead.

37. Joy Hirsch. 2005. "Raising Consciousness," Editorial, *The Journal of Clinical Investigation* 115 (5): 1102–1103.

38. American Academy of Neurology. "Practice Parameters: Assessment and Management of Patients in the Persistent Vegetative State" (Summary Statement). http://www.aan.com/professionals/practice/pdfs/pdf_1995_thru_1998/1995.45.1015.pdf. Accessed May 13, 2009.

39. Ibid.

40. Steven Laureys, Melanie Boly, and Pierre Maquet. 2006. "Tracking the Recovery of Consciousness From Coma," *Journal of Clinical Investigation* 116 (7): 1823–1825, p. 1823.

41. Ronald Cranford. 2004. "Diagnosing the Permanent Vegetative State," *Virtual Mentor* 6 (4). http://virtualmentor.ama-assn.org/2004/08/cprl1–0408.html. Accessed October 18, 2010.

A few cases of recovery after 4 months or more in the persistent vegetative state were reported in the early 1990s.[42] Were these cases of actual recovery from PVS, or were the patients misdiagnosed as PVS but actually in minimally conscious state (MCS)? Because the two states may appear identical, behavioral criteria are not reliable for distinguishing VS from MCS. Only modern neuroimaging techniques can truly distinguish between the two. In one case, a 39-year-old man who suffered a severe head injury after a car accident became comatose, and he awoke 19 years later. His case was reported into the popular media as a miraculous recovery from PVS, when actually it was determined that he had progressed to MCS before awakening. The case was also notable because it indicated that the brain in MCS is capable of some regrowth and regeneration.[43]

"Permanent VS, a prognostic term to be used with great caution, implies the prediction that the patient will not recover."[44] When brain damage is due to the brain's having been deprived of oxygen, a condition known as hypoxic-ischemic encephalopathy, the chance of any meaningful recovery is negligible after 3–6 months, and therefore permanent VS can be diagnosed at that time. After traumatic injury to the brain, permanent VS can be diagnosed after a year, because the chances of recovery are "practically nonexistent."[45]

In rare cases, patients emerge from their coma fully aware but unable to move or speak. They can communicate only by blinking. This condition, which may be mistaken for PVS, is known as "locked-in syndrome," the subject of the 1997 book, *The Diving Bell and the Butterfly*, on which the 2007 movie was based. The writer of the book, French journalist Jean Dominique Bauby, suffered a stroke and became comatose. He awoke 20 days later, but he was unable to move any part of his body except for his eyelids. He dictated the book by blinking his left eyelid for each letter. The process took 10 months, 4 hours each day.

Unlike locked-in syndrome in which there is full awareness, or minimally conscious state, in which there is some awareness, in the vegetative state, there is "wakefulness without awareness."[46] The lack of awareness can be confirmed by magnetic resonance imaging (MRI) and positron emission tomography (PET) scans, which showed a marked difference from normal brains or those in MCS. However, people in PVS are not, as is often mistakenly maintained, "brain dead." Brain death, as defined by the Uniform Determination of Death Act (a model act adopted by most U.S. states) involves the death of the whole brain. When the whole brain is dead, the functions of both the cerebral hemispheres and the brain stem, which controls vegetative functions, cease permanently. When brain

42. K. Andrews. 1993. "Recovery of Patients After Four Months or More in the Persistent Vegetative State, *British Medical Journal* 306: 1597–1600.

43. Henning U. Voss, Aziz M. Uluc, Jonathan P. Dyke, Richard Watts, Eric J. Kobylarz, Bruce D. McCandliss, Linda A. Heier, Bradley J. Beattie, Klaus A. Hamacher, Shankar Vallabhajosula, Stanley J. Goldsmith, Douglas Ballon, Joseph T. Giacino, and Nicholas D. Schiff. 2006. "Possible Axonal Regrowth in Late Recovery From the Minimally Conscious State," *Journal of Clinical Investigation* 116 (7): 2005–2011.

44. Laureys et al, "Tracking the Recovery of Consciousness From Coma" (see note 40).

45. Cranford, "Diagnosing the Permanent Vegetative State" (see note 41).

46. Steven Laureys. 2005. "The Neural Correlate of (Un)awareness: Lessons From the Vegetative State," *Trends in Cognitive Sciences* 9 (12): 556–559.

death occurs, there is no eye movement, no pupillary response to light, no cough, gag, or swallowing reflex, no spontaneous respiration. The heart can continue to beat, since this is not completely dependent on the integrity of the brain stem.[47] Once the patient is declared dead, all life-support machines are turned off, and death of the entire body ensues. However, if life support is not turned off, brain-dead patients can survive for days or weeks. There have been a few documented cases of long-term survival of brain-dead patients, including one boy who was kept alive, though brain dead, for 20 years.[48] Brain-dead women have even occasionally given birth to healthy infants.[49] Such cases lead some to argue that brain-dead patients are not really dead after all.

Despite controversy over the correct criteria of death, there are clear differences between brain death and PVS. The brain stem of patients in PVS remains relatively intact. They can breathe, often unassisted by a respirator. Their eyes are open at times, and periods of wakefulness and sleep are present. This differentiates them from comatose patients, whose eyes are shut, and who remain in a sleeplike state. The pupils of PVS patients respond normally to light. They often have an intact involuntary swallowing reflex, which theoretically allows them to be fed by mouth. However, this is extremely burdensome on those caring for them, and so most PVS patients are tube fed. They often have intact gag and cough reflexes as well, which helps account for their ability to survive for many years.[50]

Is it possible for patients who have been appropriately and reliably diagnosed as being in a persistent vegetative state to experience anything, even if they cannot communicate their experiences to us? Most neurologists (but not all) think that this is not possible. As the American Academy of Neurology expressed it in an amicus curiae brief in the Paul Brophy[51] case:

No conscious experience of pain and suffering is possible without the integrated functioning of the brainstem and cerebral cortex. Pain and suffering are attributes of consciousness, and PVS patients like Brophy do not experience them. Noxious stimuli may activate peripherally located nerves, but only a brain with the capacity for consciousness can translate that neural activity into an experience. That part of Brophy's brain is forever lost.[52]

47. Ronald E. Cranford. 1988. "The Persistent Vegetative State: The Medical Reality (Getting the Facts Straight)" (hereafter "The Persistent Vegetative State"), *Hastings Center Report* 18 (1): 27–32.

48. D. Alan Shewmon. 1998. "Chronic 'Brain Death': Meta-analysis and Conceptual Consequences," *Neurology* 51 (6): 1538–1545.

49. See, for example, "Baby Is Weak After Birth to Brain-Dead Woman," *New York Times*, http://www.nytimes.com/1986/08/16/us/around-the-nation-baby-is-weak-after-birth-to-brain-dead-woman.html. Accessed October 17, 2010.

50. Cranford, "The Persistent Vegetative State" (see note 47), p. 31.

51. *Brophy v. New England Sinai Hospital, Inc.* 1986. 398 Mass. 417, 497 N.E.2d 626.

52. *Brophy.* 1986. Amicus Curiae Brief, American Academy of Neurology, Minneapolis, MN. Cited in Cranford (see note 47), p. 31.

PVS patients sometimes grimace and cry out, and so they appear to be in pain. However, most neurologists maintain that these "stereotyped" reactions are merely reflexes, and not evidence of discomfort.

It may be objected that we cannot be certain what PVS patients experience. How can doctors be so sure that these patients do not feel pain? For years the conventional medical wisdom was that newborn infants cannot experience pain. In the last 25 years, evidence of pain in newborns became recognized as "overwhelming."[53] If doctors could confidently claim that pain behavior in newborns was not evidence of pain, maybe they are making the same mistake about PVS patients. How do they know that responses to noxious stimuli are just reflex responses?

Much of the difficulty of saying with confidence that a PVS patient experiences nothing stems from uncertainty about diagnosis. In one study, 54 patients, 23 who were diagnosed as being in PVS and 31 who were minimally conscious, showed evidence of awareness when given a functional MRI.[54] In the study, conducted between November 2005 and January 2009, the patients were asked to perform two imagery tasks while in the MRI scanner. They were asked to imagine standing still on a tennis court, and to swing their arm to hit a ball back to the tennis instructor, and they were asked to imagine navigating the streets of a familiar city, or going from room to room in their house. Five of the patients who had traumatic brain injury were able " . . . to modulate their brain activity by generating voluntary, reliable, and repeatable blood-oxygenation-level–dependent responses in predefined neuroanatomical regions when prompted to perform imagery tasks."[55] Four of the five had been diagnosed as being PVS. When they were retested at bedside, some behavioral indicators of awareness could be detected in two of them, but in two others, no evidence of awareness could be detected by an experienced clinical team, even after the results of the functional MRI were known. "This finding indicates that, in some patients, motor function can be so impaired that bedside assessments based on the presence or absence of a behavioral response may not reveal awareness, regardless of how thoroughly and carefully they are administered. In patients without a behavioral response, it is clear that functional MRI complements existing diagnostic tools by providing a method for detecting covert signs of residual cognitive function and awareness."[56]

Studies like this indicate the importance of supplementing behavioral criteria with functional MRIs, especially in cases where there has been traumatic brain injury. Although PVS can be mistaken for other conditions, and there have been a few rare cases of recovery from PVS, most neurologists believe that PVS can be diagnosed with a high degree of medical certainty (except for infants under 3 months).[57]

53. Anne B. Fletcher. 1987. "Pain in the Neonate," *New England Journal of Medicine* 217 (21): 1347–1348, p. 1347.

54. Martin M. Monti, Audrey Vanhaudenhuyse, Martin R. Coleman, Melanie Boly, John D. Pickard, Luaba Tshibanda, Adrian M. Owen, and Steven Laureys. 2010. "Willful Modulation of Brain Activity in Disorders of Consciousness," *New England Journal of Medicine* 362: 579–589.

55. Ibid.

56. Ibid., p. 589.

57. Alan J. Lerner. 2006. *Diagnostic Criteria in Neurology.* Totowa, NJ: Humana Press.

It seems, then, that we can assume that there is such a thing as PVS, that it can be reliably diagnosed, and that, if it persists long enough, it can be diagnosed as permanent and irreversible. What are we to say about the interests of those who are still alive, yet permanently unconscious? Permanently unconscious bodies, like corpses, do not have interests, a sake, or welfare of their own. Routine nursing care, such as turning over and oral hygiene, is not done for the sake of the PVS patient, who does not suffer from bedsores, a dried-out mouth, parched lips, or a swollen tongue. However, these conditions make the patient look awful. It may be assumed that the once-conscious person would not want to look grotesque, and so would prefer to have routine nursing care as long as life is sustained. Moreover, a neglected and uncared-for appearance of the patient is extremely distressing to family members. Similarly, the administration of analgesics does not reduce discomfort in the patient, since she can no longer feel pain. However, analgesics may inhibit reflex responses that resemble pain behavior and that are upsetting to family members. For this reason, pain medication may be indicated, again not for the patient's sake, but for that of the family.

The only interests patients in permanent VS have are those that have survived their permanent loss of consciousness. Antevegetative persons can have surviving interests just as antemortem persons do. However, it is unlikely that anyone has an interest in continued existence in a permanently unconscious state. Even those who opposed vociferously the removal of life support from Terri Schiavo did not claim that life in a permanent vegetative state was a good to the individual in that state. Rather, they claimed that she was not in VS, and that with adequate care, she could improve. However, her autopsy revealed that her brain had shrunk to 615 grams, about half the size of a normal human brain. It was even smaller than Karen Quinlan's brain, which weighed 835 grams after 10 years in PVS.[58] The Pinellas-Pasco Medical Examiner, Jon Thogmartin, characterized the damage to her brain as "irreversible" and said that "no amount of therapy or treatment would have regenerated the massive loss of neurons."[59]

Had Terri Schiavo's parents accepted the diagnosis of PVS, and accepted the reality that PVS patients experience nothing, they might still have wanted to keep her alive, believing that life and life alone, even with no experience of life, has value. Whether they could intelligibly claim that her life would have value *for her* without the possibility of experience is another matter. I maintain that it is the experience of life that makes life valuable to its possessor. Without the possibility of experiences, now or in the future, life no longer provides value to the one who lives. The biographical life of the PVS patient is over, even though she is not biologically dead.[60] Sustaining the person's biological life is not something we can do for her sake or to benefit her. Whatever reasons there may be for continuing treatment, or refusing to turn off the machine (such as concern for the family's feelings or fear of setting a bad precedent

58. Jamie Talan. 2005. "The Schiavo Autopsy: What Was Found." *Newsday,* June 16.

59. "Schiavo Autopsy Finds Damage Was Irreversible." http://www.ctv.ca/servlet/ArticleNews/story/CTVNews/1118842392937_114251592/?hub=TopStories. Accessed May 25, 2009.

60. The distinction between biological life (being alive) and biographical life (having a life) is drawn by James Rachels, 1986, *The End of Life: Euthanasia and Morality* (New York: Oxford University Press).

or even respecting the intrinsic value of life itself), they do not refer to the interests of the patient.[61]

Admittedly, there are a few people who would want to be kept alive if there was *any* chance, no matter how remote, of regaining consciousness. They reason that they are no worse off alive and in a PVS, since there is no pain or discomfort, and— who knows?—they just might beat the odds and regain consciousness. Such people might plausibly maintain that keeping them alive is in their interest, and that this could be done for their sake. The question then would be how to weigh their interest in staying alive, given a remote chance of recovery, against the cost to society of sustaining people in PVSs.[62] That issue aside, it should not be assumed that keeping someone alive in a PVS does not harm his (antevegetative) interests. Most people do not regard the prospect of living in a VS with equanimity. The idea of existing as a permanently nonconscious body fills many people with distress and horror. Michael Schiavo claimed that his wife had indicated to him that she would not want to live that way, and that in fighting to remove her from life support, he was simply carrying out her wishes.[63] The interest in *not* being artificially maintained belongs to the conscious individual who existed before the injury to her brain (the antevegetative person), and it survives her permanent loss of consciousness. We have as much reason to respect this sort of surviving interest as any other. As with all surviving interests, there is the difficult problem of knowing what the previously competent person wanted, but this epistemological issue does not negate the validity of surviving interests of either dead or permanently unconscious individuals.

Infants with Anencephaly

Anencephaly is the most devastating neural-tube disorder, because it involves the complete absence of the cerebral hemispheres and most of the cranial vault. Most infants born with anencephaly are blind, deaf, unconscious, and unable to feel pain (although as we will see, this claim has been questioned when there is a functioning brain stem). A variable amount of brain stem and cerebellum is present, which make reflex actions such as breathing and response to touch possible. However, most neurologists believe that "the lack of a functioning cerebrum permanently rules out the

61. This view was taken by the President's Commission for the Study of Ethical Problems in Medicine and Biomedical and Behavioral Research. 1983. *Deciding to Forego Life-Sustaining Treatment*, pp. 181–182. http://bioethics.georgetown.edu/pcbe/reports/past_commissions/deciding_to_forego_tx.pdf. Accessed October 18, 2010.

62. Not everyone thinks it is obvious we should remove PVS patients from life support. See L. Syd M. Johnson. 2010. "Withholding Care From Vegetative Patients: Financial Savings and Social Costs," *Bioethics Forum*. http://www.thehastingscenter.org/Bioethicsforum/Post.aspx?id=4789&blogid=140. Accessed October 18, 2010.

63. Susan Funaro. 2007. "Why Didn't Michael Schiavo Seek a Divorce?" http://www.legalzoom.com/planning-your-estate/living-wills/why-didnt-michael-schiavo-seek. Accessed October 18, 2010.

possibility of ever gaining consciousness."[64] The prevalence rate of anencephaly has been steadily declining over the past several decades, in part because of the discovery in the early 1990s that neural tube defects, which occur early in pregnancy, could be prevented if pregnant women and women intending to become pregnant got an adequate amount of folic acid in their diets. In 1992, the U.S. Public Health Service recommended that all women of childbearing age should get 400 micrograms of folic acid daily. This could be done by improving the diet to include leafy green vegetables, fortifying foods with folic acid, and taking dietary supplements. After mandatory fortification of cereal grain products went into effect in January 1998, the reported prevalence of neural tube defects, such as spina bifida and anencephaly, declined significantly. The other factor contributing to a decline in the prevalence rate is that maternal screening and abortion for neural-tube defects have become more common. Today, the occurrence rate of anencephaly in the United States is around 1.2 per 10,000 births.

Pregnancies of anencephalic fetuses often end in early pregnancy loss, spontaneous abortion, fetal death, or pregnancy termination. Those who are not stillborn usually die within a few days, or more rarely, weeks. What should be the moral and legal standing of anencephalic infants? Some argue that anencephalics, though live-born humans, are not persons, and therefore do not have the same moral status as other born human beings, nor should they have the same protections as other human persons. Others, who take a "higher-brain" standard of death, maintain that anencephalics are actually dead, and therefore they can be organ donors.

The meaning of death—its definition, criteria, and clinical signs—is crucial to the issue of organ donation. Although there is some live organ donation, for example, of kidneys, in general, organs can only be taken from individuals who are dead. However, traditional criteria for death—permanent and irreversible cessation of the functioning of the heart and lungs—are not compatible with organ donation. There is a rather small window of opportunity for organ transplantation once the heart stops beating and the person stops breathing. If doctors wait to ensure that the cessation of heart and lung function is permanent, the organs may deteriorate and become unusable. The need for organs for transplantation was part of the rationale for the shift from cardiopulmonary to neurological criteria.[65] The debate over the correct criteria for death continues.[66] However, even if one accepts neurological criteria, most infants with anencephaly have functioning brain stems, and therefore they do not meet the whole-brain standard of the Uniform Determination of Death Act (UDDA). If transplant physicians wait until they are brain dead, their solid

64. National Institute of Neurological Disorders and Stroke (NINDS) Anencephaly Information Page 2009. http://www.ninds.nih.gov/disorders/anencephaly/anencephaly.htm. Accessed May 27, 2009.

65. Martin S. Pernick. 1999. Brain death in a cultural context: The reconstruction of death, 1967–1981. In *The Definition of Death: Contemporary Controversies*, eds. Stuart J. Youngner, Robert M. Arnold, and Renie Schapiro. Baltimore: Johns Hopkins University Press.

66. For example, at the Pacific Division of the American Philosophical Association meetings, April 10, 2009, the Committee on Philosophy & Medicine held a Special Session on "Is 'Brain Death' Death?" featuring Bernard Gert, Ari Joffee, Don Marquis, Allen Shewmon, and Robert Truog.

organs are likely to undergo irreversible hypoxic injury and become unsuitable for donation.

The issue of using anencephalic infants[67] as organ donors was vigorously debated during the late 1980s and early 1990s. Some argued that the law should be changed to allow the organs of live-born infants with anencephaly to be used without a requirement of total brain death. The issue seems to have been resolved in favor of the legal status quo. In 1986, the only active U.S. protocol for harvesting organs from anencephalic infants (at Loma Linda University Medical Center in California) was abandoned. There appears to be consensus that any benefits that could be gained from changing the law would be outweighed by the dangers.[68] But while the policy debate over using infants with anencephaly as organ donors has ended, it is worth revisiting the arguments because they illustrate the complex medical, social and psychological factors that go into the determination of moral standing in marginal cases.

The main argument in favor of using anencephalic infants as organ donors is that, while they are certain to die quickly, regardless of what is done for them, their organs are perfectly healthy. Why let them go to waste when there are children whose lives could be saved by organ donation? There is a severe shortage of pediatric organs. "Young children rarely die in circumstances that would make them medically acceptable sources of organs. Among the children younger than two years of age registered to receive transplants, an estimated 30–50% die before an organ becomes available."[69]

In 1986, California senator Milton Marks proposed modifying the standards set forth in the UDDA and similar state laws so that they would allow organs to be taken from anencephalic infants. Apparently moved by a story of a couple frustrated by their inability to donate the organs of their anencephalic baby to an infant at the University of California Medical Center, Senator Marks introduced—but later withdrew—a bill that would have amended the UDDA by classifying an infant with anencephaly as dead. Alexander Capron succinctly states the problem with this approach:

> Adding anencephalics to the category of dead persons would be a radical change, both in the social and medical understanding of what it means to be dead and in the social practices surrounding death. Anencephalic infants may be dying, but they are still alive and breathing. Calling them "dead" will not change the physiologic reality or otherwise cause them to resemble those (cold

---

67. Sometimes the issue is framed in terms of anencephalic fetuses, because the diagnosis of anencephaly is often given during pregnancy. Parents who learn that their fetus has anencephaly may wish to donate organs after birth. The organs are taken from infants—live-born babies— although the plan to donate may be made before birth, when the infant is a fetus.

68. See D. Alan Shewmon, Alexander Capron, Warwick J. Peacock, and Barbara L. Shulman. 1989. "The Use of Anencephalic Infants as Organ Sources: A Critique," *Journal of the American Medical Association* 261 (12): 1773–1781.

69. Committee on Bioethics 1992. "Infants With Anencephaly as Organ Sources: Ethical Considerations." *Pediatrics* 89 (6): 1116–1119. This statement was reaffirmed in June 2007.

and nonrespiring) bodies that are considered appropriate for post-mortem examinations and burial.[70]

A slightly different approach is to retain the whole-brain standard of death in general, but to make an exception of anencephalics only. This approach was taken by Michael Harrison, a pediatric surgeon at the University of California San Francisco Medical Center. Harrison argues that the whole-brain definition of death was drafted to protect the comatose patient whose injured brain might recover function. This simply does not apply to anencephaly, in which the physical structure necessary for recovery is absent. This led Harrison to suggest that we might treat "brain absence" as equivalent to brain death for legal purposes.[71]

The "brain-absence" approach has been criticized on both scientific and policy grounds. Ronald Cranford and John Roberts maintain that it is medically inaccurate to call anencephalics "brain absent," as a variable amount of brain stem and cerebellum is present.[72] Other commentators argue that while anencephaly may be *clinically* distinct, it is not *conceptually* different from other devastating neurological impairments. There is no reason to limit the functional equivalence of brain death for the purpose of harvesting organs for transplantation to anencephaly. Why not take organs from infants with holoprosencephaly, hydranencephaly, and certain trisomies, as well as PVS patients?[73] Indeed, as Capron points out, hydranencephalics (whose cerebral hemispheres have been largely or entirely destroyed in utero by infection) would be more attractive sources of organs than anencephalics, because they tend to survive for longer periods of time, and so have more developed and larger organs. Shewmon et al. argue that making an exception for anencephalics could be used to justify taking organs from "incompetent patients in the final stages of a terminal illness or even prisoners on death row, whose organs would be much more suitable for transplantation than those of anencephalics and whose execution could be timed according to the availability of an optimally matched recipient." They go on to say:

> Specifically, using this kind of logic, half of all the infants who die of congenital kidney, heart, and liver disease would be better used as organ sources to preserve the lives of the other half, rather than letting them all die along with their transplantable organs. Even though this sounds preposterous, the experience at

70. Alexander M. Capron. 1987. "Anencephalic Donors: Separate the Dead From the Dying," *Hastings Center Report* 17 (1): 344–350, at p. 344.

71. Michael R. Harrison. 1986. "Organ Procurement for Children: The Anencephalic Fetus as Donor," *Lancet* 2 (8520): 1383–1386.

72. Ronald E. Cranford and John C. Roberts. 1989. "Use of Anencephalic Infants as Organ Donors: Crossing a Threshold, in Howard H. Kaufman, ed., *Pediatric Brain Death and Organ Tissue Retrieval: Medical, Ethical and Legal Aspects*. New York: Plenum, Chapter 20, pp. 191–197.

73. See John Arras and Shlomo Shinnar. 1988. "Anencephalic Newborns as Organ Donors: A Critique," *Journal of the American Medical Association* 259 (15): 2284–2285; Alexander Capron, "Anencephalic Donors" (see note 70), and D. Alan Shewmon et al. (see note 68).

transplantation referral centers indicates that the enthusiasm for using anencephalics does indeed quickly extend to other categories of dying infants.[74]

The point here is a psychological one. The suggestion is that making an exception
of anencephaly is likely to put us on a slippery slope that would endanger the lives
of other handicapped or terminally ill people. Perhaps the best answer to psychological slippery-slope arguments has been given by philosopher Samuel Gorovitz.
Speaking as an experienced skier, Gorovitz points out that it is often possible to start
down a slippery slope and then stop.[75] Instead of automatically avoiding slippery
slopes, educational and legal measures can be taken to ensure that the feared results
do not occur. For example, it could be specified that only anencephalic infants are to
be used as transplant donors.

Slippery-slope arguments can also take a conceptual form. As distinct from
the psychological issue of whether using anencephalic infants as organ donors is
likely to lead to thinking of all terminally ill infants as potential donors, the conceptual question is whether anencephaly is sufficiently different from other neurological
disorders to justify making it a unique exception to the whole-brain concept of death.
Those who regard anencephaly as unique maintain that there are several features
that differentiate the anencephalic infant from infants with less severe neurological
disorders. Anencephalic infants, it is argued, have an "utterly hopeless prognosis";
they are "permanently unconscious and terminally ill"; and "the diagnosis can
be easily established both *in utero* and at birth with an extraordinarily high degree of
certainty."[76] However, there is no consensus among the experts about any of these
characteristics.

Some commentators are positive that anencephalics lack the capacity for experience of any kind. Arthur Caplan writes, "There is no question that such children are
incapable of any cognitive activity or any form of sentience."[77] Cranford and Roberts
agree. "Because these infants are permanently unconscious and can experience no
pain or suffering, and, therefore, can never be aware of what happens to them, a strong
argument can be made that, like other permanently unconscious patients, they have
no interest in treatment, i.e., treatment can no longer benefit or harm them."[78]

However, some commentators are skeptical of the claim that anencephalics
can experience nothing. Shewmon et al. concede that while the capacity for experience is undoubtedly missing in those with craniorachischisis (a congenital fissure
of the skull and spine), such infants are invariably stillborn, and their organs unsuitable for donation. "Whether those with relatively intact brain stems have any subjective awareness associated with their responsiveness to the environment is inherently
unverifiable, but what is known about the functional capabilities of the brain stem,

74. Shewmon et al., "The Use of Anencephalic Infants as Organ Sources" (see note 68),
p. 1775.

75. Samuel Gorovitz. 1982. *Doctors' Dilemmas*. New York: MacMillan, pp. 167–168.

76. Cranford and Roberts, "Use of Anencephalic Infants as Organ Donors" (see note 72), p. 193.

77. Arthur L. Caplan. 1987. "Should Fetuses or Infants Be Utilized as Organ Donors?" *Bioethics*
1(2): 119–140, p. 122.

78. Cranford and Roberts, "Use of Anencephalic Infants as Organ Donors" (see note 72), p. 193.

particularly in newborns, suggests at least keeping an open mind."[79] They argue that decerebrate newborns are neurologically much more similar to normal infants than to decerebrate adults. Therefore, it is not possible to apply adult-derived neuro-physiological principles in support of the claim that a functioning cortex is necessary for consciousness or pain perception in newborns. In addition, according to Shewmon et al., " . . . decerebrate (anencephalic or hydranencephalic) human new-borns with relatively intact brain stems can manifest a surprising repertory of complex behaviors, including distinguishing their mothers from others, consolability, conditioning, and associative learning, although irritability and decreased ability to habituate are also common."[80]

The ability to distinguish one's mother from others is good evidence of conscious awareness. How else can this ability be explained? In addition, in light of the fact that it is only recently that physicians have acknowledged the capacity of perfectly normal newborns to feel pain, we should be cautious of claims that there is "no question" that anencephalics are nonconscious and nonsentient. In the first edition of this book, I wrote, "More research might clarify the issue. Until then, it would seem only prudent not to make radical changes in organ-donation policy." I have been unable to find any research that has clarified the issue. In part, no doubt this is because the question of subjective awareness is, as Shewmon says, unverifiable. In part, such research may not have been undertaken because of the growing consensus that anen-cephalic infants are unlikely to be a significant source of pediatric organs.

Other areas of factual disagreement concern the reliability of diagnosis, the immi-nence of death, the medical suitability of anencephalic infants to be organ donors, and the number of potential recipients. While Cranford and Roberts suggest that "hundreds or thousands" of newborns or infants can benefit from receiving organs from anencephalic infants,[81] D. A. Shewmon places the number much lower.[82] Nearly two-thirds of all anencephalics are stillborn, and their organs cannot be used. Moreover, as the use of AFP screening and amniocentesis becomes more common, more fetuses with neural-tube defects will be aborted. Taking these facts into consideration, Shewmon estimates the annual number of live anencephalic births in the United States to be just over 300.[83] (The CDC estimates the number to be considerably higher, about 1,000 babies each year.[84]) Most are born prematurely and have intrauterine growth retardation, making them unsuitable as organ donors. In addition, a number of anencephalic infants have associated gross malformations of their organs. Finally, there is the difficulty of finding an appropriate recipient. Looking 10 years into the future, even anticipating improvements in matching donors and recipients, transportation, and transplantation techniques, Shewmon

79. Shewmon et al., "Anencephalic Infants as Organ Sources" (see note 68), p. 1776.

80. Ibid.

81. Cranford and Roberts, "Anencephalic Infants as Organ Donors" (see note 72), p. 193.

82. D. Alan Shewmon. 1988. "Anencephaly: Selected Medical Aspects," *Hastings Center Report* 18 (5): 11–19.

83. Ibid., p. 13.

84. CDC. 2009. "Anencephaly." http://www.cdc.gov/ncbddd/birthdefects/anencephaly.htm Accessed October 27, 2010.

projects the annual number of infants in the country who would benefit from anencephalic organs to be fewer than 50. He concludes:

> Such present and future projections ought to be borne in mind in discussions of the impact of anencephalic organ harvesting upon the many hundreds of children who die each year from congenital kidney, heart, and liver disease, before we expend great effort in modifying diagnostic criteria for brain death, changing statutory definitions of death, or relaxing fundamental principles of transplantation ethics in order to obtain anencephalic organs.[85]

The absence of consensus on the factual issues is undoubtedly a large factor in the failure of proposals to allow organ donation from live-born anencephalic infants. If anencephalic infants are conscious and sentient, they should be treated like any other sick and dying newborns. Certainly they should not be seen as living organ donors merely because they lack cognitive potential and are certain to die soon. At the same time, if anencephalic infants are totally lacking in conscious awareness, they have no interests that can be considered. Nothing, not prolongation of life or so-called comfort care, can be done for their sake. To insist that they nevertheless be treated like other sick and dying infants who *can* be benefited and harmed is to ignore a crucial, morally relevant difference.

Alexander Capron ignores this difference when he says:

> ...if society wants to adopt a policy of sacrificing living patients for their organs, it seems very strange—and a very bad precedent—to start with the most vulnerable patients. Unconsenting, incompetent patients who have never had a chance to express their views about whether, if near death but not yet dead, they would want their bodies cut up for purposes of organ donation, are the *least* suitable source.[86]

If anencephalic infants are nonconscious and nonsentient, they are *not* "the most vulnerable patients"; they are not vulnerable at all. To be vulnerable, one must be capable of being harmed. To be capable of being harmed, one must have interests that can be thwarted, set back, or defeated. Without some form of conscious awareness, a being can have no interests and is immune from being harmed.

It might be objected that the same can be said of permanently unconscious adult patients. Capron fears that the retrieval of organs from living anencephalics would lead to the "nightmarish scenario" that took place in Robin Cook's novel *Coma*, in which vital organs were removed from comatose patients. Of course, in the novel, patients were deliberately *made* comatose in order to serve as organ sources. The nightmare is not that their vital organs were removed after they became comatose; the nightmare is that they were made irreversibly comatose. They would be no better off had they been put into a PVS but allowed to keep their vital organs.

In any event, there are important differences between PVS patients and anencephalic infants that make the analogy weak. There are reasons not to harvest organs

85. Shewmon, "Anencephaly: Selected Medical Aspects" (see note 82), p. 17.

86. Capron, "Anencephalic Donors" (see note 70), p. 8.

from PVS patients that do not apply to infants with anencephaly. To begin with, organs should not be retrieved even from *dead* bodies without consent. People often have strong feelings about what should be done with their corpses, and these surviving interests should be respected. If consent, based on the preferences of the deceased, is necessary for organ donation *after* death, how much more stringent should consent requirements be for organ donation *before* death, when there is always the possibility of misdiagnosis, and the chance of killing a patient who might have regained consciousness. This explains why even people who are happy to donate their organs after they die may not want their organs taken should they enter a PVS. Their wishes should, of course, be respected. However, the wishes of anencephalic infants cannot be respected. This is not because, as Capron suggests, they have never had a chance to *express* their views, but because they lack the capacity to *have* views on this, or any other, matter. Thus, there can be no obligation to determine what they would have wanted. Indeed, doing so does not even make sense.[87]

The conceptual version of the slippery-slope argument against using anencephalic infants as sources of organs is not terribly persuasive. A complete and irreversible lack of consciousness would differentiate infants with anencephaly from most other severely impaired newborns. It might not distinguish anencephalics from hydranencephalics or iniencephalics, if they too completely lack sentience and awareness. If they do, then hydranencephalics and iniencephalics also lack the capacity for interests and moral standing. The mere fact that they tend to survive for longer periods is not morally significant if they are completely and permanently unconscious. However, it does not follow that if we make an exception of infants with anencephaly, we are logically committed to making an exception of infants with hydranencephaly and iniencephaly, much less all dying infants, as well. The more exceptions allowed to the UDDA, the greater the danger of misdiagnosis and of confusing permanent unconsciousness with a less severe neurological condition. This is one reason for making anencephaly the only exception to the UDDA. In addition, if some physicians have doubts about the capacity for sentience in anencephalics, many more have doubts about sentience in less devastating disorders.

Sometimes it is said that infants who lack the capacity for conscious awareness are not "persons" and that this is the reason why they may be killed. In my view, the introduction of the question of personhood needlessly confuses the issue, for two reasons. First, there is no philosophical or moral consensus on the requirements of personhood. There is not even agreement on the relevant characteristics—for example, whether being human is necessary or sufficient for being a person. Some philosophers place the standard so high that even normal newborns do not qualify, while others consider fertilized human eggs to be people. It is unlikely that any argument for using infants with anencephaly as organ donors based on their lack of personhood will be successful.

Second, the term "person" is not purely descriptive, but normative, and more, honorific. When we call a newborn baby a "person," we are not so much describing its capacities as expressing the idea that it is a family member. The same is true of infants with anencephaly. Like all other babies, they have parents and a place in a network of human relationships. On this basis alone, such babies can be considered

---

87. See Allen Buchanan. 1981. "The Limits of Proxy Decision Making for Incompetents," 29 *UCLA Law Review* 321.

to be "persons." To deny that infants with anencephaly are people suggests that such babies are not important, not our children, not worthy of being treated with dignity and respect. A more accurate characterization acknowledges that they are people who, due to their devastating neurological deficit, cannot be benefited or harmed. Nothing can be done for *their* sake, although their parents can love them and mourn their deaths. The parents who have attempted to donate the organs of their infants with anencephaly have not done so because they regard their infants as worthless or undeserving of respect. Rather, they feel that respect is best shown by donating tissues and organs so that others may live. If so, then, as Caplan says, "it seems hollow sentimentality to prohibit such gifts on the grounds that it is repugnant to certain sensibilities to do so."[88] However, repugnance is not the only argument against using anencephalic infants as sources of donors. There are all the factual uncertainties mentioned earlier. In addition, such a change might create fears in the public that organs are being, or will be, taken from other humans who are not brain dead, leading to an overall decline in donations. As the bioethics committee of the American Academy of Pediatrics wrote in 1992 (and reaffirmed in 2007), "Although it is impossible to foresee its exact effects, sufficient questions exist to counsel extreme caution before adopting a policy permitting organ retrieval from anencephalic infants who retain brain stem function."[89]

FUTURE PEOPLE

The situation of future generations appears to be just the reverse of that of dead and permanently unconscious people. The interests they will have in the future can exert a claim on us now, even before they come into existence. If people today pollute the atmosphere and drinking water, despoil the environment, and deplete natural resources, this is likely to have disastrous effects on the lives of those who come later. Their actual future interests will be harmed; they will suffer because of our decisions today. The same reasons we have not to inflict harm on present existing people apply to future existing people. We can have moral obligations to them, and they can have rights against us. Because they have interests, future people qualify for moral standing.

Objections to the claim that future people have moral status are of three kinds. The first two, often not carefully distinguished,[90] are fairly easily rebutted. The third objection poses much greater problems.

The first objection is a logical argument. It maintains that future generations do not have moral standing because they do not exist. If they do not exist, nothing is true of them. They have no properties at all, and so do not have interests, moral standing, or rights. However, the fact that future people do not now exist does not deprive them of the ability to have properties. Tomorrow does not now exist, and yet all sorts of things can be said about tomorrow: it will be cloudy, it is graduation day,

88. Caplan, "Should Fetuses or Infants Be Utilized as Organ Donors?" (see note 77), p. 138.

89. Committee on Bioethics, American Academy of Pediatrics. 1992. "Infants With Anencephaly as Organ Sources: Ethical Considerations," *Pediatrics* 89: 1116–1119, p. 1119.

90. See Richard T. DeGeorge. 1978. "Do We Owe the Future Anything?" in *Law and the Ecological Challenge*. AMINTAPHIL II. Buffalo, NY: William S. Hein and Co, pp. 180–190.

it is the day we are going on a picnic, and so on. Furthermore, these features possessed by future dates can provide us with reasons for acting. ("Better buy some bread for sandwiches.") Expected events in the future can have an impact on what we ought to do now. In the same way, the needs and interests of future people can provide us with reasons for acting.

The second argument is an empirical one. It is that we cannot have obligations to future generations because we do not have sufficient information about their lives and needs. For example, we might make enormous sacrifices to conserve fossil fuels for the sake of future generations, only to learn (or perhaps we never would learn) that solar power will be the sole energy source at some point in the future. It is absurd, according to this view, to posit obligations if we cannot specify the content of those obligations. This cannot be done without detailed knowledge of the kinds of lives that will be led.

In contrast to the logical argument, this objection allows that we can make sense of obligations to future generations, or of doing things for their sake. It says only that we do not have enough information to know what to do. This point has some force. The further away future people are in time, the less we can know about their lives and needs. It would be silly to try to guide environmental policies based on the needs of people a thousand years from now. However, it is possible to predict some of the needs of the next few generations. We can reasonably expect that they will continue to drink water and breathe air. It is facetious to maintain that we have no idea what the effects of today's policies will be on future people. Admittedly, we may get it wrong. We may make unnecessary sacrifices or, worse, pursue policies that are detrimental to the interests of future people. There is always the possibility of well-meaning mistakes. But this is true of our relations with existing people as well, and so it is not a reason for denying the moral standing of future people.

So far, the claim is only that present nonexistence does not disqualify a future actual person from a place on the moral-status scale. I have not addressed the knotty problem of how much future people ought to count, or how strong their claims are, as opposed to the claims of presently existing people. My point is simply that the interests of people who will exist can have a claim on us now, so that it is possible now to do things that will harm and wrong people who do not yet exist.

It is precisely this claim that forms the basis of the third objection. This objection says that we cannot be morally required to consider the interests of people living hundreds of years from now, because it is impossible for us *to affect their interests*. This is not simply because future people do not yet exist, nor is it because we lack knowledge about the conditions of their lives. Rather, the claim is that people in the distant future are often radically inaccessible. They cannot be harmed or benefited by what we do today because their very existence may be determined by the actions we take, or fail to take, now.

THE PARFIT PROBLEM AND THE FARTHER FUTURE

This problem with future people has been explained by Derek Parfit, and thus is often termed "the Parfit problem." (Parfit himself calls it "the Non-Identity Problem"; others refer to it as "the identity problem.") To understand the problem, a distinction must be drawn between two kinds of choices. Most of our moral thinking involves what Parfit calls "Same People Choices." In Same People Choices, whatever we choose, all and only the same people will ever live. "Some of these people will be future people. Since these people will exist whatever we choose, we can either harm or benefit these people in a quite straightforward way."[91] Thus, there is no conceptual problem with having obligations to future people in Same People Choices. As Parfit notes:

> Remoteness in time has, in itself, no more significance than remoteness in space. Suppose that I shoot some arrow into a distant wood, where it wounds some person. If I should have known that there might be someone in the wood, I am guilty of gross negligence. Because this person is far away, I cannot identify the person whom I harm. But this is no excuse. Nor is it any excuse that this person is far away. We should make the same claims about effects on people who are temporally remote.[92]

However, future people differ in one crucial respect from spatially distant people. We can affect their identity. This fact produces a problem.

Suppose we are trying to decide on an energy policy. Most people agree that we should consider the long-range impact of our choices. That is, we should not think simply about the effect on ourselves and our children. We should also consider the impact of our current choices on people living hundreds of years from now, so far as we can predict this. Many people would urge that we should conserve resources now, even if this means a slight lowering in our standard of living, in order to prevent serious shortages for people in the further future. To deplete resources now will have harmful effects on generations yet to come.

However, Parfit points out, the choice we make, whether to conserve or deplete, is itself likely to affect which people get born. It is not true that, whichever policy we choose, the same particular people will exist in the further future. Over time, the choice of one policy, rather than another, is likely to affect who marries whom, and when they have children. Thus, different people will be born, depending on which policy we choose. Parfit says, "We can plausibly assume that, after three centuries, there would be no one living in our community who would have been born whichever policy we chose. (It may help to think about this question: how many of us could truly claim, 'Even if railways and motorcars had never been invented, I would still have been born'?)"[93]

We have, then, two possible sets of future people: the people who will be born in 300 years if Conservation is chosen, and the people who will be born in 300 years if Depletion is chosen. If we choose Depletion, the standard of living in 300 years will be very low, much lower than if we had chosen Conservation. However, it is not true that our choice of Depletion causes anyone to be worse off than he would have been if we had chosen differently. And, on a plausible conception of harming, to harm someone is to make him worse off than he would otherwise have been. Since choosing Depletion makes no one worse off than he would otherwise have been, the choice

91. Derek Parfit. 1984. *Reasons and Persons*. Oxford: Clarendon Press, p. 356.

92. Ibid., p. 357.

93. Ibid., p. 361.

of Depletion, paradoxically enough, *harms no one*. If we choose Conservation, the future will contain the Conservation people, living decently in a Conservation environment. If we choose Depletion, the future will contain the Depletion people, living in a not-so-nice Depletion world. The point is that they are two distinct populations. There is no way that we can choose Conservation and arrange for the same people to be born as would have been born had we chosen Depletion. The opportunity to have a decent standard of living simply is not open to the Depletion people. It's a not-so-nice life or no life at all.[94]

The Parfit problem most obviously has implications for policy planning in the areas of conservation and energy. But it also has implications for issues in this book, including abortion, "wrongful-life" cases, and assisted reproduction. Recognition of the Parfit problem forces us to reexamine the concept of harming, and to search for other principles to explain why certain choices would be morally wrong, even if, strictly speaking, they harm no one. (This issue will be examined in detail in Chapter 2.)

Same People Choices do not pose the perplexing problem raised by Different People Choices. So long as individuals will exist at a future time, regardless of what we choose, those individuals can be harmed or benefited by what we do. They have a claim to our moral concern. Futurity alone does not deprive someone of moral standing. However, all claims and rights of future people are premised on their actual future existence. It is only on the assumption that they will exist that they can have interests that exert claims on us. Merely possible future people do not have interests. Unlike future actual people, merely possible people cannot be harmed or benefited, made miserable or happy. Thus, we cannot owe it to them to bring them into existence. There is no right to be brought into existence, only a right to have one's interests considered if one comes into existence.[95]

POTENTIAL PEOPLE: EMBRYOS AND FETUSES

The ability of embryos and fetuses to have interests raises both factual and conceptual questions. The factual issue concerns the emergence of conscious mental states. Mindless, nonsentient creatures cannot have interests. Precisely when fetuses attain conscious awareness is controversial and perhaps indeterminable, but it seems unlikely that fetuses have experiences of any kind before mid-gestation (see Chapter 2). Embryos (the unborn during the first 8 weeks of gestation) at least do not have interests in the robust and morally relevant sense of interests of their own. Their interests, if one wants to call them "interests," are merely teleological, stemming from the fact that they are living organisms. They can survive or die; develop normally or abnormally;

94. Douglas MacLean. 1983. "A Moral Requirement for Energy Policies" in Douglas MacLean and Peter G. Brown, eds., *Energy and the Future*. Totowa, NJ: Rowman & Littlefield, pp. 180–197.

95. Feinberg agrees. He argues that a pact on the part of all human beings never to have children would not violate the rights of those who would otherwise have been born. "My inclination then is to conclude that the suicide of our species would be deplorable, lamentable, and a deeply moving tragedy: but that it would violate no one's rights." *Harm to Others* (see note 10), p. 493.

be healthy or sick. However, they have no stake in what happens to them. Like plants, embryos have autonomous goodness, but they do not have welfares of their own.

It might be thought that if embryos and fetuses do not have welfares of their own, then it does not matter what is done to them. In Chapter 6, I argue that this does not follow. As the earliest form of biological human life, embryos have a symbolic value that precludes using them in unnecessary experiments or for purely commercial gain. However, this symbolic value does not trump the actual interests of born human beings in life and health.

Although embryos and early fetuses do not have interests, they will acquire interests once they are born, or even late in pregnancy, once they become sentient. Their future interests can be damaged by events that occur while they are still in the womb, or even before conception. Smoking, drinking alcohol, or using drugs such as heroin or cocaine during pregnancy can cause a child to be born with serious impairments. The decision to engage in these risky activities during pregnancy is a Same People Choice. Doing these things can injure a child who otherwise would have been born healthy. Thus, to smoke or drink or take drugs is to run the risk of harming one's baby. That future baby has moral claims against its mother that she not engage in risky activities likely to cause it harm. In Chapter 4, I discuss the nature and extent of women's obligations to the children they decide to bear, as well as the question of whether any of these obligations should be legally enforced.

In the next chapter, I use the interest view to defend a pro-choice position on abortion. I argue that abortion does not harm or wrong embryos or preconscious fetuses. Lacking the capacity for awareness of any kind, early-gestation fetuses do not have interests of their own. The pro-life attempt to present embryos and early-gestation fetuses as if they were just like babies, who clearly do have interests, is therefore seriously misleading, I contend. Fetuses have only "contingent" rights and claims—contingent, that is, on future existence as interested beings.

To defend this pro-choice position, I will have to respond to those who maintain that there is a *noncontingent* right to be born, based on the humanity of the unborn and/or its potential personhood. I argue that while these features may be relevant in determining the relative moral status of beings who have moral standing, neither potential personhood nor biological humanity by itself in the absence of conscious awareness confers moral standing. At the same time, it does not follow that abortion is necessarily morally neutral. There may be moral objections to abortion, stemming from personal values and ideals concerning sexuality, marriage, and parenthood. However, such personal values and ideals should not be the basis of legal restrictions or public policy.

2

Abortion

Nearly four decades after the U.S. Supreme Court ruled in *Roe v. Wade*[1] that a woman has a constitutional right to terminate her pregnancy, and nearly two decades since the first edition of this book appeared, abortion remains one of the most divisive and emotionally charged issues in America. In 2010, at least 11 states passed laws restricting abortion, a number regarded by those on both sides of the debate as unusually high.[2] The laws ranged from the limiting of coverage of abortion by private and state insurers, to a ban in Nebraska on all abortions after 20 weeks, on the ground that the fetus at that stage might feel pain.[3] (As current abortion law gives women a constitutional right to abortion prior to viability, which occurs a month or more later, Nebraska's law may be challenged in court.) Similar measures are being introduced in Indiana, Iowa, New Hampshire, Oklahoma and other states.[4] Thirty-four states require counseling before abortions; 25 of these states require women to wait a specified amount of time—usually 24 hours—between the counselling and the abortion.[5] In March 2011, South Dakota passed a bill that would require women to wait 72 hours before an abortion, and to undergo counseling at a "pregnancy help center," which pro-choice advocates say are often run by anti-abortion groups who try to talk the women out of having abortions.[6] Seventeen states encourage the use of ultrasound in abortion, while in Alabama, Louisiana, and Mississippi, abortion providers must perform an ultrasound and offer the woman a chance to view the fetus.

1. *Roe v. Wade*, 410 U.S. 113 (1973).

2. John Leland. 2010. "Abortion Foes Advance Cause at State Level," *New York Times*, June 2. http://www.nytimes.com/2010/06/03/health/policy/03abortion.html. Accessed June 8, 2010.

3. Janice Hopkins Tanne. 2010. "Nebraska Prohibits Abortion After 20 Weeks Because of Fetal Pain," *British Medical Journal* 340:c2091. http://www.bmj.com/cgi/content/short/340/apr16_2/c2091?rss=1. Accessed June 8, 2010.

4. Erik Eckholm. 2011. "Across Country, Lawmakers Push Abortion Curbs," *New York Times*, Jan. 21. http://www.nytimes.com/2011/01/22/us/politics/22abortion.html. Accessed Jan. 23, 2011.

5. Guttmacher Institute. 2011. "Counseling and Waiting Periods for Abortion." http://www.guttmacher.org/statecenter/spibs/spib_MWPA.pdf. Accessed Jan. 23, 2011.

6. Reuters, 2011. "Group Threatens to Sue S. Dakota Over Abortion Bill." http://www.reuters.com/article/2011/03/11/us-abortion-south-dakota-idUSTRE72A84W20110311. Accessed March 16, 2011.

In Oklahoma, the Republican-controlled legislature overrode a veto by Democratic governor, Brad Henry, to enact a law that requires that women be presented with an ultrasound image, although they may avert their eyes, and with a detailed oral description of the embryo or fetus. The law was quickly challenged by two abortion providers, and it has been stayed by a state judge pending a hearing.[7]

Although laws requiring women to view ultrasound images of the fetus are often presented by their supporters as simply ensuring fully informed consent, both sides of the abortion debate regard such laws as aimed at restricting abortions. Abortion rights advocates generally oppose laws that require ultrasounds, even if viewing them is voluntary, while Focus on the Family, a Christian organization dedicated to promoting social policy "that improves the strength and health of the family, as God designed,"[8] has spent an estimated $10 million to buy ultrasound equipment and provide training for centers that steer women away from abortion.[9]

It is unclear that such laws have any effect on the number of abortions performed. In a study done in British Columbia (none has been done in the United States), two abortion clinics found that 73% of women wanted to see an ultrasound image if offered the chance, 84% said that it did not make the decision more difficult, and none reversed her decision.[10] In Alabama, which enacted its law in 2002, it is estimated that between 30% and 70% of women undergoing abortions opt to view the ultrasound. The law has had no apparent impact on the number of abortions in the state, approximately 11,300 a year. According to a provider in a Birmingham clinic, "I've never had one patient get off the table because she saw what her fetus looks like."[11] In fact, the image may be reassuring for some women, especially in an early abortion. " 'It just looked like a little egg, and I couldn't see arms or legs or a face,' said Tiesha, 27, who chose to view her 8-week-old embryo before aborting it at the Birmingham clinic. 'It was really the picture of the ultrasound that made me feel it was O.K.' "[12] But other women find the ultrasound requirement cruel and offensive for the implicit suggestion that they have not fully considered their choice. As one woman put it, "You don't just walk into one of these places like you're getting your nails done," she said. "I think we're armed with enough information to make adult decisions without being emotionally tortured."[13]

Much of the legislation passed in 2010 was made possible by a 2007 U.S. Supreme Court decision upholding a federal ban on a late-term procedure that critics call partial-birth abortion, discussed later, which gave lawmakers greater leeway to restrict abortion.[14] Although late-term abortions, those performed at 21 weeks

7. Kevin Sack. 2010. "In Ultrasound, Abortion Has New Front," New York Times, May 27. http://www.nytimes.com/2010/05/28/health/policy/28ultrasound.html. Accessed July 6, 2010.

8. Focus on the Family, http://www.focusonthefamily.com/about_us.aspx. Accessed June 8, 2010.

9. Sack, "In Ultrasound, Abortion Has New Front" (see note 6).

10. Ibid.

11. Ibid.

12. Ibid.

13. Ibid.

14. Leland (see note 2).

gestation or later, are quite rare, comprising only 1.5% of all abortions in the United States each year,[15] such abortions generate some of the most bitter battles. The very few abortion providers willing to perform late-term abortions face public opprobrium and sometimes death. On May 31, 2009, Dr. George Tiller, who performed many abortions after 20 weeks of fetuses with severe anomalies, was shot to death in church in Wichita, Kansas. His killer, Scott Roeder, who, according to members of his family, suffers from mental illness,[16] was sentenced to life in prison without eligibility for parole for 50 years.[17]

Although this was the first killing in the United States of an abortion doctor since October 1998 when Dr. Barnett Slepian was fatally shot by militant abortion opponent James Kopp, Eleanor Smeal, the founder and president of the Feminist Majority Foundation, said a survey her group commissioned in 2008 found an escalation of hostile acts toward doctors at abortion clinics.[18] This is not entirely surprising, if one takes seriously the claim that a fetus is an innocent child. If someone planned to go into a kindergarten and slaughter all the children, surely it would be morally justified to stop him, and even to shoot him, if necessary. Only a total pacifist could object, and while most pro-lifers reject violence against abortion clinics and providers, most are not pacifists.

It is often said that abortion politics in America lie behind many issues that have nothing to do with abortion, from embryonic stem cell research to assisted suicide to end-of-life care. The case of Terri Schiavo, which concerned a lengthy court battle between the husband and parents of a young woman in a permanent vegetative state, about whether to remove her feeding tube, attracted the support of the pro-life movement. As one editorial expressed the connection between the Schiavo case and abortion, "The killing of pre-born children leads to the killing of older people, people with disabilities, and people who are ill. Life is a tapestry, and when one thread has been pulled out by advocates of abortion, the rest of the threads begin to unravel. 2005, the year of Terri Schiavo's death, can be traced to 1973, the year of the infamous *Roe v. Wade* court ruling legalizing abortion for any reason during all nine months of pregnancy."[19] However, it is not only *Roe*'s critics who make connections between abortion and other life and death issues. In the first assisted suicide case decided by a federal court, *Compassion in Dying v. Washington*,[20]

15. Guttmacher Institute. 2010. "Facts on Induced Abortions in the United States." http://www.guttmacher.org/pubs/fb_induced_abortion.html. Accessed June 8, 2010.

16. Susan Saulny and Monica Davey. 2009. "Suspect in Doctor's Killing Is Tied to Vandalism Case," *New York Times*, June 3, A18. http://www.nytimes.com/2009/06/03/us/03tiller.html. Accessed July 6, 2010.

17. CNN wire staff, 2010. "Doctor's Killer Sentenced to Life in Prison," April 1. http://www.cnn.com/2010/CRIME/04/01/kansas.abortion.roeder.sentence/index.html. Accessed June 8, 2010.

18. Susan Saulny and Monica Davey, "Suspect in Doctor's Killing Tied to Vandalism Case" (see note 15).

19. Maria Vitale. 2010. "Abortion's Slippery Slope Led to Killing Terri Schiavo, We Must Never Forget," Lifenews.com, March 29. http://www.lifenews.com/bio3076.html. Accessed May 28, 2010.

20. *Compassion in Dying v. Washington*, 850 F. Supp. 1454 (WD Wash. 1994).

the judge cited another landmark abortion case, *Planned Parenthood v. Casey*, and said, "Like the abortion decision, the decision of a terminally ill person to end his or her life 'involves the most intimate and personal choice a person may make in a lifetime' and constitutes a 'choice central to personal dignity and autonomy.'"[21]

Given the influence of the abortion debate on so many areas of social policy, it is all the more crucial that we subject to philosophical scrutiny its central claims. Is the fetus a human being, with the same moral status as any born human being, as pro-lifers maintain?[22] If it is, then very few abortions, if any, could be justified, for we do not generally think that it is morally permissible to kill children because they are unwanted or illegitimate or severely disabled. On the other hand, if the fetus[23] is not a child, but only part of the pregnant woman's body, then restrictive abortion laws would be as difficult to justify in a pluralistic society as laws against contraception. This is because restrictive abortion laws impose enormous physical, emotional, and financial burdens on women. Even legal moralists, who hold that society has the right to enforce its moral beliefs through law, could not justify the imposition of such heavy burdens. Only the assumption that the unborn is a human being like any other, entitled to the law's protection, could justify the prohibition of abortion. Thus, the moral status of the unborn is central to the abortion debate.

Some writers on abortion are skeptical of any attempts to resolve the abortion question by investigations into the moral status of the unborn, because people's views on whether a fetus has moral standing are rarely independent of their opinions about abortion. Sociologist Kristin Luker argues persuasively that what really divides pro-choice and pro-life activists is not a different philosophical conception of the fetus, but rather their differing views on the meaning and value of sexuality, motherhood, and the proper role of women.[24] Their attitudes on these issues determine their views on abortion, which in turn determine how they think about the fetus. For this reason, according to philosopher Ruth Macklin, any attempt to derive the morality of abortion from a conception of the unborn is bound to be question-begging.[25]

It must be acknowledged that our conceptual views are not immune from social, political, and psychological influences. The radically different world-views of pro-choicers and pro-lifers undoubtedly affect their thinking about embryos, and

21. Ibid., 850 F. Supp. at 1459–1460.

22. As in Chapter 1, I use the term "moral standing" to refer to whether a being's interests must be considered from the moral point of view, and I have used the term "moral status" to refer to the relative weight that must be accorded its interests. All sentient beings have moral standing, in my view, but they do not all have equal moral status, since other factors, such as psychological connectedness, moral agency, and the capacity for relationships are relevant to moral status.

23. Technically, the term "fetus" refers to the unborn after 8 weeks of gestation. Many writers on abortion use the term "fetus" to refer to the unborn throughout pregnancy. I will follow this convention except where necessary to distinguish the different phases of gestation.

24. Kristin Luker. 1984. *Abortion and the Politics of Motherhood*. Berkeley, CA: University of California Press, especially Chapter 7.

25. Ruth Macklin. 1984. "Personhood and the Abortion Debate," in Jay Garfield and Patricia Hennessey, eds., *Abortion: Moral and Legal Perspectives*. Amherst, MA: The University of Massachusetts Press, p. 97.

whether they see them as clumps of cells or very small babies. But recognition of such influences does not preclude rational assessment of the arguments.

Few writers on abortion come to the topic with a fully open mind, and I am no exception. I believe that the decision to have an abortion is one that belongs to the pregnant woman—not the state, not her doctor, not her husband or partner. My pro-choice position is based on two independent considerations: the moral status of the fetus and the pregnant woman's moral right to bodily self-determination. I believe that both are necessary for an adequate treatment of abortion, yet many writers on abortion focus on only one aspect, while ignoring or downplaying the other. Thus, some opponents of abortion talk about the fetal right to live, or the wrongness of depriving a potential human being of its future life, without even mentioning the fact that a particular woman must carry and bear the fetus for it to have a future life.[26] On the other side, some feminists regard the inquiry into the moral standing of the fetus as irrelevant to the problem of abortion.[27] The central questions, from a feminist perspective, are not about the abstract individual rights of fetuses but how to create the social conditions that make possible the fulfillment of reproductive responsibilities. Sandra Harding says that we must go "beneath the surface of the abortion dispute" and ask such questions as:

> Why are adult women not treated by law or custom as full social persons with equal rights . . .? How can a woman or a child exercise her "right to life" or "freedom of choice" in the face of poverty, unemployment, racism, legal and individual sexism, and the whole gamut of material conditions attributable to these material restrictions on social personhood?[28]

But these questions, important as they are, do not go "beneath the surface of the abortion dispute." *They change the subject.* The moral issue is whether abortion is a permissible choice. This question would remain, even if poverty, racism, or sexism were eliminated. In such a world, there would presumably still be contraceptive failures and unwanted pregnancies. It goes without saying that women ought to be recognized as fully autonomous choosers; the question is whether abortion is a choice that autonomous choosers are morally permitted to make. It is hard to see how one can answer this question without responding to the claim that abortion is the killing of a human being, with a right to life.

The interest view responds to this claim by arguing that embryos and early fetuses, although biologically human, do not have moral standing. We are not morally required to consider their interests because, prior to becoming conscious and sentient, fetuses do not *have* interests. The defense of this claim requires some factual investigation as to when sentience occurs. More important, I will need to explain why sentience is essential to moral standing. After all, if allowed to grow and develop,

---

26. An example is Don Marquis, "Why Abortion Is Immoral," *The Journal of Philosophy* 76: 4 (April 1989), pp. 183–202.

27. See, for example, Sandra Harding. 1984. "Beneath the Surface of the Abortion Dispute: Are Women Fully Human?" in Sidney Callahan and Daniel Callahan, eds., *Abortion: Understanding Differences.* New York and London: Plenum Press, pp. 203–224.

28. Ibid., p. 214.

the nonconscious, nonsentient fetus will become conscious and sentient. Some maintain that its potential to acquire these characteristics gives the fetus a present interest in continued existence, endows it with moral standing, and makes abortion seriously wrong.

In the first section, I defend the sentience criterion for moral standing against its main contenders: genetic humanity and personhood. In the second section, I consider, and reject, the claim that the fetus has moral standing in virtue of its potential to develop into a person. The third section discusses Don Marquis's novel argument against abortion: the "future-like-ours account" (FLOA) of abortion. The fourth section considers the question of identity and its relevance to the morality of abortion. The fifth section takes up the moral standing of merely possible persons. I defend a "person-affecting restriction" (PAR), which maintains that we are required to consider the interests of existing beings only, whether they exist now, in the present, or at some future time. Merely possible people, that is, people who might exist, cannot be benefited or harmed, nor do they have moral claims against us. In particular, they do not have a claim to be brought into existence. One of the most significant challenges to the PAR comes from Derek Parfit. Parfit convincingly argues that our moral obligations are not limited to existing beings. We can have obligations not to do certain things, even if doing them would harm no one or make no one worse off. Such cases arise when harm can be avoided only by changing the identity of who gets born, which gives rise to the "nonidentity problem." Most of us have a strong intuition that it would be wrong to bring someone into existence in a harmful or disadvantageous condition, even if there is no way that individual could have been born without the harmful condition, if this could have been avoided by bringing a different person into existence, who does not have the disadvantageous condition. So long as the person with the harmful condition is, on balance, glad to have been born, it seems absurd to say that he or she was harmed or wronged by being born, even if we think the parents did something wrong in having *this* child rather than the child without the harmful condition. I compare Jeffrey Reiman's person-affecting, Rawlsian solution to the nonidentity problem with an approach based on an impersonal substitution principle, and argue that ultimately these approaches are not all that different from each other. Reiman's rights-based solution stems from the adoption of an impersonal stance in the original position, while the rationale for the impersonal substitution principle is to avoid the suffering experienced by real individuals. Regardless of which theoretical approach one finds more satisfactory, they both get the same and, I believe, correct normative result. Ultimately, I think that adoption of an objective, non-person-affecting, substitution principle is more defensible than an approach based on rights-violation, though I do not think that very much hinges on which approach is taken. What does matter is that the adoption of a substitution principle does not have the unacceptable implication that possible people have claims against us, including specifically a right to be born. Adoption of a substitution principle in non-identity cases does not commit us to maintaining, implausibly, that we have an obligation to bring possible people into existence, if they would have happy lives. Rather, it maintains that, other things being equal, it is objectively better not to bring someone seriously disadvantaged into the world, when this can be avoided without undue burden by substitution.

In the sixth section, I offer a pro-choice argument based on the pregnant woman's right of bodily self-determination or privacy, as it has been deemed in the law. I conceive of the right of bodily self-determination as a fundamental moral right. It includes the right to bodily integrity, as well as the right to decide what happens in and to one's body. The moral right of bodily self-determination is the basis for several common law rights, including the right to refuse medical treatment and the right to informed consent. In addition, the discovery of a constitutional right of privacy is most plausibly explained by the assumption of a fundamental moral right of bodily self-determination. The pro-choice argument I offer here has both moral and legal significance. It is based on Judith Thomson's famous and influential article, "A Defense of Abortion."[29] Thomson argues that no one is morally obligated to make large sacrifices to allow another person to use his body, not even if this is needed for life itself. I point out some problems with basing a general defense of abortion on this claim, but I suggest that these problems disappear if the fetus is not assumed to be a person, with a right to life. In other words, I combine Thomson's argument on the right of individuals to bodily self-determination and autonomy with the interest view's conception of the fetus. This results in a view very similar to that taken by the Supreme Court in *Roe v. Wade*. The seventh section discusses the significance of viability and argues that it is late gestation rather than survivability per se that has moral significance. The similarity between a late-gestation fetus and a newborn is striking, which provides some reason for giving late fetuses the same protection as newborns. However, geography plays a crucial role here; fetuses, even late fetuses, reside within the bodies of pregnant women. While states have a legitimate interest in preserving the lives of nearly born fetuses, that interest cannot be allowed to take precedence over the interests of women in their health, including their reproductive health, and their lives.

THE MORAL STANDING OF THE FETUS

The Conservative Position

The most extreme antiabortion position holds that a fertilized human ovum is a human being, with a right to life, like any other human being. This is often called the "extreme conservative" position, to contrast it with a more moderate conservative position that regards the implantation of the embryo in the uterus as the beginning of an individual human life (see later section on "Implantation"). Moderate and extreme conservatives also differ on whether any abortions are morally permissible. Moderate conservatives allow rape and threats to the woman's life, and perhaps health, as justifying abortion. By contrast, the extreme conservative, exemplified by the Roman Catholic Church, does not allow abortion even if continuing the pregnancy will cause the mother's death. This is because the Church views the mother and fetus as equal in moral status; one cannot be sacrificed to save the other. In the discussion that follows regarding the extreme conservative position, I address only the analysis of when a human life begins, and not possible justifications for abortion.

---

29. Judith Jarvis Thomson. 1971. "A Defense of Abortion," *Philosophy & Public Affairs* 1 (1): 47–66.

The argument for the extreme view has two parts. First, the conservative points to the fact that the fetus is indisputably genetically human. Moreover, it is not merely a human cell, like any cell in a human body. At the completion of fertilization, a process that can take up to 24 hours, there is a new and unique genotype, which is distinct from that of either parent. The fertilized egg, or single-celled zygote, has the full complement of 23 pairs of chromosomes, one in each pair from each parent. From this single cell develop all the different types of tissue and organs that make up the human body. Fertilization thus marks the spatiotemporal beginning of a new human being. As John Noonan expresses it, "The positive argument for conception as the decisive moment of humanization is that at conception the new being receives the genetic code. It is this genetic information which determines his characteristics, which is the biological carrier of the possibility of human wisdom, which makes him a self-evolving being. A being with a human genetic code is man."[30]

The second part of the conservative argument maintains that, after fertilization, there is no event or change in the unborn that has such moral significance that it would enable us to say, "*Now* we have a human being, but before this event it was not human." Traditionally, birth has been held to mark the beginning of human life. At birth, the fetus is separated from its mother and is no longer physiologically dependent on her. Birth as a dividing line has the advantage of being objective and definite. Your birth certificate marks the day, hour, and even minute you were born. However, the conservative denies that birth has such enormous moral significance. There is not much difference between a newborn moments after birth, and a fetus moments before it is born. How, the conservative asks, can a change in location have such a drastic effect on moral status?

The conservative then moves backward through pregnancy, dismissing other suggested landmarks. Consider, for example, viability, defined by the Supreme Court in *Roe v. Wade* as the time when a fetus is "potentially able to live outside the mother's womb, albeit with artificial aid."[31] The argument for regarding viability as having moral significance is that before the fetus can survive independently of the mother, it is really only a part of her body, like an organ or a limb. By contrast, a viable fetus, though *within* the body of the mother, is not merely a part of her body. A mere bodily part is not capable of living on its own. A viable fetus can be separated from its mother and remain alive. The conservative responds that it is a mistake to identify *independent* existence with *separate* existence. The nonviable fetus admittedly cannot exist independently of its mother, but it is nevertheless a separate individual, with its own genetic code. It is not merely a part of the pregnant woman's body. Moreover, the conservative denies that independent existence has the moral significance ascribed to it by the viability criterion. Babies and young children are also dependent on the care of others for their survival. As Noonan puts it, "The unsubstantial lessening in dependence at viability does not seem to signify any special acquisition

30. John T. Noonan, Jr. 1970. "An Almost Absolute Value in History," in John T. Noonan, Jr., ed., *The Morality of Abortion: Legal and Historical Perspectives.* Cambridge, MA: Harvard University Press.

31. *Roe v. Wade* (see note 1), at 160.

of humanity."[32] Moreover, people dependent on iron lungs or respirators are not less human, less worthy of protection, than the rest of us.[33]

Nor does the conservative find moral relevance in any earlier stages, such as quickening. Quickening refers to the mother's ability to perceive fetal movement. Probably the view that human life begins at quickening stems from the biologically inaccurate view that the fetus is not alive before it moves. Since we now know that the single-celled zygote (indeed, even the sperm or ovum) is alive, there is no reason to base moral status on the fetus's ability to move (motility), and even less reason to make its moral standing depend on its mother's alertness in detecting movement.

The fetus begins to look recognizably human between 9 and 12 weeks gestation age (g.a.).[34] The eyelids close and will not reopen until the 28th week. Its hands, still encased in an enveloping membrane, have well-demarcated fingers and thumbs. Its face is well formed, although nails, eyebrows, and lashes do not appear until about week 20. At 12 weeks, the fetus may not look much like a baby, but it is clearly a *human* fetus. By contrast, it is difficult to distinguish a human fetus at 8 weeks g.a. from a cat or pig fetus of the comparable gestational age. There is clearly a difference in appearance between an early fetus and a more developed one, but does this difference have moral significance? The conservative denies that it does, on the ground that this suggests that deformed human beings (such as the Elephant Man) who do not look like other people lack human moral status.

Finally, it has been suggested that human life begins when brain waves first appear, at about 8 weeks g.a. The rationale for this view is that it provides a symmetry between the criterion for the end and the beginning of life in that both are marked by the absence of brain function. However, as we saw in the last chapter, critics of the neurological criterion of death deny that it tracks the death of the organism, since a brain-dead body can be kept alive, sometimes for extended periods of time. Moreover, it can be argued that the emergence of brain waves has no more significance than any other developmental stage in the life of the human organism. If the embryo is not killed, it has a good chance of acquiring brain waves, human form, the capacity for movement, viability, and every other human feature. Therefore, the extreme conservative concludes, *no* stage or feature can have decisive moral significance, such that abortion is permissible before the fetus attains it, but not after. Every successive stage after conception is just development from the beginning.

As I said earlier, there are two parts to the extreme conservative position. First, it attaches moral significance to the genetic humanity of the fetus; second, it argues that this humanity is present from conception onward. Either part can be challenged independently. For example, Baruch Brody takes what might be called a modified conservative position. Like Noonan, Brody bases the moral status of the unborn on its being human. However, he does not agree that humanity begins at conception.

32. Noonan (see note 29), p. 10.

33. Richard Warner. 1974. "Abortion: The Ontological and Moral Status of the Unborn," *Social Theory and Practice* 3: 4. Revised and reprinted in Richard A. Wasserstrom, ed. 1979. *Today's Moral Problems*, 2nd edition. New York: MacMillan Publishing Company, Inc., p. 55.

34. Obstetricians date the beginning of a pregnancy from the woman's last menstrual period, which can be more reliably fixed than conception. This adds approximately 2 weeks to the fetus's age. Thus, a fetus at 14 weeks g.a. is actually about 12 weeks old.

Brody argues that a functioning brain is essential for being human. When the brain stops functioning, the person dies and goes out of existence. On the same reasoning, the fetus "comes into humanity" when its brain begins to function.[35] In other words, the beginning of brain function marks a radical discontinuity in the life of the unborn. The human being who begins when brain function starts is not identical with the embryo whose brain has not yet begun to function.

Even if one accepts the thesis of radical discontinuity (a thesis that most conservatives would reject as inconsistent with the reality of continuous physical development), it is not clear why this should be marked by the emergence of brain waves. The beginning of brain function, taken as a physiological occurrence, is not different from any other change in the fetus. The significance of brain function lies rather in its connection with mental states, such as conscious awareness. Brody suggests this when he says, "One of the characteristics essential to a human being is the capacity for conscious experience, at least at a primitive level. Before the sixth week, as far as we know, the fetus does not have this capacity. Thereafter, as the electroencephalographic evidence indicates, it does. Consequently, that is the time at which the fetus becomes a human being."[36]

The phrase "capacity for conscious experience" is ambiguous. It might refer to the physiological ability of a being to have conscious experiences *at some point* in its development. The fetus at 6 weeks after conception (8 weeks g.a.) certainly has the capacity for conscious experience in this sense, but so does the single-celled zygote. Obviously, this is not what Brody intends. In another sense of "capacity," a being has the capacity for an experience x if x occurs, given the appropriate stimulus. A frog has the capacity to feel pain if, on being subjected to certain kinds of stimuli, the frog feels pain. However, in this sense of "capacity," neither a zygote nor a 6-week-old fetus has the capacity for conscious experience.

Brain function has no significance if taken as a purely physiological development in the fetus. Brain function is significant only because it is a necessary condition for mental states, such as experiences of pain and other sensations, beliefs, memories, and the like. When someone's brain stops functioning, there are no mental states (though it is debatable that total and permanent lack of consciousness is death). However, brain function is not a sufficient condition for even the most rudimentary mental states. The brain begins to function long before there are any mental states at all. Thus, Brody's claim that the emergence of brain waves marks the beginning of human life is not tenable.

As mentioned earlier, some conservatives place the beginning of a human life at implantation. Whether a human being exists at conception or at implantation has no practical implications for abortion; an abortion cannot be performed unless a pregnancy has begun. The more moderate view does have implications for the discarding of embryos in assisted reproduction (Chapter 5) and embryonic stem cell research (Chapter 6), and it will be revisited in those chapters. Extreme conservatives oppose emergency contraception that prevents the implantation of a fertilized egg, while this is morally acceptable for moderate conservatives.

35. Baruch Brody. 1975. *Abortion and the Sanctity of Life.* Cambridge, MA: The MIT Press, p. 111.

36. Ibid., p. 83.

Fetal Sentience

The interest view places great importance on conscious awareness, the ability to have experiences, holding that this ability is essential for having interests (in the robust sense) and a welfare of one's own. It is important, then, to understand fetal development, and to understand what physiological developments, beyond simple brain function, are necessary for the experience of pain. The capacity to experience *pain* is not in itself significant, but as it is arguably the most primitive form of conscious experience, we can be confident that before the fetus is sentient, it is incapable of any other kinds of experiences, thoughts, or feelings.

The question, when does the fetus become sentient, is not solely a matter of biology. There is also the conceptual question: What do we mean when we say that a being is experiencing pain? and the epistemological question: How we can know when a being is experiencing pain? Commenting on these philosophical difficulties, Nicholas Fisk, professor of obstetrics and gynecology, writes:

> Pain as you know is a philosophical minefield. It is simply defined as "the unpleasant physical or motional response to actual or potential tissue damage." That gets us nowhere with a fetus or new-born baby. At the one extreme we have people arguing that this involves consciousness, even emotion or memory. It is possible that you then have to be three years old to feel pain. At the other extreme we got electrical responses, reflexes. Plants have profound electrical signal activity in response to trauma, yet no one seriously suggests that you give a general anaesthetic to a lawn before you mow it.[37]

I will assume in what follows that we do know, most of the time, when others are in pain, and that we know that newborn infants can feel pain, and that their facial expressions and crying are reliable evidence of this. However, we also know that "pain behaviors" are not always reliable evidence of experiences. They might be mere reflex behaviors that tell us nothing about the individual's subjective experiences. This is what most neurologists believe about persistent vegetative state (PVS) patients, because brain scans reveal that their cerebral cortexes have been destroyed. Since the cerebral cortex (also called the neocortex, because it is the last part of the brain to develop) is where pain is experienced, it seems very likely there is no experience of pain, if the cerebral cortex is absent. Can we assume that the same is true of fetuses?

Evidence for fetal sentience obviously cannot be direct. We cannot ask fetuses what they are experiencing. The evidence can only be indirect, based on what we know about the fetal nervous system, in particular, the connection between the thalamus and the cerebral cortex. Painful sensations are transmitted on nerve fibers and interpreted in the cerebral cortex. Development of the fetal cerebral cortex begins at 8 weeks of g.a., and by 20 weeks it has a normal complement of 109 neurons. The cortical neurons undergo profuse arborization and develop synaptic targets for the incoming thalamocortical fibers and intracortical connections. K .J. S. Anand and

---

37. Saulny and Davey, "Suspect in Doctor's Killing Is Tied to Vandalism Case" (see note 15).

P. R. Hickey, researchers at Children's Hospital in Boston, explain the significance of this development for pain perception:

> The timing of the thalamocortical connection is of crucial importance for cortical perception, since most sensory pathways to the neocortex have synapses in the thalamus. Studies of primate and human fetuses have shown that afferent neurons in the thalamus produce axons that arrive in the cerebrum before mid-gestation. These fibers then "wait" just below the neocortex until migration and dendritic arborization of cortical neurons are complete and finally establish synaptic connections between 20 and 24 weeks of gestation.[38]

Anand and Hickey's research was aimed at proving that neonates and preterm babies *can* feel pain, in light of the then-prevailing view that premature babies do not feel pain, and do not need anesthesia during surgery. However, their research also seemed to indicate that pain perception much earlier than the end of the second trimester is highly unlikely because the neural pathways are not sufficiently developed to transmit pain messages to the fetal cortex until 20 to 24 weeks of gestation.

The recognition that fetuses might be capable of experiencing pain after 20 weeks has potential implications both for how late abortions are performed, and whether they should be performed at all. The number of such abortions is comparatively small. Of all legal induced abortions reported to the Centers for Disease Control (CDC) in 2005, only 1.3% were performed at or after 21 weeks. However, in that year, 1.2 million abortions were performed in the United States, which means that 15,600 abortions were performed at or after 21 weeks, which is not a trivial number. If such abortions are to be performed, it is important that they not inflict severe pain. And if sentience is possible earlier, it might be advisable to administer analgesia for earlier second-trimester abortions. How early in gestation might fetal sentience occur?

In 1996, Dr. Vivette Glover and Professor Nicholas Fisk wrote:

> Studies indicate that cortical, subcortical, and peripheral centres necessary for pain perception begin developing early in the second trimester. From 14 weeks most of the body responds to touch by moving away, but this is probably a subcortical reflex response. To experience anything, including pain, the subject needs to be conscious, and current evidence suggests that this involves activity in the cerebral cortex and possibly the thalamus. We do not know for sure when or even if the fetus becomes conscious. However, temporary thalamorcortical connections start to form at about 17 weeks and become established from 26 weeks. It seems very likely that a fetus can feel pain from that stage.[39]

Might sentience occur earlier than 26 weeks? The American College of Obstetricians and Gynecologists says it "knows of no legitimate scientific information that

38. K. J. S. Anand and P. R. Hickey. 1987. "Pain and Its Effects in the Human Neonate and Fetus," *The New England Journal of Medicine* 317 (21): 1322.

39. Vivette Glover and Nicholas Fisk. 1996. "Commentary: We Don't Know; Better to Err on the Safe Side From Mid-gestation," *British Medical Journal* 313: 7 September 96: 28. http://www.bmj.com/content/313/7060/796.1.extract. Accessed October 29, 2010.

supports the statement that a fetus experiences pain at 20 weeks' gestation."[40] While it is true that no one has established that fetuses do feel pain earlier than 26 weeks g.a., some scientists are reluctant to conclude that they do not. In evidence provided in February 1996 to the Commission on Fetal Sentience, a body set up by CARE, a British Christian education charity, Professor Glover said:

... before that stage [i.e., 26 weeks] I am really much more uncertain. I do not think that one can say one can be sure before that stage what is going on. We know so little about consciousness in the adult, and we do know that the same mechanisms are taking place in the fetus. I think it is possible that there might be consciousness associated just with thalamic activity, without going through to the cortex. It is possible that there are links going through to the cortex which are not going via the thalamus. Certainly if one's thinking about distress or stress and general feelings of discomfort, not clear, sharp pain pathways, it could be going via different mechanisms. I am not saying at all we are sure that it is, we just don't know. But I would be very reluctant to say I am sure that it was not.[41]

She went on to say:

Normally scientists are very cautious and are unwilling to say beyond what they know. I think I would like to make a distinction between scientific caution and medical caution. As a scientist one always has to be very careful not to overstate one's case, but in this area I am a bit concerned that if we just say we don't know, we may be causing quite a lot of suffering. I would rather err on the safe side and say; "Well, it may be suffering and so we ought to do something about it." We don't know it is, but I think medical caution pulls one in the opposite direction to scientific caution in this area.[42]

Professor Nicholas Fisk adds, "... it is generally felt that none of the spinal pathways and cortical connections can possibly be present below 13 weeks. So it is highly unlikely that there is any central processing whatsoever. We look at a continuum between 13 and 26 weeks where connections are increasingly established and by the end of that period we are fairly confident that they are intact, but at the beginning they are very unlikely to be."[43] On the principle that it is "better to err on the safe side," Glover and Fisk recommend that anesthesia be considered after mid-gestation. "Hence until there is evidence to the contrary those conducting later terminations should try to use methods that are likely to cause as little suffering as possible. This must be balanced against the distress to the mother caused to the

40. AOL News. 2010. "Nebraska Bill Would Ban Abortions After 20 Weeks." February 25. http://www.aolnews.com/nation/article/neb-bill-citing-fetal-pain-would-ban-abortions-after-20-weeks/19373318. Accessed October 29, 2010.

41. Commission of Inquiry into Fetal Sentience 1996. Transcript of Evidence by Dr. Vivette Glover and Professor Nicholas Fisk. February 7.

42. Ibid.

43. Ibid.

method used."[44] They go on to point out that there are technical problems in delivering analgesia to fetuses, something they elaborate in their testimony to the Commission:

> ... perhaps the most challenging [thing] is to assess whether you can ablate; whether you can get rid of these [stress] responses with pain killers or analgesia. It sounds very simple, but it is actually quite a complex question. You can give these drugs to the mother but you have to give ... an awful lot [of them] because most of them cross the placenta poorly. You might have to give them such large doses that you jeopardise the mother's breathing. Or you can give it directly to the fetus. But again if you give an injection to the fetus, that is painful itself.[45]

Because there are these technical difficulties, and because physicians have to balance the pain and distress to the fetus against the welfare of the mother, it would seem that decisions to administer pain relief to the fetus in late-term abortions are best left to physicians' judgment. Legislation is likely to be a rather ham-handed method of reducing overall suffering. Yet in 2005, Minnesota became one of the few states—the others are Arkansas, Georgia, Louisiana, and Oklahoma—that required that women 20 weeks or later in pregnancy be offered analgesia for the fetus. On July 13, its legislature passed the Unborn Child Pain Prevention Act, which was signed into law by Governor Tim Pawlenty on July 14, 2005. The Act:

> Directs that prior to performing an abortion on an unborn child who is of 20 weeks gestational age or more, the physician or the physician's agent shall inform the female if an anesthetic would eliminate or alleviate pain to the unborn child caused by the method of abortion. Provides that the physician or physician's agent shall inform the woman of risks associated with the anesthetic. Provides that with the woman's consent, the physician shall administer the anesthetic.[46]

In 2004, the federal Unborn Child Pain Awareness Act was introduced into both the House and Senate by Rep. Chris Smith (R-NJ) and Sen. Sam Brownback (R-KS). (It was defeated in the House of Representatives in December 2006.[47]) The legislation would have required abortion providers to tell pregnant women, at any stage of pregnancy, that Congress has determined that the "unborn child has the physical structures necessary to experience pain." The bill also required providers to offer anesthesia to women. Critics pointed out that there is no established procedure for administering anesthesia to a fetus during an abortion. The position of the

---

44. Glover and Fisk, "Commentary: We don't know; better to err on the safe side from mid-gestation" (see note 36).

45. Commission of Inquiry into Fetal Sentience (see note 40).

46. Minnesota Citizens Concerned for Life 2009. Unborn Child Pain Prevention Act. http://www.mccl.org/Page.aspx?pid=363. Accessed June 5, 2009.

47. Zimmerman, L. 2007. "The Unborn Child Pain Awareness Act: Bad Medicine on the Hill," *Litmus* 1 (2), Jan. 22. http://www.litmuszine.com/sin/1.22.07.html. Accessed June 5, 2009.

National Abortion Foundation (NAF) is that anesthesia should not be offered to the fetus outside of a clinical trial, because doing so poses a risk to the woman.[48]

A striking feature of the Unborn Child Pain Awareness Act is that it would have required abortion providers to offer women anesthesia for the fetus, at *any* stage in pregnancy. The vast majority of abortions in the United States—approximately 9 in 10 (88%)[49]—take place in the first 12 weeks of pregnancy, when none of the spinal pathways and cortical connections necessary for pain perception are present, and experts agree that the fetus is not sentient. Given this, it seems that the intention of the bill was not to enable women to make an informed choice about how the abortion is performed, but rather to bully them into not choosing abortion.

There is a parallel between the issue of anesthesia during abortion and moral standing. If a fetus is too undeveloped to feel pain, it is pointless to offer pain relief. If a fetus has no interests, it is impossible to do anything out of considerations for its interests, or for its own sake. Moral standing is limited to beings who have a sake or welfare of their own. Since presentient fetuses lack interests, and therefore a sake or welfare of their own, they do not have moral standing. However, even if they lack moral standing, they have moral value, which limits what may be done to them. Their moral value could derive from the stake others have in their well-being, or from their being a form of developing human life. (See Chapter 6 for further discussion of the distinction between moral standing and moral value.)

It might be argued that fetuses *do* have interests, even before they become sentient. The interests a non-sentient fetus possesses now are the interests of the person it will become or could become, if it is not killed. It has those interests in virtue of its identity with the future person. I consider and argue against this possibility in the section "The Argument From Potential."

Implantation

Another moderate conservative position places the beginning of human life at implantation of the embryo into the lining of the uterus. The process of implantation begins approximately on the sixth day following fertilization, and it takes about a week. The chances of an embryo's developing into a fetus improve significantly after implantation occurs. This is one reason for choosing implantation as "the decisive moment of humanization," as Noonan calls it (although implantation is not "a moment" but a process that takes about a week). Another reason for regarding implantation as the beginning of a new human being is that it coincides with gastrulation, or the formation of the "primitive streak," the precursor of the spinal cord and the nervous system. After gastrulation, embryonic fission, which produces identical twins, cannot occur. As Mary Warnock put it in a television interview,

48. Chinue T. Richardson and Elizabeth Nash. 2006. "Misinformed Consent: The Medical Accuracy of State-Developed Abortion Counseling Materials," *Guttmacher Policy Review* 9 (4) Fall: 6–11. http://www.guttmacher.org/pubs/gpr/09/4/gpr090406.html. Accessed October 29, 2010.

49. Guttmacher Institute. 2010. "Facts on Induced Abortion in the United States." http://www.guttmacher.org/pubs/fb_induced_abortion.html. Accessed June 16, 2010.

"Before fourteen days the embryo hasn't yet decided how many people it is going to be."[50] It could become two individuals or three or four or five (as in the case of the Dionne quintuplets in Canada in 1934). Therefore, at fertilization, there is not one unique human being. However, once the primitive streak has formed, and implantation has taken place, there is only one, unique individual.

Implantation also marks the beginning of what is called a "clinical pregnancy." The hormone, human chorionic gonadotropin (hCG), enters the blood stream as soon as implantation happens, and it can be detected by a blood test about a week after conception, or more commonly, by a urine test approximately 2 weeks after conception, or when the woman's period is due. Is a woman pregnant prior to implantation? This depends on how the terminology is used. Most commonly, the term "pregnant" is used to refer to the start of a clinical pregnancy, which can be detected only after implantation. However, those who regard fertilization as the start of a new human life consider the pregnancy to begin prior to implantation, as soon as conception occurs. This is sometimes called a "chemical pregnancy."

The debate over when pregnancy begins has implications for the permissibility of emergency contraception (EC), also known as emergency birth control, backup birth control, the morning-after pill,[51] and the brand name Plan B. The active ingredients in morning-after pills are similar to those in birth control pills, except in higher doses. Some morning-after pills, such as Plan B, contain only one hormone, levonorgestrel, while others contain two, progestin and estrogen. Progestin prevents the sperm from reaching the egg and keeps a fertilized egg from attaching to the wall of the uterus (implantation). Estrogen stops the ovaries from releasing eggs (ovulation) that can be fertilized by sperm.

Insofar as EC works by preventing ovulation or fertilization, it is clearly a form of contraception, and it is acceptable to those who oppose abortion, but not contraception. However, since EC may prevent implantation, some who believe that pregnancy begins at conception regard it as a very early abortifacient, and therefore morally unacceptable. Others who adopt the conception criterion find EC morally acceptable, at least in some cases (e.g., pregnancy due to rape), because one cannot be sure that conception has occurred.[52]

So far, we have looked at two challenges to the conservative claim that there is no nonarbitrary, morally relevant postfertilization event that marks the beginning of a human life. One challenge argues that the beginning of brain function marks a morally significant event, on the ground that the fetus after brain function begins is

50. Cited in Michael Lockwood. 1988. "Warnock Versus Powell (and Harradine): When Does Potentiality Count?" *Bioethics* 2 (3), p. 190.

51. The name "morning-after pill" is actually a misnomer, because the pills are licensed for use up to 72 hours after intercourse, and they can be used up to 5 days after contraceptive failure. http://www.plannedparenthood.org/health-topics/emergency-contraception-morning-after-pill-4363.htm. Accessed June 9, 2009. A new pill, "ella," which appears to be more effective than Plan B, and can prevent pregnancy if taken as late as 5 days after unprotected sex, was recommended for FDA approval by an advisory panel on June 17, 2010. http://www.nytimes.com/2010/06/18/health/policy/18pill.html. Accessed July 6, 2010.

52. Julie Cantor and Ken Baum. 2004. "The Limits of Conscientious Objection—May Pharmacists Refuse to Fill Prescriptions for Emergency Contraception?" *New England Journal of Medicine* 351 (19): 2008–2012.

not identical to the fetus prior to brain function. The other challenge maintains that implantation has moral significance, because the numerical identity of the unborn is decided then.

A quite different objection to the conservative position maintains that the assumption that genetic humanity is relevant to moral status is radically confused. I will refer to this objection, and the stance on the status of the fetus that comes out of it, as "the person view."[53]

The Person View

WARREN: THE IRRELEVANCE OF GENETIC HUMANITY

Proponents of the person view maintain that the conservative position is based on a conceptual error, a confusion between two senses of the word *human*. A human fetus is undeniably genetically human. However, this sense of *human* lacks moral relevance, according to person-view proponents, such as Mary Anne Warren.[54] It is not genetic human beings who have a special moral status and a right to life, but *persons*. As a matter of fact, all the people we know are genetic human beings. This leads us to confuse the moral and genetic senses of the word *human*. The confusion is cleared up when we realize that there could be nonhuman persons, such as the eponymous hero of the movie *E.T. E.T.* is a person because he resembles us in morally important ways. He is conscious, self-conscious, rational (indeed, far more rational than humans), a moral agent, and a language user. It is in virtue of his possession of these characteristics that he deserves the respect due to persons and cannot be treated as a mere thing. The person view goes on to maintain that personhood, and the special moral status it involves, cannot be based on anything so arbitrary as species membership, but instead it must be defined in terms of the possession of certain psychological and cognitive capacities, including consciousness, self-consciousness, reasoning, self-motivated activity, and language. Warren concedes that possession of all these capacities may not be necessary for personhood, but she maintains that a being who possessed none of these characteristics is clearly not a person. So a fetus, at least in early or mid-gestation, is clearly not a person. Even a late-gestation fetus, which has some degree of conscious awareness, has fewer of the person-making characteristics than does a mammal or even an adult fish. Warren concludes that it is not seriously wrong to kill fetuses. In fact, abortion is "morally neutral," comparable to having one's hair cut.[55]

53. I borrow this term from Rosalind Hursthouse, *Beginning Lives* (Oxford: Basil Blackwell in association with the Open University), 1987.

54. Mary Anne Warren. 1973. "On the Moral and Legal Status of Abortion," *The Monist* 57 (1): 43–61.

55. Ibid., p. 109. Warren later repudiated this analogy in conversation. Her book, *Moral Status: Obligations to Persons and Other Living Things* (New York: Oxford University Press, 2000), while still denying moral standing to fetuses, gives a more nuanced view of the morality of abortion than her 1973 article.

This comparison outrages many people, even those who support a woman's right to choose abortion. Warren seems to be saying that the decision to have an abortion is "no big deal," and this trivializes the complex feelings many woman have had in connection with abortion, especially late abortions. To compare abortion to having one's hair cut is to ignore the physical, emotional, and cultural significance of pregnancy. Nevertheless, one could argue that, whatever the *psychological* significance of the decision to terminate a pregnancy, the decision is still not a matter of *moral* concern. This suggests that actions have moral significance only if they harm or wrong persons. If the fetus is not a person, then the decision to abort it is not a moral one. This seems to me to be an excessively narrow conception of morality. A wider conception views morality as being about the right way to live, or about being the right sort of person. In making certain choices or acting on certain reasons, one might be acting as a shallow, thoughtless, uncaring kind of person would act. To act in such ways is not morally neutral, even if one's choice does not harm or wrong any person.

A more worrisome objection to the person view is that it apparently justifies not only abortion but also infanticide. A newly born infant is not significantly different from a late fetus in terms of person-making characteristics. A newborn is conscious and sentient, but then, so is a late-gestation fetus. More important, so are many nonhuman animals. Advocates of the person view are thus faced with the following choice. If they set the requirements for personhood low enough to include newborns, they will have to acknowledge the personhood of late-gestation fetuses and most animals. Infanticide will be wrong, but so will killing animals for food. On the other hand, if they require more than mere sentience for personhood, neither animals nor human babies will be persons. This accords with the commonsense view about animals, but it conflicts strongly with most people's views about the wrongness of killing babies.

Warren attempts to get out of this dilemma by arguing that the opposition to infanticide, but not abortion, can be justified on consequentialist grounds. Parents ought not to be allowed to opt for the death of a newborn, even if they do not want to raise it, because there are other people ready and willing to adopt the child and who would be "deprived of a great deal of pleasure" if the child were destroyed. Even if a child is considered to be unadoptable because she is severely physically or mentally handicapped, it is still wrong in most cases to kill her, because most people would prefer to pay taxes to support orphanages and state institutions for the handicapped rather than to allow unwanted infants to be killed. By contrast, a previable fetus cannot be put up for adoption, and requiring women to go through pregnancy and put their babies up for adoption is unlikely to be justified on consequentialist grounds.

This consequentialist attempt to placate ordinary moral thinking about babies is unsatisfying. If killing babies is seriously morally wrong, the reason cannot be merely that most people in fact prefer that babies live. What if the market for adoptable babies vanished because new reproductive technologies enabled anyone who wanted a child to have one of her own? What if people stopped being willing to spend money on orphanages and state institutions for handicapped infants? It seems that Warren would have to agree that under such conditions it would be perfectly all right to destroy unwanted infants, a conclusion that is enormously counterintuitive. Warren's attempt to explain what's wrong with killing babies leaves out entirely the idea that infanticide, like other homicides, is a wrong to the child who is killed, because it deprives the child of his life. It treats the destruction of an infant as if it were merely the destruction of a valuable commodity. As Jean Elshtain suggests, this puts infanticide "about on the level of having one's stereo and Beatles' albums stolen."[56]

Of course, the mere fact that a conclusion is counterintuitive does not prove an argument wrong. Perhaps there really is nothing wrong with killing babies, aside from the distressing effect on sensibilities. This is the approach favored by Michael Tooley, another proponent of the person view. He maintains that the opposition to infanticide is not based on rational principle. It is a mere taboo, like the taboo against masturbation or oral sex. These practices are not morally wrong simply because some people—or even the majority of people—are revulsed by them. However, while I acknowledge that feelings are no substitute for reasons, the existence of strong and widely held feelings against the implications of a view provide us with a motivation for finding an argument against it.

An objection to Warren's analysis is that it suffers from the same defect she discovered in the conservative position. Just as there is ambiguity in the word *human* between its genetic and moral senses, so there is ambiguity in the word *person* between its descriptive and normative senses. In its descriptive sense, the word *person* refers to a being with certain psychological traits, such as consciousness, self-consciousness, and rationality. In its normative sense, a person is someone with full moral standing, and, in particular, a right to life. Warren simply assumes that all and only descriptive persons are normative persons; indeed, she takes it as "self-evident." Missing from her account is an explanation of the moral significance of the capacities that make someone a descriptive person. Without this explanation, the person view is as arbitrary as the genetic-humanity criterion.[57]

We need an argument that justifies the special moral standing of descriptive persons. Such an argument might go like this. The moral significance of rationality and self-consciousness lies in their connection with moral agency. A moral agent is someone who is responsible for his or her own actions, who can be held accountable, praised, and blamed. This requires the ability to consider the merits of possible courses of action, decide which is the best thing to do, and to act on that judgment. Such activity is possible only for intelligent, reflective, and self-aware beings. In addition, moral agents are capable of moral reasoning, which involves detachment from one's own personal perspective and interests. Because of their ability to engage in moral discourse, to modify their behavior in response to rational considerations, to refrain from injurious behavior if others are likewise willing to refrain, moral agents occupy a unique moral status. H. Tristram Engelhardt, Jr., defends the superior moral standing of descriptive persons, or "persons in the strict sense," as he calls them, this way:

> This central place of persons in the strict sense in moral reflection flows from the very notion of a moral community. If one views ethics as a means of resolving

---

56. Jean Bethke Elshtain, "Commentary to Chapter 5," in Sidney Callahan and Daniel Callahan, eds., *Abortion: Understanding Differences* (see note 26), p. 139.

57. Joel Feinberg makes this point in "Abortion," in Tom Regan, ed., *Matters of Life and Death: New Introductory Essays in Moral Philosophy*, 2nd edition (New York: Random House, 1986), p. 259. See also Don Marquis, "Why Abortion Is Immoral" (note 25).

moral disputes in a fashion not based upon force, but rather upon peaceable nego-
tiation, in a context where the participants are held accountable for their actions,
the only original members of that community, of the moral world, will be persons
in the strict sense: entities who are self-conscious, rational, and self-determining
and therefore accountable for their choices, and who have interests.[58]

This argument links descriptive and normative personhood. It provides a rationale for treating all descriptive persons, whatever their species, as normative
persons, entitled to respect and moral concern. But it does not follow that *only*
descriptive persons have this moral status. There may be good reasons for extending
the moral status of descriptive persons to all human beings. Conservatives who insist
that a human embryo is a person need not be *confused* about the distinction between
genetic humanity and moral humanity. Instead, they could be maintaining that
genetic humanity is sufficient for normative personhood. Ruth Macklin comments,
"If there is any confusion here, it is to be laid at the door of those like Warren who,
apparently forgetting her avowal that the concept of a person is in part a moral concept, treats it as a purely descriptive notion. . . What antiabortionists are doing . . . is
proposing that the fetus be considered a person, and therefore, a creature to be treated
as a member of the moral community."[59]

The most likely basis for the conservative proposal that fetuses be treated as
members of the moral community is some version of the argument from potential.
The argument from potential says that fetuses deserve to be treated now as if they
were persons because if they are allowed to grow and develop—in other words, are
not aborted—they eventually will acquire all the properties of descriptive persons.
This differentiates human fetuses and newborns from, say, guppies. Potentiality arguments pose the greatest difficulty for pro-choicers; I will return to this subject shortly.
But first I want to consider another attempt to show that abortion is not seriously
morally wrong, based on an argument that fetuses cannot have a right to life.

The Right to Life

Like Mary Anne Warren, Michael Tooley maintains that all and only descriptive
persons have a right to life. But whereas Warren takes this to be self-evident,
Tooley has an argument. Tooley begins by espousing Feinberg's interest principle
(see Chapter 1). According to the interest principle, all and only beings that can
have interests can have rights. Tooley takes the interest principle one step further,
arguing that particular rights are connected with specific sorts of interests. That is,
an individual cannot have a particular right R unless that individual is capable of
having some interest I that is furthered by its having right R. Tooley calls this the
"particular-interests principle."

58. H. Tristram Engelhardt. 1983. "Viability and the Use of the Fetus," in W. B. Bondeson,
H. Tristram Engelhardt, Jr., S. F. Spicker, and D. H. Winship, eds., *Abortion and the Status of
the Fetus*. Dordrecht, Holland: D. Reidel Publishing Company, p. 185.

59. Macklin (see note 24), p. 97.

The particular-interests principle is supposed to explain and defend certain widely held moral views. For example, most people would maintain that it is worse to kill a normal adult human being painlessly than to torture one for 5 minutes. Though both acts are seriously wrong, they are not equally wrong. But most people would regard it as much worse to torture a newborn kitten for 5 minutes than to kill it painlessly. How is this difference to be explained? The particular-interests principle suggests an explanation: "Though kittens have some interests, including, in particular, an interest in not being tortured, which derives from their capacity to feel pain, they do not have an interest in continued existence, and hence do not have a right not to be destroyed."[60]

To have an interest in not feeling pain, a kitten need only have the desire that a particular sensation cease. "The state desired—the absence of a particular sensation—can be described in a purely phenomenalistic language, and hence without the concept of a continuing self."[61] By contrast, the desire protected by a right to life is a desire for one's own continued existence. To have this desire, one must possess a bundle of fairly complex concepts, including the concept of something's continuing to exist and the concept of a continuing subject of experiences. In addition, the desire for one's own continued experience is a desire that *this* subject of experiences should continue to exist. Thus, to have the desire for continued existence, one has to be able to think of oneself as a subject of continuing experiences. Tooley concludes that only beings that have this concept can have a right to life.

Two responses might be made to this argument. It might be argued that a desire to live does not require the concept of oneself as a continuing subject of experiences. All that is necessary is the capacity to have desires in general, and a preference for survival, which can be expressed behaviorally. Plants cannot have a desire to live, because they do not have desires at all. But conscious, sentient beings that struggle |to avoid death may be said to want to live, and so to have an interest in continued existence.

Or perhaps not. An animal's struggle to avoid death might be just a struggle to cease the pain or terror associated with what is happening to it.[62] How are we to determine what the behavior—the struggling—means? In Chapter 1, I rejected as implausible the view that animals and prelinguistic children lack beliefs and desires, simply because they lack language. Nevertheless, I must acknowledge that it may be difficult to specify the content of the desire in such beings. It seems reasonable to me to ascribe a desire to go on living to an animal that behaves in ways that will preserve its life, but as other interpretations of the behavior are possible, agnosticism about the nature of the animal's desire is probably safest.

A different response makes use of the distinction noted in Chapter 1 between two senses of "interest." Whatever promotes a being's good or welfare is *in* its interest; I called these interests$_1$. By contrast, the things one wants or pursues, the things in which one *takes* an interest, are interests$_2$. Keeping this distinction in mind, one might respond to Tooley's argument by agreeing that only a being with a concept of

60. Michael Tooley. 1983. *Abortion and Infanticide*. Oxford: Clarendon Press, p. 100.

61. Tooley. 1984. "A Defense of Abortion and Infanticide," in Joel Feinberg, ed., *The Problem of Abortion*. Belmont, CA: Wadsworth, p. 73.

62. I owe this objection to David Shoemaker.

itself as a continuing subject of experiences can want to go on existing as the being it is. Only beings with self-concepts can have an interest$_2$ in continued existence. But it does not follow that only beings with a self-concept can have an interest$_1$ in continued existence. Rights can surely protect interests$_1$, as well as interests$_2$. So if continued existence is *in* a being's interest, it can have a right to life, even if it cannot *take* an interest in its own continued existence. Is there any reason to deny that life can be in the interest of animals, babies, and other individuals without self-concepts?

Tooley responds with a version of the radical-discontinuity argument. Imagine, Tooley says, a preconscious embryo that develops into a person, Mary. Mary has a happy life and is glad her mother did not abort her. So it may be said that it was in Mary's interest that the embryo from which she developed was not destroyed. However, Tooley argues, it is a mistake to think that therefore nondestruction is in the *embryo's* interest. The embryo is not a subject of consciousness. It does not have any interests at all, and so cannot have an interest in its own continued existence.

Now consider a human baby that is sentient and has simple desires but is not yet capable of having a desire for its own continued existence. If it will develop into an individual with a happy life, can we not say that it is in the baby's interest not to be killed? Tooley denies this. He says that we mistakenly attribute to the baby an interest in continued existence because we wrongly identify the baby with the adult person she becomes. We then think that because it is in the adult Mary's interest that she was not destroyed when she was a baby, it must also be in the baby Mary's interest not to be destroyed. After all, baby Mary just *is* adult Mary, when she was younger. However, Tooley maintains that such an identification is justified only if there are causal and psychological connections between adult Mary and baby Mary. In the absence of any such connections, it is "clearly incorrect to say that Mary and the baby are one and the same subject of consciousness, and therefore it cannot be correct to transfer, from Mary to the baby, Mary's interest in the baby's not having been destroyed."[63]

Tooley's argument is open to several objections. First, it assumes, implausibly, that there are no causal and psychological connections between a baby and the adult person she becomes. Presumably this is because adult Mary does not remember being a baby. But memory is not the only kind of causal and psychological connection. Most psychologists believe that the treatment one receives as an infant affects the development of one's personality. Parents who were once warned against "spoiling" babies are today encouraged to meet their infants' needs not only for food, but for comforting and loving.[64] It is believed that this creates not only happier *babies*, but happier, more secure, more well-adjusted *adults*. This would be impossible if there were not causal and psychological connections between the infant and the adult she becomes.

Second, even if there is a radical discontinuity between a baby and the adult it becomes, it does not follow that the baby cannot have an interest in its own continued existence. Granted, the baby cannot *take* an interest in its continued existence, in the sense of thinking abstractly about continuing into the future, and hoping that it continues to exist in the future. Babies lack the concepts necessary for that sort of desire.

---

63. Tooley, "A Defense of Abortion and Infanticide" (see note 60), p. 120.

64. Benjamin Spock. 2004. *Dr. Spock's Baby and Child Care*, 8th edition, updated and revised by Robert Needlman. New York: Pocket Books.

Still, life can be *in* the baby's interest. Life is in a being's interest if the experiences that comprise its life, now and in the future, are and are expected to be, on the whole, enjoyable ones. Such a life is a good to the being in question. Infants, even very young ones, can enjoy their lives. They can take pleasure in a variety of activities and experiences. This being the case, we can certainly preserve their lives for their own sake. The same is true for animals and severely mentally retarded humans. It is only when life is miserable, and suffering cannot be alleviated, that we begin to doubt whether continued existence is a benefit. If this is right, then a self-concept is not necessary to have an interest (an interest$_1$) in continuing to exist. All that is necessary is the ability to enjoy one's life.

A conscious, sentient newborn ordinarily has a life worth living, a life he enjoys, a life that is a good to him. Continuing to live is certainly *in* the baby's interest, because of the value to him of his life *right now*. A right to life protects his interest$_1$ in his life. I conclude that there is no conceptual bar to ascribing to newborns a right to life.[65] Nor is there any conceptual bar to ascribing a right to life to the nearly born fetus. A late-gestation fetus is conscious and sentient. It is very likely that it can experience pain, and presumably, it has pleasurable experiences. If so, it has an interest in continuing to live and in having those pleasurable experiences, an interest that can be protected by a right to life. By contrast, embryos and preconscious fetuses do not have lives that they value, lives that are a good to them, because they are unaware of everything around them. To put it another way, they do not have a stake in what happens to them. They lack interests$_2$. But since interests$_2$ are what comprise interests$_1$, they also do not have interests$_1$. (See Chapter 1.) Life is no more a good to an embryo than it is to a plant or a sperm. Thus, the importance of sentience is not primarily that abortion causes pain to the sentient fetus. That problem might be taken care of with an anesthetic. The relevance of sentience is that a sentient being can have a life it values, and that we can protect for its own sake.

Some antiabortionists consider it callous and unfeeling to deny moral status to the preconscious fetus. But the charge of callousness makes sense only if we persist in thinking of embryos and fetuses as being just like babies, only smaller. In fact, I think that this is how many opponents of abortion do regard the fetus. For example, the 1984 video *The Silent Scream* purported to show a 12-week fetus struggling to get away from the abortionist's scalpel, and opening its mouth in "a silent scream." Critics of the film charged that normal fetal movements were speeded up to make it look as if the fetus were recoiling in pain. But even if the film was not doctored, such movements are not by themselves evidence of pain. A mimosa plant shrinks from touch, but no one claims that the mimosa feels pain. The reason is that a plant lacks the nervous system necessary for the experience of pain. Similarly, the fetal nervous system at 12 weeks is not sufficiently developed to carry and transmit pain messages. Insofar as opposition to abortion is based on factual error, or worse, deliberate misrepresentation of the facts, it must be rejected out of hand.

A more sophisticated conservative position acknowledges that embryos and early fetuses do not *suffer* from being aborted, nor does death deprive them of lives they now value and enjoy. Nevertheless, it maintains that even a zygote (on the conception criterion) or an embryo (on the implantation criterion) has an interest in not

---

65. A similar argument is made by Carson Strong, "Delivering Hydrocephalic Fetuses," *Bioethics* 5:1 (January 1991), pp. 7–11.

being killed. This interest in continued existence does not derive from the kind of life it has *now*, but rather on the kind of life it *will* have, if it is allowed to grow and develop. Such arguments are known as arguments from potential. If successful, they can support the conservative proposal that genetic humans ought to be treated as normative persons.

THE ARGUMENT FROM POTENTIAL

There are different versions of the argument from potential, but the basic idea is that it is wrong to kill, or otherwise prevent the development of, a human fertilized egg because it possesses the potential to be a descriptive person. As Stephen Buckle expresses it, "It is, potentially, just like us, so we cannot deny it any rights or other forms of protection that we accord ourselves."[66] A fertilized egg does not now have any of the properties of a person. It is not even sentient. But this does not matter because, left alone and allowed to develop, the zygote will become a person. Buckle says, "The fertilized egg is not 'just like us' only in the sense that it is not *yet* just like us. Therefore, the argument concludes, we should not interfere with its natural development towards being a rational, self-conscious being. On its strongest interpretation, the argument is thought to establish that we should treat a potential human subject as if it were already an actual human subject."[67]

The Logical Problem

A standard objection to the argument from potential is that it involves a logical mistake. The mistake consists in thinking of a "potential person" as a kind of person, and, on this basis, ascribing to "potential persons" the rights of other persons. But potential persons are not persons; they do not now have the characteristics of persons. As Stanley Benn makes the point, "For if A has rights only because he satisfies some condition P, it does not follow that B has the same rights now because he *could* have property P at some time in the future. It only follows that he *will* have rights *when* he has P. He is a potential bearer of rights, as he is a potential bearer of P. A potential president of the United States is not on that account Commander-in-Chief."[68]

It is a logical error to think that potential personhood implies possession of the rights of actual persons. However, the argument from potential need not be based on this logical mistake. Like the defender of the genetic humanity criterion, the defender of the argument from potential can be understood as making a normative proposal: that potential persons *ought* to have the same rights as actual persons. Understood this way, the argument is not based on a logical confusion, but is rather in need of defense. Why should beings who are potentially "just like us" be entitled to the same protection as we are?

66. Stephen Buckle. 1988. "Arguing From Potential," *Bioethics* 2 (3): 226–253, p. 227.

67. Ibid.

68. Stanley Benn, "Abortion, Infanticide, and Respect for Persons," in Feinberg (see note 60), p. 143.

Contraception and the Moral Standing of Gametes

The strongest objection to the argument from potential is that it seems to make contraception, and even abstinence, prima facie morally wrong. Why aren't unfertilized eggs and sperm also potential people? John Harris makes the point this way:

> To say that a fertilized egg is potentially a human being is just to say that if certain things happen to it (like implantation), and certain other things do not (like spontaneous abortion), it will eventually become a human being. But the same is also true of the unfertilized egg and the sperm. If certain things happen to the egg (like meeting a sperm) and certain things happen to the sperm (like meeting an egg) and thereafter certain other things do not (like meeting a contraceptive), then they will eventually become a new human being.[69]

So if abortion is seriously wrong because it kills a potential person, then the use of a contraceptive is equally seriously wrong. In using a spermicide, one commits mass murder! Indeed, even abstinence is wrong, insofar as it prevents the development of a new human being. Very few defenders of the potentiality principle are willing to accept this conclusion.[70] They must then give reasons why a zygote, but not a sperm or ovum, is a potential person.

Defenders of the potentiality criterion sometimes appeal to an enormous difference in probabilities. John Noonan points out that the chances of any particular sperm becoming a person are remarkably low. There are about 200 million spermatozoa in a normal ejaculate, of which only one has a chance of developing into a zygote. By contrast, he estimates the chances of a zygote developing into a person to be about 80%. The difference is still impressive, even if we adjust Noonan's estimate to reflect more recent information on the miscarriage rate. About 30% to 40% of all conceptions result in pregnancy loss,[71] usually in the early weeks of pregnancy and often before women even know they are pregnant. This suggests that a given zygote's chance of becoming a person is about 60% to 70%, rather than the 80% chance Noonan gives it. Still, these odds are a lot better than a sperm's 1-in-200-million chance. The odds of an ovum developing into a person are better than those of a sperm, but still much worse than those of a fertilized egg. If we think of potential in terms of statistical likelihood, a zygote has greater potential than a gamete. But it is not clear that the odds matter. Although the chances of any particular sperm becoming a person are infinitesimal, why should that prevent its being a potential person? Is not every entrant in a lottery a potential winner, even if the odds of winning are

69. John Harris. 1985. *The Value of Life: an Introduction to Medical Ethics.* London: Routledge & Kegan Paul, pp. 11–12.

70. R. M. Hare may be the only potentiality theorist who does not base his argument on a morally significant difference between embryos and gametes. On his version of the argument from potential, abortion is prima facie morally wrong, but so are contraception and abstention from procreation, and the prima facie wrongness of all of these is easily overcome by the interests of people in not having children. See "Abortion and the Golden Rule," *Philosophy & Public Affairs* 4:3 (Spring 1975): 201–222.

71. Thomas C. Michels and Alvin Y. Tiu. 2007. "Second Trimester Pregnancy Loss," *American Family Physician* 76 (9): 1341–1346, p. 1341.

extremely low? Every gamete, it may be said, has the potential to develop into a person, even though very few do.

Rosalind Hursthouse maintains that thinking about potentiality in terms of the chance or opportunity to become a human being embodies "a confusion about the concept of potentiality."[72] It is not the odds of a fetus's becoming a human being that make it a potential human being, but rather the fact that this is the result of "natural development" or what the fetus will become if nothing external intervenes. Richard Warner makes a similar point: "All things being equal, the zygote will grow into a person. On the other hand, the ovum or sperm qua itself is neither growing nor developing no matter in what sort of environment one should find it or put it into. A gamete will not, by itself, grow into anything other than what it already is—a gamete."[73]

The notion that an X is a potential Y only if an X will grow into a Y "all by itself" does not seem generally applicable. The orange powder known as "Tang" has the potential, when mixed with water, to become an orange-flavored drink. However, the powder does not turn into a drink all by itself. Someone has to intervene and add the cold water. So why should the fact that a gamete cannot become a person without external intervention deprive it of potential personhood? This seems especially so in light of the new reproductive technologies, such as in vitro fertilization, or IVF (see Chapter 5), in which fertilization takes place outside the body, in a petri dish. The resulting embryo is then transferred to the uterus of a female. The IVF embryo cannot become a person without considerable human intervention. Yet surely the embryo created in a laboratory is as much a potential person as the embryo produced by the normal human reproductive process.

Defenders of a potentiality principle sometimes try to differentiate between a gamete and a zygote by saying that, prior to fertilization, no particular individual exists. It is at conception, not before, that the particular human being *who I am* comes into existence. The child's question "Where was I before I was born?" has an answer: you were in your mother's womb. But the question "And where was I before that?" has no answer. Before I was conceived, I did not exist. Had the sperm and egg that combined to make me fused with any other egg or sperm, I would never have existed at all. So the zygote is identified with me, in a way that neither the egg nor the sperm is.

To this it might be retorted that while neither the egg nor the sperm is a particular potential person, each is potentially *some* person—namely, the person it will develop into if it fuses with another gamete. Why should its potential personhood be diminished by the fact that it is impossible to say, in advance, *which* person it will be? As Peter Singer and Karen Dawson say, "Potentiality is one thing: uniqueness is something quite different."[74]

Stephen Buckle argues that, on one conception of morality, potentiality and uniqueness are connected. He suggests that those who debate the moral relevance of potentiality often seem to be at cross purposes because they are appealing to different

72. Hursthouse, *Beginning Lives* (see note 52), p. 80.

73. Warner, "Abortion: The Ontological and Moral Status of the Unborn" (see note 32), p. 57.

74. Peter Singer and Karen Dawson. 1988. "IVF Technology and the Argument From Potential," *Philosophy & Public Affairs* 17(2): 87–104, p. 96.

interpretations of the concept of potentiality. The consequentialist conception of potentiality focuses on future outcomes: the production of future persons. Consequentialists who accept the argument from potential maintain that abortion is prima facie wrong, though justifiable if the alternative (not having an abortion) produces a worse state of affairs, all things considered. For example, terminating *this* pregnancy may enable a woman to have a child at a time when she could care for it better. The argument also applies to contraception and even abstinence, as ways of preventing future people from coming into existence. From a consequentialist standpoint, there is no crucial difference between the fertilized egg, on the one hand, and the sperm and unfertilized egg, on the other. "This is so because the sperm and unfertilized egg, when considered jointly, also have the potential *to produce* a future human subject, even though that potential is not *activated* until fertilization occurs."[75]

A different conception of potentiality, and a different reason for regarding it as morally significant, is associated with a deontological approach to ethics. Buckle refers to this version of the argument from potential as the "respect for capacities of individuals" argument. According to this version, ". . . respect is due to an existing being because it possesses the capacity or power to develop into a being which is worthy of respect in its own right; and respect is due to such a being because it is *the very same being* as the later being into which it develops. The already-existing being is a being which has the potential *to become* a being worthy of respect in its own right."[76] It is the identification of the zygote with the later person that both makes the zygote a potential person and entitles it to respect and concern. Neither the sperm nor the egg has the same genetic code as the being who develops from their union, so neither is the same being as the fertilized egg.

It might be objected that, although the sperm and egg do not individually have the potential to become a person, when considered together, they do. Why must a potential entity be composed of a single object? We can speak of the potential of a team or an army; why not the potential of the sperm and the egg? Buckle argues that this response is misplaced. It works if we take potential to refer to the potential *to produce*, but it will not do as an argument about the potential *to become*.

This is because the potential *to become* attaches only to distinct individuals that preserve their identity over time. It therefore attaches only to entities that, if they are composed of distinct parts, nevertheless can be classed as a distinct single individual. To satisfy this condition, the several and distinct parts must in some way constitute a complex *whole*. Where a collection of discrete entities is not organized into a whole, there is no individual to possess the potential *to become*, no individual that develops through the actualization of the potential.[77]

"In the case of the sperm and egg," Buckle says, "there is no complex unity, no overarching organization. Such unity or organization arises only with fertilization (in fact, only with the completion of the fertilization process at syngamy)."[78] Although the

75. Buckle, "Arguing From Potential" (see note 65), p. 241.

76. Ibid., p. 230.

77. Ibid., p. 237.

78. Ibid., p. 238.

sperm and egg, considered jointly, have the potential *to produce* a human subject, they do not have the potential *to become* a human subject.

Is there any reason to prefer one conception of potentiality over another? An argument against the consequentialist conception is that it is objectionably broad; it does not distinguish potentiality from mere possibility. Feinberg suggests that the reason for holding the line at conception is that if we acknowledge the sperm to be a potential person, this may lead to the view that the entities that combined still earlier to form that spermatozoon are also potential people. "At the end of that road is the proposition that everything is potentially everything else, and thus the destruction of all utility in the concept of potentiality. It is better to hold this particular line at the zygote."[79] There are, it seems, conceptual reasons for adopting the "becoming," rather than the "producing," notion of potentiality. But does this conception have the moral significance the conservative thinks it does? What makes it seriously morally wrong to kill entities that can *become* persons, but not at all morally wrong to destroy entities that can *produce* persons?

At this point, the debate seems to be at a standstill. Antiabortionists are convinced that there is an enormous moral difference between the product of conception and the ingredients of conception. Their opponents are convinced that the difference is one of degree, and lacking in moral importance. Neither side is obviously right or wrong. Yet the success of the argument from potential hinges on differentiating the zygote from its component gametes.

The interest view rejects the argument from potential as providing a basis for moral standing. Potential people have no more moral status than merely possible people. Just as there is no obligation to bring possible people into existence, there is no obligation to enable potential people to develop into actual people. Does this mean that embryos and presentient fetuses are valueless, that they have no more moral significance than gametes? Michael Tooley takes this position:

> ... the destruction of a human organism that is a potential person, but not a person, is prima facie no more seriously wrong than intentionally refraining from fertilizing a human egg cell, and destroying it instead. Since intentionally refraining from procreation is surely not seriously wrong, neither is the destruction of potential persons.[80]

For Tooley, abortion and contraception are morally equivalent.

Many people will reject this equivalence as obviously wrong. There is no question that abortion is for most women psychologically and emotionally different from contraception. Few women experience abortion as just another way to avoid motherhood. While relief is the most common reported feeling after having an abortion, some women feel sadness or guilt,[81] even when the abortion is felt to be necessary. Pregnancy affects a woman's body in concrete, noticeable ways, preparing her to

79. Feinberg, "Abortion" (see note 56), p. 267.

80. Tooley, *Abortion and Infanticide* (see note 57), p. 193.

81. Guttmacher Institute. 2008. "Abortion and Mental Health." http://www.guttmacher.org/media/evidencecheck/2008/10/08/Advisory_Abortion_Mental_Health_2008.pdf. Accessed June 12, 2010.

carry and bear a child. The child she would have, if she did not abort, is thus likely to have for her a reality that no merely possible person can have. Some women are pleased at finding that they *can* bear a child, even if they realize that having a child at this point in their lives is unwise. In ending the pregnancy, they are likely to have mixed feelings. In addition, pregnancy is imbued with certain cultural meanings. It is ordinarily a joyous experience, and one that is associated with congratulations, gift giving, and special treatment. As one woman expresses it, "Sadness at not being able to celebrate pregnancy, to enjoy the sense of specialness it brings, is an understandable response."[82] Once we understand this, we can see why so many women (and men) do not have the same attitude toward abortion as they do toward contraception. Unless one's religion forbids it, contraception is likely to be regarded as morally neutral, a sensible preventive health habit, like flossing your teeth. It has none of the sadness or sense of loss that often accompanies abortions. A view that equates abortion and contraception is remote from the experiences of most people.

Does this matter? Some philosophers deny that it does. They argue that people's intuitions or felt convictions have no moral significance. They remind us that some people "experience" blacks and women to be inferior to whites and men. They maintain that we should not try to account for such feelings in our moral theories. The appropriate response to feelings that do not accord with moral theory is, "So what?"

I do not agree with this total rejection of moral feelings. It *may* be that a feeling is mere prejudice, incapable of being supported by good reasons. I think that this can fairly easily be shown of racist and sexist views. But from the fact that some strong convictions are indefensible, it does not follow that all are. A morality that is radically divorced from our deepest feelings, and disconnected from our experiences and emotions, cannot be practical or action guiding. For all the reasons I have given earlier, I think we are justified in regarding abortion as morally more serious than contraception, and for thinking that abortion is a moral issue in a way that contraception is not. Still, I would not go so far as Rosalind Hursthouse, who argues that abortion is a choice that a completely wise and virtuous person would rarely make, because it usually displays a callous and light-minded attitude toward life.[83] This is unfair. A great many abortions occur because of contraceptive failure. A woman who is responsibly using a reliable contraceptive, and nevertheless gets pregnant, should not be accused of having a callous or light-minded attitude toward life. At the same time, this characterization might fit a woman who does not use contraceptives, repeatedly becomes pregnant, and has several abortions. I knew a 16-year-old girl who was about to have her third abortion. I asked her what seemed to be the problem. "Oh," she responded, "I can never remember to put in a diaphragm, and the pill makes me fat." We can acknowledge that her attitude toward sexuality, pregnancy, and potential human life is immature and superficial, without implying that the unborn has moral status. Abortion may be morally undesirable, in a way that contraception is not, without its being a *wrong to* the unborn.

---

82. Angela Neustatter, with Gina Newson. 1986. *Mixed Feelings: The Experience of Abortion.* London: Pluto Press, p. 10.

83. Hursthouse, *Beginning Lives* (see note 52).

I will return to the moral significance of potential personhood in sentient beings later. But first I will consider what is widely regarded as the most interesting and successful of attempts to show that abortion is seriously wrong, Don Marquis's future-like-ours account (FLOA).

THE FUTURE-LIKE-OURS ACCOUNT

Don Marquis argues that abortion is seriously immoral, for the same reason that killing an innocent adult human being is immoral.[84] What makes killing wrong is not primarily the effects on other people, or the threat to the fabric of society. What makes killing wrong is the effect on the victim. The loss of one's life is one of the greatest losses one can suffer. The loss of one's life deprives one of all the experiences, activities, projects, and enjoyments that would otherwise have constituted one's future. When I am killed, I am deprived of all of the value of my future. But exactly the same is true when a fetus is killed. Abortion deprives the fetus of its future, a future just like ours. Hence, abortion is prima facie seriously morally wrong.

In his original 1989 article, Marquis said very little about what a future of value is, only that it is a future "sufficiently like ours."[85] In later articles,[86] he elaborates on the idea, saying that a future of value contains the goods of life, and that these are what make life worth living. They will vary somewhat from person to person, but include "friendships, loves, absorption in various projects, aesthetic experiences, identification with larger causes seen as valuable, such as one's team winning a victory, and physical pleasures."[87]

Is the FLOA a version of the argument from potentiality? In the first edition of this book, I thought that it was, primarily because of what he says in his 1989 article to distinguish the FLOA from a potentiality argument:

> This argument does not rely on the invalid inference that, since it is wrong to kill persons, it is wrong to kill potential persons also. The category that is morally central to this analysis is the category of having a valuable future like ours; it is not the category of personhood.[88]

However, if what makes the FLOA not a potentiality argument is the absence of the category of personhood, the argument fails. Even if it is the category of FLO that is central to his argument, not the category of personhood, personhood is

84. Marquis, "Why Abortion Is Immoral" (see note 25).

85. Ibid., p. 191.

86. Don Marquis, "An Argument That Abortion Is Wrong," in Hugh LaFollette, ed., *Ethics in Practice* (Oxford: Blackwell Publishers, 1997). Reprinted in John Arthur, ed., *Morality and Moral Controversies*, 7th edition (Englewood Cliffs, NJ: Prentice-Hall, 2005), pp. 204–212; Don Marquis, "Abortion Revisited," in Bonnie Steinbock, ed., *The Oxford Handbook of Bioethics* (Oxford: Oxford University Press, 2007), pp. 395–415.

87. Don Marquis, "Abortion Revisited," (see note 85), p. 399.

88. Marquis, "Why Abortion Is Immoral" (see note 25), p. 192.

clearly implicit in his account, since the only kinds of beings who can have valuable futures like ours are beings capable of abstract thought, complex relationships, and future plans and goals—that is to say, *persons.* Nevertheless, the FLOA is not an argument from potentiality, because it does not maintain that it would be wrong to kill a fetus because of a characteristic it has only *potentially,* such as personhood. It says that it would be wrong to kill a fetus because of a characteristic it has right now: namely, a valuable future. It has that future because it is identical with the future person. A fetus now has a future in the same way that any of us now has a future, of which we would be deprived if we were now killed.

While Marquis does not give a traditional potentiality argument, his view is also vulnerable to the objection that it makes contraception as wrong as abortion. If a fetus has a valuable future like ours, why don't gametes? Specifically, why don't the egg and sperm before they conjoin have a future of value which they lose because of the use of contraception? Marquis acknowledges that if the ethic of killing he gives implies that contraception is seriously wrong, that would be a difficulty with the analysis. However, he maintains that it entails no such thing. Considering the possibility that contraception deprives both the sperm and the ovum separately of a future of value, Marquis says, "On this alternative, too many futures are lost. Contraception was supposed to be wrong because it deprived us of one future of value, not two."[89] But why can't the sperm and egg jointly share one future of value?

This possibility is pursued by David Shoemaker, who maintains that Marquis fails to distinguish between two distinct notions: identity and ownership. Neither the sperm nor the egg is identical with the fetus; that must be granted. However, what makes killing a fetus seriously wrong is that the fetus is deprived of its valuable future. The relevant concept here, Shoemaker notes, is ownership, not identity: the valuable future of which the fetus is deprived is *its own.* But whereas identity is unique, ownership need not be. "To say that some property is mine, in other words, does not mean that X is mine *exclusively.* Just as one may jointly own property with another, so too one may jointly own a valuable future with another."[90] If ownership is the relationship that matters morally, and ownership doesn't entail numerical identity, then there's no reason in principle why an egg and a sperm couldn't jointly own a valuable future, even though neither of them is identical to the future person. Contraception would deprive them of this valuable future, just as abortion deprives the fetus of its valuable future, making contraception just as seriously wrong as abortion. To avoid this reduction, Marquis has to show that ownership in fact entails numerical identity.

A different, though related, objection to the FLOA concerns the harm of being killed, which both Marquis and I agree is the basis for the wrongness of killing. Where I differ from Marquis is that I maintain that presentient fetuses are not harmed by being killed. The death of an early-gestation fetus is no more a misfortune for it than the death of a sperm or egg is a misfortune for it.

---

89. Ibid., p. 201.

90. David Shoemaker. 2009. "The Insignificance of Personal Identity for Bioethics," *Bioethics* 24 (9): 481–489, pp. 485–486.

The idea that only conscious, sentient beings can be harmed by death is expressed in two different versions. The first Marquis calls the *desire account*, originally given by Michael Tooley, and updated by David Boonin. The desire account says that killing is wrong because it interferes with the fulfillment of a strong and fundamental desire, the desire to live. Since fetuses have no desires, they have no desire to live; killing them does not frustrate any of their desires, and so it is not wrong. "One problem with the desire account," Marquis says, "is that we do think that it is seriously wrong to kill those who have little desire to live or who have no desire to live, or, indeed, have a desire not to live. We believe it is seriously wrong to kill the unconscious, the sleeping, those who are tired of life and those who are suicidal."[91]

Boonin has a response to this objection, or rather two responses. The first has to do with the wrongness of killing those who are temporarily unconscious, whether comatose or merely asleep, and requires a distinction between two kinds of desire, occurrent and dispositional. Occurrent desires are the ones of which we are presently aware. These are but a fraction of all the desires we have. Many are dispositional; that is, we are not currently aware of them, or thinking about them, but they are still things we want, and we would attest to this if asked and if we could respond. Someone who is asleep has no occurrent desire not to be killed, but nevertheless has that desire dispositionally. That is, prior to falling asleep, he wanted not to be killed, and he continues to have this desire even after falling asleep. To think otherwise is to think, implausibly, that every night all our desires go away, and we have to regain them in the morning. It is his dispositional desire to continue to live that makes it wrong to kill him. Marquis calls Boonin's dispositional desire strategy for dealing with the wrongness of killing temporarily unconscious individuals "reasonable."[92]

However, he thinks that Boonin's strategy for explaining the wrongness of killing people who are suicidal fails. In such cases, Boonin appeals to ideal desires. It would be wrong to kill a person who is suicidal, Boonin says, because often the person's desire to die is distorted by a temporary mental impairment, such as depression. The suicidal person wants to die because, in his present emotional state, he cannot imagine things ever being better or wanting to live. We know that, with medication and therapy and time, he will feel differently. What matters morally is not his actual desire, but the desire he would have, if his perspective were not clouded by emotion or mental illness. The trouble with the ideal desire strategy, Marquis says, is that it is dependent on the future of value account. That is, a person's ideal desires are those that a rational and fully informed person would have. A rational and fully informed person would judge that the suicidal person's ideal desire is to go on living just in case he or she has a future of value. It is the objective future of value that is doing the work in explaining the wrongness of killing the suicidal person, not his or her desires.[93] Since fetuses have futures of value, it is seriously prima facie wrong to kill them.

However, the central idea in Boonin's account is that the suicidal person's desire not to go on living has been *distorted* by extreme emotion or psychopathology or misinformation. There is no comparable distortion of fetal desires, since the presentient

91. Marquis, "Why Abortion Is Immoral" (see note 25), p. 196.

92. Marquis, "Abortion Revisited" (see note 83), p. 409.

93. Marquis makes a similar point in "Why Abortion Is Immoral" (see note 23), p. 196.

fetus has no desires at all. We can ask of an individual who has desires what his or her wants would be, if not distorted. It makes no sense to ask of an individual incapable of having desires what its desires would be, if it could have desires.

It might be objected that this move does not work. It does not matter whether the desire is distorted, as in the case of the suicidal teenager, or nonoccurrent, as in the case of an early fetus, because Marquis has shown that the desire account is parasitic on FLO, the more fundamental normative idea.[94] If it is the possession of a valuable future that is doing the work, the presence or absence of desires about that future is irrelevant to the wrongness of killing. This appears to be a decisive objection to the desire account.

The second version of the wrongness of killing is the *discontinuation account*. On the discontinuation account, what makes killing wrong is the discontinuation of the *experience* of having a life worth living. Since fetuses have no experiences at all during early gestation, prior to becoming sentient, they do not experience the discontinuation of living, and so killing them is not wrong.

Marquis concedes that the discontinuation account is intelligible but holds that it is inferior to his FLO account of the wrongness of killing. The value of one's present life is irrelevant, he argues. What matters is the future of which one is deprived by death. He says:

> It makes no difference whether the patient's immediate past contains intolerable pain, or consists in being in a coma (which we can imagine is a situation of indifference), or consists in a life of value. If the patient's future is a future of value, we want our account to make it wrong to kill the patient. If the patient's future is intolerable, whatever his or her immediate past, we want our account to allow killing the patient. Obviously, then it is the value of that patient's future which is doing the work in rendering the morality of killing the patient intelligible.

This being the case, it seems clear that whether one has immediate past experiences or not does no work in the explanation of what makes killing wrong. The addition the discontinuation account makes to the value of a human future account is otiose.[95]

However, the existence of past experiences clearly does "no work" only in cases where the victim is an experiencing subject. Of course, it makes no difference to the wrongness of killing if the person is in a temporary coma. Someone's life does not lose all value simply because he or she is temporarily unconscious, any more than someone loses the desire to go living whenever temporarily unconscious. Death is clearly a harm to someone who already has a life worth living and will continue to have that life after waking up. That has no relevance to the question of whether death can be a harm to a nonsentient being in virtue of its potential future sentience. The intuitive idea behind the discontinuation account is that it is not biological life per se that has value, but biographical or narrative existence, for which

94. I am grateful to David Shoemaker for pointing this out.

95. Marquis, "Why Abortion Is Immoral" (see note 25), p. 197.

sentience is a necessary condition. Prior to the onset of sentience, a fetus cannot value its life or anything else.

Peter McInerney[96] argues that the inability of the fetus to have experiences prevents it from having a future in the same way that you and I have futures. You and I have personal futures, that is, futures to which we are connected through psychological states, such as memories, character traits, habits, and the like. A fetus, having no psychological states at all, has no personal future. This differentiates the fetus from a temporarily unconscious person, who still has the beliefs, desires, memories, and even intentions she had prior to losing consciousness. "Since a temporarily unconscious person is still strongly related to her future, to kill her while she is unconscious is to deprive her of her future."[97] The same cannot be said of the nonsentient fetus. McInerney concludes that the fetus does not have a personal future, only the potential to develop a personal future, and this, he says, makes killing a fetus very different from killing a normal adult human. I think this is right. Although a fetus has a future in the biological sense, that is, it develops from the fetal stage to infancy to childhood to adulthood, its psychological connection to the later stages is completely absent. For this reason, it has no stake in its future, and therefore, killing it is morally very different from killing a being already psychologically connected to its future.

It must be admitted that certain examples pose serious difficulties for the interest view. Consider the following example. Imagine that an infant is born in an unconscious condition. Her brain stem is intact, and so she breathes on her own. However, the part of the brain controlling consciousness is damaged. The baby cannot suck and needs to be tube fed. The rest of her brain is structurally normal. Imagine further that there is a treatment that can cause the damaged part of the brain to regenerate, allowing the baby to become conscious. If she is treated, she will go on to a normal babyhood. If she is left untreated, she will die within a few weeks. Would we not regard such treatment as *in the best interest* of the child? Does she not have a right to the treatment? If she is allowed to die, is she not harmed, and indeed wronged?

The answer seems to be "yes" and yet an affirmative answer conflicts with the sentience criterion of the interest view. For the brain-damaged baby is not, and never has been, sentient. She does not have a life that is a good to her; she does not have any enjoyable experiences. Yet the ability to have pleasurable experiences was the basis for ascribing to a normal newborn an interest in its own continued existence. If we think that treatment that enables the brain-damaged baby to become conscious is in her interest, this seems to imply that she has an interest$_1$ in becoming a being with interests$_2$. Why is this not also true of the embryo? Neither the baby nor the embryo has a biographical life yet, but both have the potential for one. If we think that the unconscious baby can be a victim, how can we deny "victimizability" to the embryo?[98]

96. Peter McInerney. 1990. "Does the Fetus Already Have a Future-Like-Ours?" *Journal of Philosophy* 87 (5): 264–268.

97. Ibid., p. 266.

98. Paul Bassen. 1982. "Present Sakes and Future Prospects: The Status of Early Abortion," *Philosophy & Public Affairs* 11 (4): 314–337. Bassen argues on grounds similar to mine that embryos are not the sorts of things that can be victims.

One possibility is to accept the conclusion that the baby has no interests, and hence no sake or welfare of her own. Life is not in *her* interest, though there are plenty of other reasons to sustain her life and give her the treatment that will enable her to become conscious. For example, this would be in her parents' interest. They have an interest in having a normal, healthy child, but the child herself has no interest in her own coming to exist as a conscious, sentient being.[99]

This seems very counterintuitive. It is hard to think of a fully developed, otherwise healthy baby as not having a welfare of her own, simply because she is temporarily unconscious. Moreover, treating the baby might conceivably not be in the interest of her parents. They might have their own reasons for refusing treatment—if they were Christian Scientists, for example. If they refused treatment, allowing the baby to die, would they not be guilty of child neglect, just as they would be for refusing lifesaving medical treatment for a conscious child?

Another possibility is to look for differences between the unconscious baby and embryos that justify different moral status and treatment, differences that allow us to regard the baby, but not the embryo, as victimizable. The most obvious differences between the baby and the embryo are physiological. A fetus is still in the process of becoming a human being, and an embryo is in the very first stage. By contrast, the unconscious neonate in our example is a fully developed baby, physically similar to any other baby. Moreover, the baby in our example could easily be a normal baby. Everything is already in place. She is not merely a potential person, as is an embryo or a fetus. She is a *baby*, albeit one who needs treatment. Because she is physiologically almost a normal baby, it is virtually impossible to treat her as anything else. In other words, although, strictly speaking, she does not have interests of her own, we treat her as if she did, because she is so close to having them. We extend human moral status to the temporarily unconscious neonate because she is like a normal infant in all respects save one, and that deficiency can be easily remedied. A zygote, at the other extreme, is nothing like a baby. As the biologist Clifford Grobstein says, "Biologically, the preembryo [the fertilized egg prior to implantation] and the newborn are so different—separated by nine months of development but a billion years of evolution—that it seems almost bizarre to think of them having the same status."[100] The same is true of a newly implanted embryo. Indeed, throughout the first trimester of pregnancy, in terms of its actual capacities and abilities, a fetus is closer to a gamete than it is to a late-gestation sentient fetus, much less a born baby.

There is another difference between the brain-damaged infant and the fetus that is relevant to moral status. In order for the fetus to achieve consciousness, it needs the woman to act as its life-support system. The brain-damaged baby is already born. It needs medical attention to become conscious, but this can be provided without making another person into a life-support system. Society can therefore recognize

99. Considering a similar example, Jeff McMahan suggests that while it may be impersonally better if a fetus with cerebral deficits has those deficits corrected (that is, the world is a better place), it is difficult to maintain that correcting the deficits is done for the sake of the fetus or interest, given the fetus's weak time-relative interest in realizing its potential to become a person. See *The Ethics of Killing: Problems at the Margins of Life* (Oxford: Oxford University Press, 2002), pp. 316–329.

100. Clifford Grobstein. 1988. *Science and the Unborn*. New York: Basic Books, Inc., p. 76.

the baby as a human person and member of the moral community without infringing on anyone's privacy or bodily self-determination.

Thus, there are reasons to extend human moral status to the unconscious neonate that do not exist in the case of zygotes, embryos, or preconscious fetuses. It is not until the fetus becomes sentient that it has serious moral claims on us. This explains the considerations offered to justify terminating a pregnancy should be stronger at the end of pregnancy than at the beginning, something the FLOA cannot explain.

I conclude that Marquis has not shown the discontinuation account of the harm of death to be inadequate. What about the claim that the fetus, at every stage of gestation, has an interest$_1$ in its future? The motivation for this claim is the view of gestation as just one stage in a person's natural history. According to Marquis, if my life and my future existence are something I value, then it is rational for me to be glad that I was not killed at an earlier stage, for example, when I was a fetus. My valuable future is its valuable future. Having that future (that is, not being killed) is as much in its interest as it is in mine. Or rather, not being killed is as much in my interest when I was a fetus as it is in my interest now.

This depends on the assumption that "we all were fetuses once."[101] In the next section, I examine a challenge to that assumption.

IDENTITY

The Embodied Mind Account

According to Marquis, the basis for ascribing to a nonsentient fetus a valuable future like ours is that the fetus is identical with the adult it will develop into, if it is not aborted. This is precisely what Jeff McMahan denies.[102] He acknowledges that a new human life begins at conception, as the resulting entity—the zygote—is not identical with either the sperm or the egg. It is indisputably alive and it is genetically human:

> But from the fact that something living and human begins to exist around the time of conception it does not follow that you or I began to exist at conception. even if we grant that a new human organism begins to exist at conception, it follows from this fact that *we* began to exist at conception only if we *are* human organisms—that is, only if each of us is numerically identical with, or one and the same thing as, the human organism he or she animates. if I *am* a human organism, I began to exist when this organism did. But the assumption that I am numerically identical with the organism with which (to put it as neutrally as possible) I coexist is hardly uncontroversial.[103]

101. Marquis, "Abortion Revisited" (see note 85), p. 399.

102. Jeff McMahan, *The Ethics of Killing* (see note 98).

103. Ibid., p. 4.

Thus, the question of whether the fetus that developed into me is identical to me, and thus shares my future, is the question of when I began to exist. This in turn, McMahan argues, depends on what is necessarily involved in my continuing to exist over time, or the problem of personal numerical identity. Numerical identity is a matter of recognizing something as the same being over time. It is sometimes contrasted with narrative identity, which concerns questions about the individual's personality and character: who he or she really is. In what follows, the term "identity" is shorthand for "numerical identity."

If what I am essentially is a conscious or minded being, as McMahan wants to argue, then I cannot have existed as a preconscious fetus, for whatever essentially is a minded being must always exist as a minded being. *I* came into existence when my organism began having conscious experiences, probably between the 20th and 28th week of gestation. If this is right, then I am not identical with the embryo or early-gestation fetus that developed into me, and my valuable future is not its future. Indeed, an early fetus does not have a future at all, for it is not anyone, but rather an "unoccupied human organism."[104] According to McMahan, "An early abortion does not kill anyone; it merely prevents someone from coming into existence. In this respect, it is relevantly like contraception and wholly unlike the killing of a person. For there is, again, no one there to be killed."[105] Thus, from the fact that it would be wrong to kill me, we cannot conclude that it is wrong to kill an embryo or early-gestation fetus.

McMahan's view belongs to a tradition going back to Locke, and which has dominated the literature on personal identity since the 1980s.[106] This psychological approach asserts that our identity—or continuing existence over time—is (at least partly) a function of psychological continuity. McMahan differs from a Lockean approach in that he thinks that minds are—or are caused by—brains functioning in certain ways. And we can plausibly individuate minds not in terms of their mental contents, but by individuating brains. "Thus his 'mind essentialism' suggests that we are essentially *embodied* minds—a thesis that apparently avoids reifying minds."[107] The strongest arguments for the psychological approach are certain thought experiments, some realistic, as in "What would happen to you if you entered PVS?" and some highly fanciful, as in the case of one's brain being removed from one's dying body, and transferred into the healthy body of a different person from which the brain had been removed. Most people, contemplating this scenario, would think that they would continue to exist in the other person's body. The intuition is that you would go where your mind—your brain—goes.[108]

104. Ibid., p. 268.

105. Ibid., p. 267.

106. David DeGrazia. 2003. "Identity, Killing, and the Boundaries of Our Existence," *Philosophy & Public Affairs* 31 (4): 413–432, p. 417.

107. Ibid., p. 419.

108. David DeGrazia. 2005. *Human Identity and Bioethics*. New York: Cambridge University Press, p. 52.

McMahan offers support for this initial intuition by asking people who adopt the organism view of identity to consider what they would really prefer if given the following choice:

> Suppose that you have an identical twin whose brain has been destroyed but whose body has until now been kept in a healthy state through intensive artificial support. Serendipitously, you discover today that you have an invariably fatal condition. If your entire brain were transplanted into your twin's body, it is estimated that that body could support life for another thirty years. But this option must be seized immediately . . . [or else] the organs in your twin's body will in a matter of days begin a precipitous process of deterioration. Alternatively, you can continue for about a year in an unimpaired state, whereupon you will die painlessly from rapidly developing complications of the fatal condition. I think that one could be said to accept the implications of the view that we are organisms *only* if one would *really* prefer death within a year to having one's brain sustained alive in a different organism for thirty years.[109]

If I am not my organism, but a separate substance, then what is the relationship between me and my organism? According to McMahan, it is the relation of part to whole. That is, the organism which I am associated—my organism—has, as one of its parts, a mind. The organism is conscious by virtue of having a mind that is conscious. This seems to imply the existence of two conscious beings, me and my organism, but McMahan shows that this is not disturbing by giving an analogy. "In the same sense in which the tree grows because its limb does, and in which the car honks because its horn does, my organism may be said to think, feel, and perceive because I do. This is just another case in which a whole (the organism) has certain properties by virtue of having a part (the mind or person) that has those properties."[110]

Identity plays an important role in a person's special concern about his or her own future (egoistic concern), but it is not the whole story. Another part of McMahan's theory is the Time-Relative Interests Account (TRIA). It maintains that one's interest in staying alive is not simply determined by the amount of good in one's future but also by the degree of psychological connectedness between oneself now and oneself in the future. Psychological connectedness is a matter of both the richness of the subject's mental life and the number of internal connections within the subject's narrative, including memories of past experiences, anticipations of future experiences, plans, intentions, and goals.

An early fetus is literally no one, on McMahan's account. A late fetus is someone, namely, it is identified with the person it would become if not aborted, but its interest in staying alive is weak. McMahan explains:

> The developed fetus cannot envisage or contemplate its future and hence cannot have future-directed psychological states, such as intentions; it would, if it were to become a person, be unable to recall its life as a fetus; and it now has no

---

109. McMahan, *The Ethics of Killing* (see note 98), pp. 31–32.

110. Ibid., p. 92.

psychological architecture—no beliefs, desires, or dispositions of character—to carry forward into the future. It is, in short, psychologically cut off or severed or isolated from itself in the future. Its future is, figuratively speaking, relevantly like someone else's future. It is for this reason that, despite the great good in prospect for it, the developed fetus has only a comparatively weak, time-relative interest in continuing to live.[111]

The Biological View

David DeGrazia considers McMahan's embodied mind account to be perhaps the most promising version of the psychological approach, but it too is ultimately unsatisfying. Like McMahan, DeGrazia embraces essentialism, but he differs on what we are essentially. For DeGrazia, we are essentially organisms, specifically, human animals. He calls this the biological view.

DeGrazia's main reason for rejecting the embodied mind account is its implication that we are not animals. He comments, "I cannot believe this. I do not think that biology teachers systematically misinform students when they teach them that each of us is an animal."[112] A major defect in the embodied mind account, according to DeGrazia, is that it is not consistent with scientifically informed common sense. For example, McMahan's claim that early fetuses cannot *become* or *develop into* minded beings, like you and me, seems contrary to the biological facts of embryology, which teaches us that at some stage in its development, a fetus becomes sentient and begins to have conscious experiences. McMahan would undoubtedly deny that his view is incompatible with science. Instead, his *metaphysics* demands that we describe what happens biologically by referring to the life history of the organism, which is distinct from me. As we saw earlier, the organism becomes conscious when the brain becomes capable of generating conscious experiences. But, according to McMahan, the early fetus does not become or develop into a conscious being; rather, with the onset of consciousness, an entirely new individual comes into existence. For McMahan, this is no odder than saying that I cease to exist when I die, even though my corpse still exists.

It does not seem, then, that the embodied mind account is necessarily contrary to science. Nevertheless, it is at odds with scientifically informed common sense, which sees continuous development in the same being from conception through birth. There is something odd in identifying a fetus at 21 weeks with me, but maintaining that it is not me at 19 weeks. The intuition that an infant was once a fetus, and indeed, an embryo before that, is held by most people, regardless of their position on the morality of abortion. For example, in the preface to *A Defense of Abortion*, David Boonin, notes that among his pictures of his son, Eli, one is a sonogram taken 24 weeks before Eli was born. Boonin writes, "There is no doubt in my mind that this

111. Ibid., pp. 275–276.

112. DeGrazia, *Human Identity and Bioethics* (see note 107), p. 71.

picture, too, shows the same little boy at a very early stage in his physical development."[113]

To recap, Marquis thinks that abortion throughout gestation is seriously wrong because it deprives the fetus of its valuable future. McMahan rejects the assumption on which the FLO account rests, namely, the identification of the early fetus with the later person, and therefore the claim that they have the same future. Rejecting the embodied mind account, DeGrazia agrees with Marquis that we all were once fetuses. However, he does not accept Marquis's conclusion that abortion is seriously wrong because DeGrazia adopts the TRIA, which he considers superior to either Boonin's desire-satisfaction or Marquis's whole-lifetime approach because it better accounts for our considered judgments about the harm of death.

According to DeGrazia, the TRIA is independent of the embodied mind view, and this has important implications for the morality of abortion. The TRIA can be used to defeat the whole-lifetime approach, which is the heart of Marquis's FLOA, regardless of which view of our numerical identity and essence is correct.

> If we are essentially embodied minds, or beings of some other psychological kind, then the FLOA rests on a false assumption about our identity over time and therefore lacks any ontological footing. If we are essentially human animals, then while the FLOA has an ontological footing, my appeal to the TRIA will trip it up.[114]

DeGrazia agrees with Marquis that no later than about 2 weeks after conception (when implantation occurs), there is a human organism with a future like ours. "*But the utter lack of psychological unity between the presentient fetus and the later minded being it could become justifies a very substantial discounting of the harm of the fetus' death.*"[115] While future sentience gives the fetus some interest in staying alive, the absence of psychological unity makes that interest ". . . too weak to ground a right to life or, equivalently, a very strong presumption against killing it."[116] Thus, DeGrazia, like McMahan and me, can justify a pro-choice position on abortion. The disagreement between DeGrazia and McMahan is not moral, but rather metaphysical.

Which view of numerical identity ought we to adopt? The question implies that essentialism is true, that there is something that we are essentially, but I find this questionable. Why assume that there is one property, whether that of embedded consciousness or that of being a human animal, that we are essentially? Why can't we be both?

DeGrazia responds to this challenge in the following way. The fact that I can survive some, but not all, transformations, implies that there are criteria for my identity and that the basic kind that determines those criteria also determines my essence. In general, a thing's basic kind or substance concept also tells us, in a fundamental way, what that thing is, and not just what it does, where it is, or some other inessential fact about it. For example, I was once an adolescent. That is not essential to my existence,

113. David Boonin. 2003. *A Defense of Abortion.* New York: Cambridge University Press, p. xiv.

114. Ibid., p. 71.

115. Ibid., p. 72.

116. Ibid., p. 73.

but only a phase. We know this since I continued to exist when I turned 20 years old. Or I can say that I am a Democrat and a philosopher. But neither of these is a criterion of my identity, since I existed before I was a Democrat and a philosopher and will continue to exist even if I become a Republican and give up philosophy. The argument for essentialism is basically this: everything, including human persons, must have an essence, or essential properties, for without such properties, we could not identify things over time or know when they come into or out of existence.

There are two points to make in response.[117] First, DeGrazia's argument in favor of essentialism—that it is necessary for identification—does not work. Essential properties are not required for identification, because they may not be what we use to identify a thing over time. For example, water is essentially a combination of two atoms of hydrogen and one of oxygen, but people were able to identify something as water long before they knew anything about hydrogen and oxygen. Its essence, then, is not doing the work of identification.

Whether something has essential properties is an open question, depending on context. One can be an essentialist about water, but not about, say, chairs. There are many phenomena that do not lend themselves to essentialist analysis. Consider the current (as of this writing) recession. Economists want to know when it ends. But there are multiple and sometimes conflicting criteria: unemployment, stock market dropping, consumer spending, housing market, and so on. Not only is it not true that there is one essential property, but it may be impossible to state the identification criteria in advance. I think the same is likely to be true about people, so I am a skeptical agnostic about essentialism, at least the kind of one-property essentialism advocated by both McMahan and DeGrazia, in the case of persons. Rather, I would say that we are or have minds; we are human animals; we may even have immortal souls (though this seems unlikely). Why think that we can, much less have to, choose between these different criteria with their different persistence conditions? DeGrazia's answer is that we all believe that an individual will persist through some changes but not others. Without an essence, we would be unable to judge when someone has gone out of existence. However, that just begs the question. It assumes that there is *a* correct answer to the question, which is just what the essentialist skeptic denies. Instead of assuming that there is only one characteristic underlying identity, there might be several. The question about existence then depends on which criteria we have in mind. For example, qua embedded mind, Terri Schiavo ceased to exist when her brain stopped functioning, sometime in 1990. Qua organism, she died March 31, 2005. And if she has an immortal soul, she continues to exist today.

The Interest View and the Time-Relative Interests Account

However, even if I am wrong about this, and essentialism (or one-property essentialism) is true of persons, it does not have much, if any, moral significance. For while McMahan and DeGrazia disagree about what we essentially are, and therefore about numerical identity, they agree that abortion is morally permissible, because both adopt the TRIA: the discounting of interests where there is little or no

---

117. I owe a great debt to my colleague, Ron McClamrock, for helping me to articulate my objections to essentialism.

psychological connectedness. What is doing the work is psychological unity, not numerical identity.[118] It seems to me that the TRIA is both consistent with the interest view and a welcome addition to it. The interest view, as I originally developed it in the first edition of this book, focuses only on the necessity of conscious awareness, or a mental life of some kind, for the possession of interests, and therefore, for moral standing. The TRIA enables us to explain why sentient fetuses, which have some interests, specifically in avoiding pain, do not have equal moral status with more developed human beings, and specifically, why they do not have a right to life. Interested beings have an interest in continued life in the future that would be the basis for a right to life only if they have some psychological unity over time. Lacking a mental life and psychological unity, the presentient fetus has no interests at all and thus cannot be harmed. Even after the onset of sentience, when it has a rudimentary mental life, but no psychological unity, the fetus has very little stake in remaining alive and is not seriously harmed by death.

The TRIA can also explain some of our intuitions about the relative harm of death. DeGrazia gives the example of a lifeboat which contains several human beings and a dog.[119] Someone must be sacrificed to prevent the lifeboat from sinking. Everyone—even those who believe that humans and nonhumans should be accorded equal concern—agrees that the dog should be sacrificed. Why is this? DeGrazia considers several plausible candidates: that the dog's life is subjectively less valuable than that of the humans, that we have closer ties to other humans than to dogs, that dogs cannot desire their continued existence. None of these approaches is satisfactory. A dog may have a terrific life, filled with as many pleasures as a dog can have. The dog might have stronger social bonds with other people than some of the humans on the boat. And while a dog cannot desire its own continued existence, at least on one interpretation of desire, neither can a human infant. Yet everyone agrees that it would be wrong to sacrifice one of the human beings instead of the dog. The TRIA explains why death is a greater harm to the human than to the dog. The difference between the human and the dog is that the human being is much more psychologically invested in and connected to her possible future than the dog is to hers. A human being has a well-developed, nuanced sense of herself as a protagonist in a life story—a narrative—that dogs do not have.

The TRIA is superior to either the desire-satisfaction or the whole-lifetime approach because it better accounts for our considered judgments about the harm of death. On the desire-satisfaction account, one is harmed by death only if one can desire to stay alive. Given the primitive nature of infant conceptions, infants seem to lack this sort of desire, but it is implausible to think that they are not harmed by death. The whole-life perspective can explain why death is a harm to an infant, but it has the implausible implication that death is a greater harm to an infant (who loses more life) than it is to a child or young adult. The TRIA steers between these two extreme positions:

> Thus, this approach delivers a plausible verdict here while satisfyingly explaining precisely what factor justifies discounting the harm of death, in cases like

---

118. This point is made by Shoemaker (see note 89), p. 484.

119. Ibid., p. 57.

the infant's, as it would be understood from a whole-lifetime perspective: degree of psychological unity over time. The desire-satisfaction view is correct that caring about or appreciating (and therefore desiring) one's future is relevant to the harm of death, but incorrect that one who does not appreciate or desire one's future loses nothing from having that future snatched away. The whole-lifetime approach is correct that appreciating one's own future is not necessary for having a stake in that future, but incorrect in thinking that such appreciation is irrelevant to the magnitude of the harm of death. The TRIA, meanwhile, gets right what these polar views get right while avoiding their errors.[120]

In the first edition, I appealed to potential personhood to explain why it is worse to kill a human infant than a nonhuman animal.[121] I now think that the TRIA provides a better explanation for why it is worse to kill a human infant than to kill a nonhuman animal. If potential personhood is what makes an infant's life more valuable than that of an animal, then it is unclear why potential personhood is irrelevant prior to the onset of sentience. And even if that can be explained, there is another problem. Both the sentient fetus and newborn are equally potential persons. This suggests that late abortions and infanticide are morally comparable, which is hard to accept. By contrast, the TRIA can explain why infanticide is in general more seriously objectionable than late abortion. A newborn infant's time-relative interest in continuing to live is normally stronger than that of a developed fetus. Once born, the infant is bombarded with stimuli and its psychological development proceeds at a rapid pace. Therefore, As McMahan puts it, ". . . the newborn infant's time-relative interest in continuing to live is stronger than it was when the infant was a fetus, and it will continue to increase in strength as the infant continues to mature psychologically."[122] However, it must be acknowledged that some infants, because of birth defects, may never acquire sufficient psychological continuity to develop strong time-relative interests in remaining alive. Where should we place such infants on a moral-status scale? Is the fact that they are *human* of any moral significance, when humanity is severed from the potential to become a descriptive person? Are there good reasons, in other words, to extend normative personhood to humans who will never have the complex capacities of descriptive persons? There are several things that should be said in response. First, the moral standing of newborns is based in part of the special relations that develop between the infant and others, in particular, its parents. These relations, which may begin before birth in the case of a wanted pregnancy, but which certainly obtain and intensify after birth, provide additional reasons for others not to frustrate the infant's time-relative interest in continuing

120. Ibid., p. 67.

121. Here is the relevant passage: "Human babies are not just sentient beings. They are also potential persons. Their potential descriptive personhood is a good reason for regarding their lives as more important, morally more valuable than the lives of sentient beings who are not potential persons, such as animals. Just as it is reasonable to value the life of a person over a nonperson, it is equally justifiable to value the life of a sentient potential person over the life of a sentient being who lacks this potential. So potential personhood, while it cannot get someone onto the moral-status scale, so to speak, can determine one's relative place on that scale." *Life Before Birth*, p. 68.

122. McMahan, *The Ethics of Killing* (see note 98), p. 343.

to live.[123] A disability, even a very severe one, does not take away an infant's status as *someone's child*. The fact that an infant may never develop into a complex, reasoning being should not, and usually does not, lessen the parents' love and concern for the child. The relationship of parent creates a duty of care, a duty that may be taken over by others if the parents are not available or capable of performing it.

Second, it is not always easy to know at birth what the psychological capacities of an infant are. Consider the case of Keri-Lynn—Baby Jane Doe—(discussed in Chapter 3) whose doctors predicted that, if she survived, she would never learn to speak, recognize her parents, or enjoy life. She not only survived, but she did all of these things and more. Third, it is easy, but mistaken, to assume that personhood is solely a matter of intellectual ability. Eva Kittay[124] writes movingly of her daughter, Sesha, a young woman in her 30s, who never learned to walk or talk or read, but whose taste in music became more complex as she grew up. This suggests psychological development, despite profound developmental disabilities, which might provide the kind of psychological connectedness that grounds a robust time-relative interest in continued existence.

When it is clear that the infant has no stake in continued existence, the decision not to prolong life is not a difficult one, although it may still be heart-rending for the parents. To take the most extreme example, life-sustaining treatment should not be given to infants with anencephaly, because it is pointless to sustain the life of someone who will never become conscious. Most doctors believe that infants with anencephaly are incapable of experiencing anything. If this is correct, then such infants do not have interests at all, and so nothing can be done in their interest or for their sake. Some think that they may be capable of experiencing pain. If so, then analgesics should be given during their brief lives, but prolonging their lives still is not warranted.

Another relatively "easy" case occurs when the infant's life is filled with irremediable pain, followed by an early death, as in severe cases of dystrophic epidermolysis bullosa (EB)[125] "Affected infants are typically born with widespread blistering and areas of missing skin, often caused by trauma during birth. Most often, blisters are present over the whole body and affect mucous membranes such as the moist lining of the mouth and digestive tract. As the blisters heal, they result in severe scarring. Scarring in the mouth and esophagus can make it difficult to chew and swallow food, leading to chronic malnutrition and slow growth."[126] In the most severe cases, the

123. Ibid.

124. Eva Feder Kittay. 1999. *Love's Labor: Essays on Women, Equality, and Dependency.* New York: Routledge.

125. Jonathan Glover uses this example in "Future People, Disability, and Screening," in Peter Laslett and James Fishkin, eds. 1992. *Justice Between Age Groups and Generations.* New Haven, CT: Yale University Press, pp. 127–143.

126. Genetics Home Reference: Dystropic Epidermolysis Bullosa, http://ghr.nlm.nih.gov/condition/dystrophic-epidermolysis-bullosa. Accessed May 31, 2010. It should be noted that epidermolysis bullosa, like virtually every medical condition, can be more or less severe, complicating medical decision making.

death rate is as high as 87% in the first year of life.[127] In the worst cases, the constant pain suffered by the baby deprives him or her of the ordinary pleasures of infancy, while death at an early age prevents the child from acquiring compensating interests. In such cases, it seems that acting in the child's best interest means allowing him or her to die. It may even mean killing the child, although this is not a legal option in most countries. To acknowledge that acting in the child's best interest may mean allowing or seeking the child's death is not to say that infants do not have the same right to life as other persons. It is rather to say that their right to life is not violated if they are genuinely "better off dead." (See Chapter 3 for a discussion of "wrongful life.")

Cases where infants can be said to have no interests or where death is seen as clearly in their best interest are relatively rare. It is much more often the case that it is difficult to say what is in the child's best interest. Sometimes aggressive treatment is warranted, as in the case of Keri-Lynn, whose disabilities might have been less severe if a shunt had been implanted right away. It is very unlikely that any neonatologist practicing today would give the same advice that Keri-Lynn's parents were given in 1983: infants with spina bifida are almost always treated aggressively. The difficulty of predicting the outcome complicates decision making for newborns. This is especially true for very premature infants who, if they survive, could be entirely normal or could have profound disabilities. This uncertainty leads some to advocate extremely aggressive treatment for such babies. In my view, this unduly discounts the suffering that can be inflicted on the child. As one parent put it, her child was being "tortured to life." The relatively weak time-relative interests of newborns in continuing to live supports allowing parents and doctors to opt against aggressive life-sustaining treatment, in cases where the child is unlikely ever to have a stake in his or her own future, and when such treatment is likely to inflict considerable suffering.

Sentient Fetuses

What is the moral status of sentient fetuses? They have begun to have experiences, and so it is at least possible that they enjoy their lives. Obviously, the range and nature of their enjoyment is not very great, but perhaps late fetuses, like babies, are capable of sensuous pleasure, from sucking their thumbs, from the warmth of the womb, from the sound of their mothers' heartbeats, from motion as the mother moves around. Certainly in newborn nurseries the temperature is kept quite high, on the ground that this is what the baby was used to before birth. The ability to calm infants by motion is often attributed to this being a replication of the uterine environment. Studies have been done correlating fetal activity with extrauterine sound, leading researchers to claim that fetuses can not only hear inside the womb, but that they enjoy some kinds of sounds more than others.[128] If all of this is right, then it seems plausible to say that late fetuses have, or have begun to have, lives in the

127. Google Health, Epidermolysis Bullosa. https://health.google.com/health/ref/ Epidermolysis+bullosa. Accessed May 31, 2010.

128. A researcher at Queen's University School of Nursing, Dr. Barbara Kisilevsky, did a study that allegedly proves that fetuses can hear at 30 weeks.

biographical sense. Death deprives them of their lives, and so is a harm to them. Thus, it seems that life is *in* the interest of the conscious fetus, and it, like a newborn, can have a right to life.

On the other hand, fetuses, unlike born babies, dwell inside pregnant women. This has been dismissed by conservatives as "mere geography," but the geography is not insignificant. As Mary Anne Warren puts it, "Normally, a being's location makes no difference to its moral status; but this case is unique. So long as the fetus remains within the woman's body, it is impossible to treat it as if it were already a person with full and equal moral rights, without at the same time treating the woman as if she were something less."[129] Any attempt to protect the life of a fetus may conflict with, or even endanger, the interests of the pregnant woman, including her life or health. There is a possibility of conflict that simply does not exist in the case of the newborn. For this reason, we cannot simply extend the right to life possessed by all human newborns to sentient fetuses.

To summarize, sentience is sufficient for minimal moral status. The interests of all sentient beings—persons, animals, conscious fetuses, and babies—must be considered. When a sentient being has a life it enjoys, death is a harm to it. However, the harm of death is greater for sentient beings with greater psychological connectedness, because their time-relative interests in continued existence are stronger. This makes it worse to kill a newborn human infant than a full-grown dog, and worse to kill a newborn human infant than to kill a late fetus. In addition, although conscious fetuses are substantially similar to newborns, and thus entitled to moral consideration, they are located inside the pregnant woman's body. This makes it impossible to give them full protection without violating her right to privacy or bodily self-determination (see the section, "The Argument From Bodily Self-Determination").

Embryos and preconscious fetuses are potential persons, but this is not relevant to their moral standing, nor is it relevant to the decision to bring them to term. A pregnant woman who wishes to be responsible and conscientious in making a decision about abortion is not required to consider the child who might have been born. In particular, she does not have to claim that her child would be miserable in order to justify having an abortion. She can acknowledge that, if she does not abort, the resulting child might well have a very happy life. Pro-lifers are quite right to cast scorn on the notion that all unplanned pregnancies result in unwanted children, or that all unwanted children necessarily have unhappy lives. Instead, pro-choicers should respond that the happiness of the potential child is not determinative— indeed, not even relevant to the decision to abort. There is no obligation to bring happy people into the world, only an obligation to try to give the children one decides to bring into the world a decent chance at happiness.

It may seem obvious that there is no obligation to bring happy people into the world. How can someone who does not exist have any claim to our attention and concern? However, future people do not exist either and, as I argued in Chapter 1, this does not prevent them from having claims against us. For this reason, philosophers like R. M. Hare have argued that merely possible people do count. We can harm people in the future by using up all the world's resources or by destroying the ozone layer, Hare notes; why can't we harm them by preventing them from

129. Mary Anne Warren. 1985. *Gendercide: The Implications of Sex Selection*. Totowa, NJ: Rowman and Allenheld, p. 102.

being conceived? In the next section, I will argue that it is only future actual people who can be harmed, not merely possible people.

POSSIBLE PEOPLE

Nonexistence admittedly does not cause anyone to *suffer*. Nor can a nonexistent person be *deprived* of existence, in the sense of having it taken away. But it may be argued that someone who is prevented from being conceived or born is *denied* existence, denied the chance to enjoy life. R. M. Hare puts the point this way:

> . . . if it would have been a good for him to exist (because this made possible the goods that, once he existed, he was able to enjoy), surely it was a harm to him not to exist, and so not to be able to enjoy these goods. He did not suffer; but there were enjoyments he could have had and did not.[130]

The point may be put another way. If death—no longer existing—can be a harm to the one who dies, why isn't nonexistence a harm to someone who never exists? Why should we have an interest in continuing to exist, but no interest in coming to exist in the first place? There seems to be an asymmetry that needs explanation.

Such an explanation can be given if we think about why we consider death to be a harm. Death is not merely nonexistence, but the termination of someone's life. Death ends all of one's plans, projects, concerns, and desires. Feinberg explains why death is a harm this way: "To extinguish a person's life is, at one stroke, to defeat almost all of his self-regarding interests: to ensure that his ongoing projects and enterprises, his long-range goals, and his most earnest hopes for his own achievement and personal enjoyment, must all be dashed."[131] None of this is true of never-existing people. The failure to bring them into existence does not thwart their plans, end their relationships, or destroy their hopes of achievement and happiness. Admittedly, it forecloses the possibility of there ever being these plans, hopes, and relationships, but that is a tragedy for no one. There is literally no one to feel sorry for, or guilty about, when people who might have existed are not brought into existence.

However, there remains an issue that requires investigation. I have been arguing that we have obligations to actual sentient beings, existing now and in the future, but no obligations to merely possible people. Actual people count; merely possible people do not.[132] Derek Parfit characterizes this as a "person-affecting view." Person-affecting principles maintain that only actions that harm actual people are wrong. Such principles can explain many of our moral views, because ordinarily the choices we face are Same People Choices (see Chapter 1). We run into difficulties, however, with Different People Choices, where our choice itself affects *who* will exist. The recognition

130. Hare, "Abortion and the Golden Rule" (see note 69), pp. 220–221.

131. Joel Feinberg. 1984. *Harm to Others.* Oxford: Oxford University Press, pp. 81–81.

132. This view is also taken by John Bigelow and Robert Pargetter in "Morality, Potential Persons and Abortion," *American Philosophical Quarterly* 25:2 (April 1988), pp. 173–181.

of Different People Choices may force us to reconsider the adequacy of person-affecting principles, and this could have implications for abortion.

The Nonidentity Problem[133]

A Different Person Choice we discussed in the last chapter concerned a 14-year-old girl who chooses to have a baby. There seem to be compelling reasons why this would be a bad idea; some have to do with the likely effects on the girl's life, but others refer to the effect on the child. Teenage mothers tend to have babies who are low birth weight, which is associated both with a significantly higher mortality rate than that for full-term babies, and with learning disabilities in the future. The child of a teenage mother is also unlikely to get adequate mothering, because her mother is still a child herself. These considerations incline us to urge the 14-year-old to wait and have a baby when she can give it a good start in life. Suppose she pays no attention and goes ahead and has a child. Parfit points out that it is simply not true that it would have been better *for that child* if she had waited. If she waits, and has a child later on, it will be a different child.

The same problem arises with another kind of example, which Don Locke calls "the Fated Child."[134] In this example, a woman learns that if she conceives at a certain time, the resulting child will inevitably die of a heart attack around the age of 25. If she waits a month, she will have a child with a normal life expectancy. Most of us would agree that it would be wrong to conceive the Fated Child. But why, exactly, would it be wrong? The answer cannot be that the child is disadvantaged by being conceived at that time. If the woman waits, she will have a different child. (It will be a child from a different ovum and sperm.) Assume that the Fated Child has a worthwhile life, despite his premature death, that he does not object to his mother's decision. He is glad to be alive. So how is her decision wrong?

In both of these cases, there is a crucial factor that differentiates them from other instances of prenatal or preconception harming, namely, that nothing can be done to prevent the disadvantageous condition, except to prevent the child's birth altogether. To capture this unique feature, David Heyd terms these cases "genesis problems."[135] We can see the unique philosophical issue raised by genesis problems if we contrast them with other examples of prenatal harming, where something can be done to prevent the harm to the child (see Chapter 4). For example, a pregnant woman can reduce the risk of prematurity or low birth weight (which are associated with various health risks) in her baby by not smoking or drinking alcohol. She can lessen the risk her child will have a neural tube disorder by getting enough folic acid in her diet. In fact, she can do this even before she gets pregnant. The fact that the

133. Some of the material in this section comes from my article "Wrongful Life and Procreative Decisions" in Melinda A. Roberts and David T. Wasserman, eds., *Harming Future Persons: Ethics, Genetics and the Nonidentity Problem* (New York: Springer, 2009), pp. 155–178.

134. Don Locke. 1987. "The Parfit Population Problem," *Philosophy* 62 (April), pp. 131–157, at 137.

135. David Heyd. 1992. *Genethics: Moral Issues in the Creation of People.* Berkeley, CA: University of California Press.

child does not yet exist is not the relevant factor. What is important is that the harm can be prevented. By contrast, in genesis cases, nothing can be done to prevent the harm to this child. It's life with the disadvantage or no life at all. And that makes the question of whether bringing the child into existence in a harmful condition is "unfair to the child" a much more difficult one.

It is also important to stress at the outset just how strong most people's intuitions regarding genesis problems are. Virtually every professional society or national commission or oversight group that has considered the matter takes for granted that expected impact on offspring must be taken into consideration in determining the permissibility of a reproductive treatment or arrangement. For example, the main objection to reproductive cloning in the National Advisory Bioethics Commission's report, "Cloning Human Beings," was an unacceptable level of risk of serious defects in offspring.[136] The suggestion that this child would not exist without reproductive cloning was briefly mentioned, only to be rejected as morally irrelevant. The strength of most people's intuitions makes genesis problems particularly vexing because, while our intuitions go one way, the arguments seem to go another. This is obviously undesirable and provides a motive for attempting to resolve this disconnect between intuitions and moral arguments. Another motive for examining genesis problems is that they have profound implications for ethical theory in general, in particular, the explanation of why wrong acts are wrong. On one plausible ethical view, acts that are wrong must be wrong *for someone*. Moral principles, on this view, must concern the interests of individuals; they must be "person affecting."[137] Genesis problems pose a challenge to this assumption because they seem to provide examples of wrong acts that are not a wrong or a harm *to* anyone.

This is especially problematic for a view of abortion such as I am defending, which is based on the idea that abortion deprives no one of anything and makes no one worse off. In genesis cases, we seem to have to appeal to what Don Locke terms "the Possible Persons Principle": "the principle that in judging the rightness or wrongness of an action or decision we need to take account not merely of those who actually do, or will, exist, but also of those who would have existed if there had been a different action or decision."[138] So, for example, it is wrong to conceive a Fated Child, one with a limited life expectancy when, with a little restraint or foresight, one could have had a healthy child. But if we adopt the Possible Persons Principle (PPP) in order to explain what is wrong with conceiving a Fated Child, we will have to give up the Person-affecting Restriction (PAR). The PPP is, in effect, the rejection of the PAR, which requires that actions and decisions be judged only by their effect on those people who actually exist, now or in the future. And if we give up the PAR, then we cannot say that abortion is morally permissible because it affects no actual

136. National Bioethics Advisory Commission. 1997. "Cloning Human Beings," Executive summary, p. ii. http://bioethics.georgetown.edu/nbac/pubs/cloning1/executive.pdf. Accessed October 29, 2010.

137. I use the term "person affecting" because it is prevalent in the literature. I do not mean to imply that interests are limited to persons, or that morality concerns only the interests of persons. "Person affecting" is simply more graceful than "interested individual affecting."

138. Locke, "The Parfit Population Problem" (see note 133), p. 138.

person (or more accurately, no individual with moral standing), and only actual persons count.

There are several possible responses to the nonidentity problem.[139] We can retain the PAR, and accept the inference that the nonidentity problem seems to support, namely, that in the acts in question, no one is harmed or wronged or made worse off, and therefore, these acts are not wrong. Or we can reject the view that all of morality is person affecting, and we can argue that acts can be morally wrong even if no one was harmed or wronged or made worse off. We can appeal to impersonal principles to explain the wrongness of some genesis cases. Or we can insist that the people brought into existence in a harmful condition have been wronged, not because they have been made worse off than they would otherwise have been, but because their rights were violated.

John Robertson is an example of the first approach. Perhaps the best-known advocate for procreative liberty, he has argued that banning risky procreative technologies or arrangements *out of concern for the welfare of offspring* makes no sense.[140] As Robertson puts it, "But for the technique in question, the child never would have been born. *Whatever psychological or social problems arise, they hardly rise to the level of severe handicap or disability that would make the child's very existence a net burden, and hence a wrongful life.*"[141] His view has two notable features. First, it suggests that life can be a net burden to a child if the disadvantage is severe enough. In such cases, it makes sense to characterize the child's life as wrongful, that is, to claim that the child would be better off unborn. Second, it maintains that procreative decisions can harm or wrong offspring *only* in such cases. If the child has or is likely to have a life that is or will be, from the child's own perspective, on balance worth living, then, whatever disadvantages it has, its life logically cannot be regarded as wrongful, that is, as a harm or wrong to the child. Procreative decisions are not wrong, on this view, unless the child himself or herself would choose or prefer nonexistence. Let us call this standard for morally permissible procreation "the nonexistence condition."

It cannot be overemphasized how permissive this standard is. No matter how limited the child's life, no matter how filled with suffering, or how empty of the things that make life worth living, so long as the child finds life barely worth living, he or she has not been harmed or wronged by birth. Moreover, regardless of their motives for bringing the child into existence, so long as the child is not harmed or wronged or made worse off, his parents have done nothing wrong in conceiving him for this purpose. This, I submit, is absurd. As I have explained it elsewhere:

> A more plausible criterion for "rightful" birth than the nonexistence condition
> is one in which life is actually a benefit to the child, as opposed to a life that is

---

139. These are outlined in the Introduction to Melinda A. Roberts and David T. Wasserman, *Harming Future Persons* (see note 132), pp. xx–xxiii.

140. There might be other reasons to prohibit such technologies or arrangements, including the interests of prospective parents or society at large. The issue here is whether the interests of the child justify preventing his or her birth.

141. Robertson. 1994. *Children of Choice: Freedom and the New Reproductive Technologies.* Princeton, NJ: Princeton University Press, p.122. Emphasis added.

wretched, although still marginally worth living. For life to be a positive benefit, certain minimal conditions must be satisfied, and therefore we can call this criterion for responsible procreation the "decent minimum standard." A decent minimum is reached only if life holds a reasonable promise of containing the things that make human lives good: an ability to experience pleasure, to learn, to have relationships with others. If someone's life will be inevitably and irremediably bereft of many of these goods, then we do that person no favor by bringing him or her into existence; indeed, knowingly and voluntarily to conceive a child under such conditions is a harm and a wrong to the person. This aspect of the decent minimum standard focuses on the child's capacities for a good human life. In addition, the ability to be a good enough parent is also part of the decent minimum. I maintain that it is wrong, irresponsible procreation, to have a child if one knows that one lacks either the ability to love the child or the capacity to care properly for him or her.[142]

The intuition behind the decent minimum standard is that children have a right to something more than lives that are barely worth living. The child whose life falls below a decent minimum is deprived of that to which he or she has a right, and thus is wronged.

The decent minimum standard is consistent with the person-affecting intuition because it maintains that a child who is brought into existence below a decent minimum has been wronged. However, there are cases where the child's predicted life, although disadvantaged in some way, is not so bad as to fall below a decent minimum standard, and yet the decision to procreate is morally problematic because the prospective parents could have had a different child without the disadvantage.

To see this, consider the following pair of examples, which I have adapted from Derek Parfit and Dan Brock.[143]

1. Angela is pregnant. Her doctor discovers that she has a condition that will result in mild retardation in her baby. The doctor prescribes a medication that will prevent the retardation. But Angela does not want to take the medication, because a side effect of the medication is that it can cause mild acne. So she does not take it and, as predicted, her baby is born mildly retarded.

2. Betty wants to get pregnant. However, she is on medication that has the following side effect: if she gets pregnant while on the medication, her baby will be born mildly retarded. Going off the medication is not a feasible option, as it would adversely affect her health as well as her fertility. Fortunately, she only needs to take the medication for a few months. Her doctor advises her to wait to get pregnant until she is off the medication. But Betty does not want to wait. She plans to visit her family during her summer vacation, and so she wants to have the baby in June at the latest.

142. Steinbock, "Wrongful Life and Procreative Decisions" (see note 132), p. 163.

143. Derek Parfit. 1976. "On Doing the Best for Our Children," in Michael Bayles, ed., *Ethics and Population*. Cambridge, MA: Schenkman Company; Dan Brock. 1995. "The Non-Identity Problem and Genetic Harms: The Case of Wrongful Handicaps," *Bioethics* 9 (3/4): 269–275.

She gets pregnant right away and has a baby in June who, as predicted, is born mildly retarded.

Many people would regard both Angela and Betty as having acted wrongly, and indeed equally wrongly. I certainly do. Both give birth to a mildly retarded child, when this easily could have been prevented, and for reasons that are morally trivial. Morally, there seems to be no difference between what Angela does and what Betty does. Those who agree accept the "No-Difference View."[144]

However, there is a difference in the two cases, a difference that ordinarily would affect our judgments of wrongdoing. The difference is that Angela, but not Betty, has harmed her baby. By not taking the prescribed medication, Angela has caused her baby to be born retarded, when he could have been born with normal intelligence. She has caused him to be worse off than he otherwise would have been, which is the ordinary straightforward conception of harming. But the same is not true of Betty. She has not made her baby worse off than he would have been or could have been. There is no way that the child she had in June could have been born with normal intelligence. There was nothing Betty could do to make *him* mentally normal. Waiting would have enabled her to have a child with normal intelligence, but it would have been a *different child*, one conceived from a different egg and a different sperm.

If mild mental retardation could be seen as making the child's life fall below a decent minimum, we could argue that Betty, as much as Angela, harms her child. But mild mental retardation clearly falls above that standard. Individuals who are mildly retarded can go to school, make friends, get jobs, and generally have lives that are well worth living, even if limited in various ways. This being the case, I think we have to admit that Betty has not harmed her baby. Defenders of the PAR insist that it follows that Betty has done nothing wrong. For example, Melinda Roberts argues that Betty acts wrongly only if there was something she could have done to make the life of the child she has in June better. Since that is not the case, she has done nothing wrong. Indeed, she has done the best she could have done for that child.

Roberts is willing to acknowledge this counterintuitive result in order to retain the PAR. This, it seems to me, is too high a price to pay. It seems to me perverse to maintain that Betty does nothing wrong or that her act is morally significantly different from Angela's. Another possibility is that both Angela and Betty wrong the children they bear and for the exact same reason: they violate their rights. This possibility is

---

144. Derek Parfit. 1986. *Reasons and Persons*. Oxford: Oxford University Press, p. 367. By the No-Difference View, I mean simply the claim that there is no *moral* difference between what Angela does and what Betty does. One does not act more wrongly than the other. The more generalized version of the No-Difference View holds that the wrongness of both acts must have the *same explanation*. Thus, if person-affecting reasons cannot explain the wrongness of Betty's act, it cannot explain the wrongness of Angela's act either. This leads Parfit to reject person-affecting reasons altogether in the area of morality concerned with beneficence and human well-being. For an excellent critique of the generalized version of the No-Difference View, see Jeff McMahan, "Wrongful Life: Paradoxes in the Morality of Causing People to Exist," in John Harris, ed. 2001. *Bioethics*. Oxford: Oxford University Press, pp. 445–475. I agree with McMahan that both kinds of reasons, person affecting and impersonal, are necessary in moral discourse, and that neither can be reduced to the other.

explored by Jeffrey Reiman in "Being Fair to Future People: The Non-Identity Problem in the Original Position."[145] Reiman uses the theory of John Rawls[146] to defend the commonsense judgment that, in choosing a policy that will have a negative effect on future people, though not so negative as to make their lives not worth living, one has wronged the future people who are negatively affected as a result— even though the alternative is that those people would not have existed at all, if one had chosen a different alternative. They are wronged not because they are made worse off than they otherwise would have been, but because they have a right that has been violated: a right to normal functioning. They have this right because it would follow from the choices of rational agents in the original position.

The original position, as Reiman explains it, is a mental experiment for choosing principles of justice. The individuals (or parties, as Rawls call them) who are choosing the principles must consider to what principles of justice governing their treatment of one another they can rationally agree. The device for ensuring that the principles are fair is the "veil of ignorance," which deprives them of knowledge of their specific circumstances, such as their sex, race, age, talents, social class, wealth, or to what generation they belong. Parties in the original position must chose principles thinking that they may turn out to be *anyone* in the society governed by those principles. The veil of ignorance prevents them from tailoring principles to their own advantage, and thus it builds fairness into the conditions of choosing in the original position.

What duties to future people would parties in the original position accept? It seems reasonable, Reiman says, for the parties in the original position to agree to a general duty of living people to provide for future generations' normal functioning since the parties want to safeguard their ability to pursue their goals whatever they turn out to be and normal functioning does this. Deprived of knowledge about the generation to which they belong, it would be irrational for them to refuse to acknowledge any duty to generations yet to come. At the same time, the standard of normal functioning limits the duty to future people. We currently living people do not have the obligation to make the lives of future generations as good as they could be, but only to make reasonable sacrifices to ensure they will have normal functioning.

Crucial to Reiman's argument is the distinction between the properties individuals have, whether their own personal properties or the properties of the world in which they live, and their existence as particular individuals. When we are considering how to act or what policies to choose, we are morally required to consider the effects on future people's properties, but not, Reiman argues, which particular people they turn out to be. And the reason we are not morally required to think about which particular people they turn out to be is that this is not an interest of theirs. Nonexistent possible people do not have an interest in coming into existence as a particular individual; that is an interest that is restricted to actual living people. Once we understand this, we see that the morally relevant interests of future people are different in form from those of present people. "Their morally relevant interests are a function of

145. Jeffrey Reiman. 2007. "Being Fair to Future People: The Non-Identity Problem in the Original Position," *Philosophy & Public Affairs* 35 (1): 69–92.

146. John Rawls. 1999. *A Theory of Justice*, revised edition. Cambridge, MA: Harvard University Press.

what we can do now to improve or worsen their lives in the future, and that is a matter of what properties they are born with or into, not which particulars they are apart from that, since they are not yet particular individuals."[147]

This way of thinking about future generations coheres with our intuitions about how people ought to reason and how most people do think about their duties to future people. If the 14-Year-Old-Girl considers the cost to her future child of getting pregnant now, as opposed to waiting a few years, she is considering the properties of the future child, not who the child will be. This is also true in what Reiman calls the Preconception Wrongful Disability case (the case of Betty). However, Reiman does not think that the 14-Year-Old-Girl and Betty merely act wrongly; he maintains that the choice to have a child who is impaired, when this could have been prevented by changing the timing of conception, violates the right of the future person to reasonable efforts to ensure normal functioning. Reiman summarizes his position by saying, ". . . choosing to do actions that adversely affect interests of future people wrongs them by violating their rights to our efforts to ensure them a normal level of functioning. This is so even though the alternative would be that those particular people would not have existed, because the interests harmed are the interests of people considered *as if which particulars they are is irrelevant.*"[148] In other words, from the stance of the original position, it is morally irrelevant which particular people come into existence. It is a fact that the parties in the original position are morally required to ignore, and that we currently existing people are morally required to ignore in making reproductive decisions.

The rights of future people are violated, according to Reiman, when present people make choices that result in future people being deprived of normal functioning. Moreover, even if, under the threat of nonexistence, people would waive this right, such a waiver would be illegitimate, Reiman says, because it would have been performed under duress. "A person who waives a right in the face of an unjust threat of not existing, however, does not make a free and morally binding choice. Thus, even if the future people in the non-identity cases would waive their rights, that waiver would not be valid."[149] The fact that the child now has a life worth living, and that this could have been predicted, does not get the person responsible for his impaired existence off the moral hook.

I agree with Reiman that it is wrong to bring people into the world in an impaired condition when this can be avoided with reasonable precautions. I agree with him that when we are making decisions that affect future people, considerations about which people will get born are morally irrelevant. Betty's refusal to delay conception was wrong—indeed, just as wrong as Angela's refusal to take medication. Both women had a mentally handicapped child when this could have been easily prevented, and their reasons for doing what would have prevented this outcome were trivial.[150] However, even if individual reproductive choices (and social policies

147. Reiman, "Being Fair to Future People" (see note 144), p. 85.

148. Ibid., p. 86.

149. Reiman, "Being Fair to Future People" (see note 144), p. 88.

150. Reiman eliminates the woman's motivation in his account of "Preconception Wrongful Disability," because he thinks that a frivolous motive interferes with objective consideration of the case. On the contrary, I think that the more frivolous the motivation, the more likely we

about conservation) ought not to be influenced by who will come into existence, and even if the choice can be criticized as immoral or wrongful, it is difficult to see how the particular person who comes into existence as a result of that wrongful decision has been wronged, so long as the individual has a life above a decent minimum. Even though it is only existing people, not future possible people, who have an interest in existing as the particular people they are, once the child is born, he or she will be a particular person who has an interest in continuing to exist as that person. On Reiman's view, the child claims both that he personally was wronged by the procreative decision that led to his birth, and that he is glad his mother made that wrongful decision. This may not be inconsistent, but it certainly seems odd.

A third alternative is to give up the PAR and acknowledge that not all wrong acts are bad for someone. We can instead adopt a substitution principle, narrowly tailored to genesis cases:

> Individuals who face reproductive decisions are morally required not to bring into the world children who will experience serious suffering or limited opportunity or serious loss of happiness, if this outcome can be avoided, without imposing substantial burdens or costs or loss of benefits on themselves or others, by bringing into the world different individuals who will be spared these disadvantages.[151]

This principle is an impersonal principle. It is not person affecting because the failure to substitute does not harm anyone or wrong anyone, or cause anyone to be worse off than he might have been. There is no victim of a failure to substitute. And yet, in another sense, the principle is person affecting: namely, that it is based on the badness of avoidable human suffering and limited opportunity. Concern to prevent human suffering can be seen as person affecting in that, as Dan Brock notes, "suffering and limited opportunity must be experienced by some person—they cannot exist in disembodied form. . . ."[152] Jonathan Glover makes a similar point when he says that comparative impersonal principles, that is, those that compare amounts of suffering in the world, are "rooted in people and their lives, rather than derived from mere abstract rules."[153] This makes the incorporation of comparative impersonal principles into our morality more palatable than it otherwise might be.

are to judge that the woman acted wrongly, whereas if the motive for being unwilling to delay pregnancy is a serious one, we may decide that she did nothing wrong, assuming that the child has a life worth living. For example, a woman may want to become pregnant in a particular month because her husband is a soldier on home on leave. It is far from clear to me that she is morally required to forego the chance of getting pregnant while he is home to prevent the birth of a child with a mild disabling condition, given that he may be away for years, or perhaps not come home at all.

151. This is a simplification of a principle offered in Allen Buchanan, Dan Brock, Norman Daniels, and Dan Wikler. 2000. *From Chance to Choice: Genetics and Justice.* Cambridge: Cambridge University Press, p. 249.

152. Brock, "The Nonidentity Problem and Genetic Harms" (see note 142), p. 273.

153. Glover, "Future People, Disability, and Screening" (see note 124), p. 142.

From the perspective of meta-ethics, it matters whether wrongful procreative decisions are matters of rights violations or impersonal wrongs. From the perspective of normative ethics, it matters very little. What matters is that we are morally required not to bring people into existence in disadvantageous conditions, where this could have been avoided with reasonable precautions.

What are the implications for abortion? At the beginning of this section, I said that the nonidentity problem seemed to threaten the defense of abortion provided by the interest view. On the interest view, we should be concerned with the happiness or unhappiness of actual interested beings, existing now or in the future. So it is prima facie wrong to make people miserable, and equally wrong to cause them to exist, if this can be reasonably avoided, if their lives are likely to fall below a decent minimum. By contrast, not causing a child to exist is not a wrong to that child, and the happiness of the child who might have been does not have to be considered to justify either contraception or abortion.[154]

I then acknowledged that there are cases, like that of Betty, where a procreative decision is morally wrong, and it seems as if the wrongness cannot be explained in terms of harming or wronging or making an actual future person worse off. Nevertheless, we can explain the wrongness by appealing to an impersonal substitution principle. Does the acceptance of a substitution principle require us to consider the interests of possible people, and thus undercut the interest view's defense of abortion?

I do not think it does. When we say that Betty acts wrongly in bringing into existence the June baby, who will have a disability, we are not saying that this is because she owed it to the July baby to bring him into existence. Neither possible child has an interest in getting born. To think otherwise is to be susceptible to what Reiman calls the Woody Allen illusion, the idea that possible people are waiting in the wings, so to speak, to get born. There is no right on the part of possible people to come into existence, which is why it would be entirely morally acceptable for Betty to decide not to have *any* child. The normative claim is rather that *if* Betty decides to have a child, she

154. In *Abortion and the Moral Significance of Merely Possible Persons* (Dordrecht, The Netherlands: Springer, 2010), Melinda Roberts argues that it is a mistake to say that merely possible people do not count. They do matter morally, in the same way that we matter morally. But that's just to say (according to Roberts) that some of their losses, and some of ours, matter morally and some do not. According to her view, which she calls Variabilism, while the merely possible person counts, the loss to that person does not matter morally, unless that loss is incurred in a world where the person in fact comes into existence. "Incurred in a circumstance, or possible future or *world*, where a person does or will exist, a loss will have *full moral significance*. Incurred anywhere else, a loss will have *no moral significance whatsoever*, not even the littlest bit" (p. 45). Thus, Roberts accepts the asymmetry which says that the choice not to bring into the world a child who would be happy is permissible, while the choice to bring into the world a child who would be miserable is impermissible. I of course agree with this normative judgment (subject to the constraints discussed in this chapter and Chapter 4). My difficulty is first in understanding what it means to say that merely possible people suffer losses. That seems to me simply false. Even if that is accepted, I have difficulty understanding the claim that these losses have no moral significance, unless suffered in a circumstance in which the person comes into existence. How exactly does this differ from the view I hold, which is that possible people do not count? If an individual's *losses* matter morally only if that individual comes into existence, that seems to me equivalent to saying that the *individual* matters morally only if he or she comes into existence.

ought to think about the quality of that child's life. She ought, if possible, to avoid having a child who will be disadvantaged from the outset. Whether this is conceived in terms of violating the rights of a future person, or as an impersonal wrong, it does not give moral standing or rights to any possible person, and therefore it does not undercut the interest view or its defense of abortion.

Asking people to think about the lives their children will have does not imply an implausible perfectionism. I am *not* arguing that only well-educated, perfectly healthy, and materially well-off people should have children. Nor am I saying that it is wrong to have children who are less than "perfect." The morality of having children who will foreseeably be disadvantaged depends on whether the parents are able and willing to compensate for the disadvantages, to give the child a decent shot at a happy life. I doubt very much whether the average 14-year-old girl will be able to do this. On the other hand, many people are able to give children with serious disabilities the love and attention necessary to make their lives worth living. Society too has an obligation to provide the children with the medical care and educational opportunities they need. Acknowledging this is entirely consistent with recognizing a societal obligation to reduce the incidence of preventable disability.

Becoming a parent is not solely, or even primarily, a right. It is also, and primarily, an awesome responsibility. Prospective parents must think not simply of their own reproductive interests but also of the welfare of their offspring, and this means thinking about the kinds of lives their children are likely to have. At the very least, procreative responsibility means avoiding having children if they will not have minimally decent lives, and it may mean delaying procreation until one can give one's child a better start in life. While reasonable people can disagree about what a decent minimum is, at the least it requires a commitment to love and care for the child created. Finally, the morality of procreation, and the obligation to avoid procreation, is based partly on an objective assessment of the likely quality of the future child's life but also on the reasons, intentions, and attitudes of those who would have children.

On the interest view, abortion might conceivably be morally obligatory, if it were certain that the nonexistence condition would be met. As I indicated earlier, this is rarely the case. In light of the moral and psychological differences between abortion and contraception that I discussed earlier, an attempt to derive from the moral obligation to avoid conception an obligation to abort seems unwarranted. Making abortion legally mandatory could not be justified because of the woman's right to bodily integrity, which is discussed in the next section.

THE ARGUMENT FROM BODILY SELF-DETERMINATION

Thomson's Defense of Abortion

In 1971, Judith Jarvis Thomson published a genuinely novel, and now classic, defense of abortion.[155] She noted that most debates about abortion center on the moral status of the fetus: whether it is a person with a right to life. This is because people have generally thought that if we accept the premise that the fetus is a person, it follows that abortion is always wrong. The argument goes like this: All persons have a right

---

155. Thomson, "A Defense of Abortion" (see note 28).

to life. The fetus is a person, and so it has a right to life. The mother has the right to decide what happens in and to her body, but the right to life is stronger and more stringent than the mother's right to decide, and so outweighs it. So the fetus may not be killed; an abortion may not be performed.

It is this argument that Thomson wants to challenge. She argues that even if we grant the personhood of the fetus, abortion is not necessarily wrong. For it is possible that in at least some cases abortion does not violate the fetus-person's right to life. This is initially puzzling. If the fetus has a right to life, and abortion kills it, then how can abortion fail to violate its right to life? Thomson suggests that our perplexity stems from a failure to understand the nature of rights in general and the right to life in particular. In a nutshell, her argument is that having a right to life does not entitle a person to whatever he or she needs to stay alive, and in particular does not entitle him to the use of another person's body.

To illustrate this point, Thomson creates the following example:

> You wake up in the morning and find yourself back to back in bed with an unconscious violinist. He has been found to have a fatal kidney ailment, and the Society of Music Lovers has canvassed all the available medical records and found that you alone have the right blood type to help. They have therefore kidnapped you, and last night the violinist's circulatory system was plugged into yours, so that your kidneys can be used to extract poisons from his blood as well as your own.[156]

The director of the hospital, while acknowledging that it was very wrong of the Society to kidnap you, nevertheless refuses to unplug you, since to unplug you would be to kill him. Anyway, it is only for 9 months. After that, the violinist will have recovered and can be safely unplugged. Thomson questions whether it is morally incumbent on you to accede to this situation. It would be very nice of you, of course, but do you *have* to stay plugged in to the violinist? What if it were not 9 months, but 9 years? Or longer still? What if the director were to maintain that you must stay plugged in forever, on the ground that the violinist is a person, and all persons have a right to life? Thomson suggests that you would regard this argument as "outrageous" and says that this suggests that something really is wrong with the plausible-sounding right-to-life argument presented earlier.

The violinist example, fantastic though it is, preserves some of the features of the pregnancy situation without making at all doubtful the personhood of the "victim." Given that the violinist is a person, with a right to life, do you murder him, do you violate his right to life, if you unplug yourself? If not, then we have, it seems, a case of terminating the life of an innocent person that is not a case of violating his right to life.

The violinist example is intended to demonstrate Thomson's central theme: that the right to life does not necessarily include getting whatever you need to live. To take a less fanciful example, I may need your bone marrow in order to live, but that does not give me a right to it. Even if you *ought* to be willing to donate, even if your refusal is selfish and mean, it does not follow that I have a right to your bone

---

156. Ibid., pp. 48–49.

marrow or that you may legitimately be compelled to donate.[157] The right to life does not imply a right to use another person's body.

However, it may be objected that the fetus *does* have a right to use the pregnant woman's body because she is (partly) responsible for its existence. By engaging in intercourse, knowing that this may result in the creation of a person inside her body, she tacitly gives the resulting person a right to remain. This argument would not apply in the situation most closely aligned with the violinist example—pregnancy due to rape. A woman who is pregnant due to rape does not voluntarily engage in sexual intercourse, and so she cannot be said to have given the fetus even tacit permission to use her body.

On this analysis, even if abortion is ordinarily a grave wrong, it is permissible in the case of rape. Many antiabortionists wish to make such an exception, but they have been hard-pressed, on their own argument, to account for it. For antiabortionists maintain that the fetus is an innocent person. How can it be right to kill the fetus because its father is a rapist? The Thomson argument gives an answer: the fetus whose existence is caused by rape has no right to use the pregnant woman's body. Killing it does not violate its right to life.

But what about most pregnancies, which do not result from rape but from voluntary intercourse? Given that the presence of the fetus is due in part to the woman's own voluntary action, can she now eject it at the cost of its life? Thomson responds by saying that even where the woman voluntarily engages in sex, she may not be responsible for the presence of the fetus. She argues that responsibility for an outcome depends on what one has done to prevent it. She suggests that if a person has taken all reasonable precautions to prevent something from happening, then she has not been negligent and should not be held responsible for its having occurred. So whether the woman can be said to have given the fetus a right to use her body would depend on such variables as whether she was using a reliable contraceptive that happened to fail, or whether she was not using any contraception at all. Not surprisingly, defenders of the right to abortion find such an account wanting. Mary Anne Warren writes, "This is an extremely unsatisfactory outcome, from the viewpoint of the opponents of restrictive abortion laws, most of whom are convinced that a woman has a right to obtain an abortion regardless of how and why she got pregnant."[158] David Boonin agrees. He points that Thomson's response to the tacit consent objection not only makes morally impermissible for a woman to have an abortion if she was not using contraception—which is the case in a significant number of abortions—but may make it immoral even where the woman was using contraception that failed, since contraceptive devices are known to be imperfect. If this is right, then a Thomson-type approach provides at most a defense of abortion

---

157. The claim that individuals do not have a legal obligation to donate body parts to others, even when they are needed for life itself, has been upheld in several cases. The first recorded case, to my knowledge, is *Shimp v. McFall*, 10 Pa. D. & C.3d 90, 1978 WL 255, Pa. Com. Pl., July 26, 1978 (No. GD78-17711), which I discuss in Chapter 4.

158. Warren, "On the Moral and Legal Status of Abortion" (see note 53), p. 50.

in the case of rape.[159] Ironically, this means that Thomson's argument is most useful, not for defenders of the right to abortion, but for critics of abortion who would like to make an exception in the case of rape, something that has seemed impossible to do if one grants that the fetus is an innocent human being with a right to life.

Some critics of Thomson have taken her to task for concentrating exclusively on rights. The real question, they say, is not what constitutes giving the unborn person a right to use one's body, but rather the conditions that make aborting the fetus morally permissible. Thomson responds by saying that since her intention was to examine the right-to-life argument, she can hardly be faulted for concentrating on rights. However, she acknowledges that we can have moral obligations to help people, even when they do not have rights against us. Suppose that the violinist needed your kidneys only for an hour, and that this would not affect your health at all. Even though you were kidnapped, even though you never gave anyone permission to plug him into you, still you ought to let him stay: "it would be indecent to refuse."[160] Similarly, if pregnancy lasted only an hour, and posed no threat to life or health, the pregnant woman ought to allow the fetus-person to remain for that hour. She ought to do this even if the pregnancy was due to rape, and the fetus has no right to use her body. This conclusion is based on the principle (which Thomson calls "minimally decent Samaritanism") that if you can save a person's life without much trouble or risk to yourself, you ought to do it. In the real world, however, pregnancies do not last for only an hour, and they do involve considerable sacrifices.[161] Thomson concludes, "Except in such cases as the unborn person has a right to demand it—and we were leaving open the possibility that there may be such cases—nobody is morally *required* to make large sacrifices, of health, of all other interests and concerns, of all other duties and commitments, for nine years, or even for nine months, in order to keep another person alive."[162]

As indicated earlier, Thomson's analysis has been criticized by those who take a pro-choice stance as justifying abortion only in a relatively narrow range of cases. Many unwanted pregnancies occur because contraception was not used at all, or only occasionally. In such cases, the woman has not act responsibly or reasonably. She *is* (partly) to blame for the pregnancy, and so the resulting fetus may be said to have been given the right to use her body. If so, then abortion violates its right to life, and thus it is impermissible. It appears that a defense of abortion cannot be based solely on the woman's moral right to decide what happens in and to her body, because this yields a defense of abortion in a relatively narrow range of cases—namely, those in which the woman is absolved of responsibility for the presence of the unborn.

---

159. Boonin, *A Defense of Abortion* (see note 112), pp. 150–151. Boonin thinks that a better response to the tacit consent objection is available, one that turns on the distinction between a state of affairs one brings about voluntarily, and a state of affairs which foreseeably arises from one's voluntary action. See pp. 148–167.

160. Thomson, "A Defense of Abortion" (see note 28), p. 60.

161. The burdens of pregnancy are well detailed by Donald Regan, "Rewriting *Roe v. Wade*," *Michigan Law Review* 77 (1979): 1569–1646.

162. Thomson, "A Defense of Abortion" (see note 28), p. 61.

Even if Thomson ultimately fails to provide a general defense of abortion, the philosophical importance of her article remains. For that lies in her critique of the right-to-life argument, and her demonstration that a right to life is not necessarily a right to whatever one needs to stay alive. A full-fledged defense of abortion is not necessary for that purpose. All she needs to show is that, even if we concede that the fetus is a person, with a right to life, there are at least some cases in which abortion is not unjust killing, and so is not murder.

Despite David Boonin's valiant attempt to shore up Thomson's Good Samaritan argument,[163] it seems to me that the strongest argument in favor of a liberal abortion policy must rest on both the woman's right to bodily self-determination and the claim that the fetus lacks full moral and legal standing. This was the approach taken by the U.S. Supreme Court in *Roe v. Wade*.

Roe v. Wade

The legalization of abortion in *Roe v. Wade* was based on two factors: the woman's right to privacy and the status of the unborn. First, the Supreme Court held that the unborn have never been recognized in the law as persons in the whole sense: "In areas other than criminal abortion, the law has been reluctant to endorse any theory that life, as we recognize it, begins before live birth or to accord legal rights to the unborn except in narrowly defined situations and except when the rights are *contingent upon live birth*."[164] Because the unborn is not a person within the language and meaning of the Fourteenth Amendment, it therefore does not have the right to life specifically guaranteed by that Amendment. So states are not permitted to prohibit abortion to protect the fetus's right to life. On the other side, the woman's constitutional right of privacy entitles her to make this most personal of decisions, without state intervention, at least throughout the first two trimesters. At the same time, the Court recognized legitimate state interests in protecting maternal health, in maintaining medical standards, and in protecting potential human life. "At some point in pregnancy, these respective interests become sufficiently compelling to sustain regulation of the factors that govern the abortion decision. The privacy right involved, therefore, cannot be said to be absolute."[165]

In the second trimester, states may regulate the abortion procedure in ways that are reasonably related to maternal health but may not forbid abortion. This changes after the fetus becomes viable, or capable of surviving outside the womb, albeit with artificial aid, sometime around the 28th week of gestation, possibly as early as the 24th week. "If the State is interested in protecting fetal life after viability, it may go so far as to proscribe abortion during that period, except when it is necessary to preserve the life or health of the mother."[166]

163. Boonin, *A Defense of Abortion* (see note 112), especially Chapter 4, "The Good Samaritan Argument."

164. *Roe v. Wade* (see note 1), p. 161.

165. Ibid., p. 154.

166. Ibid., pp. 163–164.

Since it was announced, *Roe v. Wade* has been controversial. Some critics (such as Judge Robert Bork, the unsuccessful candidate for the Supreme Court in 1987) object to the "creation" of a right of privacy nowhere mentioned in the Constitution. Others, who accept a constitutional right of privacy, deny that the Constitution protects a woman's right to abort. They maintain that the right to abortion is "judge-made" and one upon which the Constitution is silent. An adequate discussion of these claims would take us far afield into the topic of constitutional interpretation and judicial decision making.[167] I will simply say that I agree with those who maintain that the right of privacy is a fundamental right and a central American value that is implicit in the concept of ordered liberty.[168] Moreover, as Justice Brennan said in *Eisenstadt v. Baird*, "if the right to privacy means anything, it is the right of the individual, married or single, to be free from unwarranted governmental intrusion into matters so fundamentally affecting a person as the decision whether to bear or beget a child."[169]

Not all of *Roe*'s critics oppose the right to abortion. Rather, they think that the constitutional analysis in *Roe* is shaky. For example, Donald Regan claims that the right to abortion would have been given a sounder footing if it had been based on the right to "equal protection" instead of a right to privacy.[170] Regan uses Thomson's "Defense of Abortion" to make an equal protection argument that says that it is unfair to require pregnant women to become "Good Samaritans" when similar burdens are not imposed on other members of society. This provides an argument against restrictive abortion laws that does not depend on a right to privacy nowhere mentioned in the Constitution.

The problem with basing the right to abortion solely on an "equal-protection" basis is that it implies that restrictive abortion laws are unconstitutional only if comparable burdens are not imposed on other members of society. Some have argued that restrictive abortion laws do not pose unique burdens on women: the law can impose comparable or greater burdens on men, for example, a military draft in time of war. Others think that all citizens *should* be legally required to undergo burdens or make sacrifices to save lives. They support Good Samaritan statutes that, if enacted, would undercut an equal-protection basis for the right to abortion. Moreover, basing the right to abortion solely on "equal protection" completely leaves out the element of governmental intrusion into one of the most private, most personal decisions a woman may ever face. In my view, such intrusion by the state is unjustified even if the pregnancy is relatively trouble-free and even if others in society are legally required to be Good Samaritans.

It is not necessary to choose between the argument from privacy and the equal-protection argument. They can be used together to support a constitutional right to abortion. Indeed, it seems to me that this is implicit in the approach taken by Justice

167. See, for example, Ronald Dworkin, "The Great Abortion Case," *New York Review of Books* 36 (11), June 29, 1989, pp. 49–52.

168. See, for example, George J. Annas, Leonard H. Glantz, and Wendy K. Mariner, "Brief For Bioethicists For Privacy as *Amicus Curiae* Supporting Appellees," *American Journal of Law and Medicine* 15(2–3), 1989: 169–177.

169. *Eisenstadt v. Baird.* 405 U.S. 438, 453 (1972).

170. Regan, "Rewriting *Roe v. Wade*" (see note 160).

Blackmun in *Roe v. Wade*. For while Blackmun explicitly mentions only the right to privacy, he elaborates the physical and psychological harms that the state would impose upon the pregnant woman by denying the choice of abortion as part of his defense of the claim that there exists a right of privacy "broad enough to encompass a woman's decision whether or not to terminate her pregnancy."[171]

At this writing, *Roe* is still the law of the land, despite numerous attempts by state legislatures to restrict the right to abortion. An important post-*Roe* case was *Planned Parenthood of Southeastern Pennsylvania v. Casey*.[172] Five abortion clinics and a physician challenged as unconstitutional several provisions of Pennsylvania's Abortion Control Act of 1982, including an "informed consent" provision that required doctors to provide women with information about the health risks and possible complications of having an abortion, a 24-hour waiting period, the consent of at least one parent before abortion is performed on a minor (although with a judicial bypass procedure), and spousal notification. Pennsylvania defended the Act by urging the Court to overturn *Roe v. Wade* as wrongly decided, and many people thought that the Supreme Court would use *Casey* to overturn *Roe*. This seemed especially likely because of the composition of the court. Two liberal justices, William Brennan and Thurgood Marshall, had been replaced by David Souter and Clarence Thomas, both appointed by President George H. W. Bush. All but one of the justices in 1992 were Republican appointees, and the only Democratic appointee, Byron White, was one of two dissenters in *Roe v. Wade*.[173] However, to the surprise of many, Justice Souter joined Justices Sandra Day O'Connor, John P. Stevens, and Harry Blackmun. *Roe* was still in danger of being overturned, as it would have left a five-justice majority in favor of upholding the abortion restrictions, composed of Chief Justice William Rehnquist, Byron White, Antonin Scalia, Anthony Kennedy, and Clarence Thomas. However, although Justice Kennedy voted at the justices' conference to uphold Pennsylvania's law, he changed his mind and cast a fifth vote to reaffirm *Roe v. Wade*.[174] Writing for the majority, Justice O'Connor said, "After considering the fundamental constitutional questions resolved by *Roe*, principles of institutional integrity, and the rule of *stare decisis*, we are led to conclude this: the essential holding of *Roe v. Wade* should be retained and once again reaffirmed."[175] Although the justices recognized that the fate of the fetus is of great personal concern to many Americans, they said that decisions about abortion nevertheless deserve special constitutional protection because such decisions involve "the most intimate and personal choices a person may make in a lifetime."[176]

171. *Roe v. Wade* (see note 1), p. 153.

172. *Planned Parenthood of Southeastern Pennsylvania v. Casey*, 505 U.S. 833, 112 S. Ct. 2791, 1992.

173. Wikipedia, http://en.wikipedia.org/wiki/Planned_Parenthood_v._Casey. Accessed July 5, 2010.

174. Charles Lane, "All Eyes on Kennedy in Court Debate on Abortion," *Washington Post*, November 8, 2006. http://www.washingtonpost.com/wp-dyn/content/article/2006/11/07/AR2006110701333_pf.html. Accessed July 5, 2010.

175. *Casey* (see note 171), p. 833.

176. Ibid., p. 851.

The major difference between *Roe* and *Casey* is that *Casey* substituted the "undue burdens" doctrine for *Roe*'s trimester analysis, which the plurality said was not an essential part of *Roe*. The "undue burdens" test says that a state regulation of abortion is unconstitutional if either its purpose or its effect is to create an "undue burden" on a woman who chooses abortion prior to viability. The plurality acknowledged that the state has legitimate interests from the outset of pregnancy in protecting the woman's health and the life of the fetus. It cannot put substantial obstacles in the way of a woman seeking an abortion, prior to viability, but it can take steps to ensure that her decision is thoughtful and informed, because ". . . there is a substantial state interest in potential life throughout pregnancy."[177] That interest justifies "rules and regulations designed to encourage her to know that there are philosophic and social arguments of great weight that can be brought to bear in favor of continuing the pregnancy to full term"[178] and information about the alternative of adoption. The informed consent provision, the waiting period of 24 hours (a requirement that excludes medical emergencies), and consent from one of the parents of a minor (with a judicial bypass option) were all upheld as consistent with *Roe*'s central premises. The husband notification requirement was struck down on the ground that some women might be battered or otherwise intimidated, and thus prevented from exercising their choice of abortion.

Casey agreed with *Roe v. Wade* that viability is the correct cutoff point after which states may, if they choose, prohibit abortion. This raises the following question: why viability?

THE MORAL AND LEGAL SIGNIFICANCE OF VIABILITY

The *Roe* court offered the following as justification: "With respect to the State's important and legitimate interest in potential life, the 'compelling' point is at viability. This is so because the fetus then presumably has the capability of meaningful life outside the mother's womb. State regulation protective of fetal life after viability thus has both logical and biological justifications."[179] *Casey* reiterated the justification of viability given in Roe, supporting it largely on grounds of *stare decisis*.

A number of commentators have pointed out that *Roe*'s justification of viability is no justification at all. The capacity for independent life does not *explain* the significance of viability; it merely gives the meaning of viability. As John Hart Ely has argued, ". . . the Court's defense seems to mistake a definition for a syllogism . . ."[180] In fact, it could be maintained that viability's logical significance is the opposite of

177. Ibid., p. 876.

178. Ibid., p. 872.

179. *Roe v. Wade* (see note 1), p. 163.

180. John Hart Ely. 1973. "The Wages of Crying Wolf: A Comment on *Roe v. Wade*," *Yale Law Journal* 82: 920–949, p. 924.

what the Court implied: "Why should a fetus' capacity to live independently be a reason to forbid the mother from forcing it to live independently?"[181]

At the time *Roe* was decided, viability was usually placed at about 7 months (28 weeks g.a.), although the Court acknowledged that it might occur earlier, even at 24 weeks. While the point of viability may be somewhat earlier than the one cited in *Roe v. Wade*, medical science appears to have reached a biological limit in its ability to save premature infants. If a baby is born before 23 or 24 weeks of pregnancy, it simply cannot survive, because its lungs are too immature to function, even with the help of respirators. While rates of survival between 23 and 25 weeks of gestation have improved significantly since the 1980s,[182] rates of survival before 23 weeks remain very low. There have been reports of fetuses surviving at 22 or even 21 weeks, although these are difficult to confirm, because of doubts about gestational age. In any event, such events are truly rare. In 1986, Nancy Rhoden wrote, "Many experts believe that because of the extreme immaturity of a fetus of less than about 23 weeks, 22 or 23 weeks represents an absolute lower limit on fetal viability absent development of an artificial placenta."[183] This remains the case today for virtually all fetuses.

What if an artificial placenta were invented? Viability might then be pushed back into the first trimester. Would that give it the moral and legal significance assigned to it by the Court in *Roe v. Wade*? Nancy Rhoden presents a compelling argument that it would not. She suggests that the reason the Supreme Court focused on viability as the point at which states might prohibit abortion is that, in 1973, the capacity for independent existence *coincided with* late gestation. The Court did not realize the possibility of divergence between viability and late gestation because "in 1973 it was virtually inconceivable that a viable fetus would be anything other than one that was substantially developed and had survived to the last stage of pregnancy."[184] Rhoden argues that where ex utero survivability is divorced from late gestation, survivability no longer has moral significance.

Rhoden distinguishes between viability as simple technological survivability (which she calls "Viability$_1$") and viability as a normative concept ("Viability$_2$"). She says, "Viability as a normative concept thus has at least two major components. It is not merely technological, but rather encompasses the idea that the fetus is so substantially developed that it has a claim to societal protection."[90] Rhoden argues that Viability$_2$—"the complex, value-laden notion that once a fetus can survive ex utero and is substantially developed, its claim to societal protection increases"—is a necessary, although unarticulated, component of the *Roe* viability standard. She recommends that the *Roe* decision be revamped, and that legal protection be

181. Norman Fost, David Chudwin, and Daniel Wikler. 1980. "The Limited Moral Significance of 'Fetal Viability,'" *Hastings Center Report* 10 (6): 10–13, pp. 12–13.

182. H. Emsley, S. Wardle, D. Sims, M. Chiswick, and S. D'Souza. 1998. "Increased Survival and Deteriorating Developmental Outcome in 23 to 25 Week Old Gestation Infants, 1990-4 Compared with 1984-9," *Archives of Diseases in Childhood: Fetal and Neonatal* 78 (2): F99–F104. http://www.ncbi.nlm.nih.gov/pmc/articles/PMC1720768/. Accessed July 5, 2010.

183. Nancy K. Rhoden. 1986. "Trimesters and Technology: Revamping *Roe v. Wade*," *Yale Law Journal* 95 (4): 639–697, p. 661.

184. Ibid., p. 658.

extended to the *late-gestation*, rather than technologically viable, fetus. She acknowledges that "late gestation" is a fuzzy concept, but she believes it certainly does not occur before the midpoint of pregnancy (week 20). She believes that the point at which states can prohibit elective abortions "should remain approximately what it is today, and in no event should it creep earlier than the week 21–24 range."[185]

Rhoden's analysis is supported by the interest view, which explains more fully the significance of late gestation. It is only after the fetus has a fairly developed nervous system that it becomes conscious and sentient. The most important similarity between the newborn and the late-gestation fetus is sentience, because of the conceptual connection between sentience and interests. As we have seen, some researchers think the onset of sentience might be as early as 17 weeks. Should the bare possibility of fetal sentience justify banning abortion altogether at this stage?

I do not think we need to take this position, for three reasons. First, the claim is not that fetuses are sentient at 17 weeks, only that it is not possible to rule this out. Second, even if there is some level of awareness, the fetus's time-relative interest in staying alive is extraordinarily weak. Third, the fetus is inside a pregnant woman. These factors give strong reasons not to extend *equal* protection to even fully developed fetuses. The question, therefore, is not simply whether the fetus counts, but how much of a stake it has in its continued existence, as well as how much the state can require of the pregnant woman. This raises the question of the justification for time limits on abortion.

Late Abortions

As discussed in the beginning of this chapter, postviability abortions are extremely rare. In 2006, 62% of abortions took place in the first 8 weeks of pregnancy, with an increasing number occurring earlier than 6 weeks; only 1.3% of abortions occur after 21 weeks. One reason for late abortions is the age of the woman; late abortions are had disproportionately by teenagers. Adolescents obtain approximately 25% of all abortions performed after the first trimester.[186] "The very youngest women—those under age 15—are more likely than others to obtain abortions at 21 or more weeks gestation."[187] Adolescents tend to find out that they are pregnant later than older women, often because their periods are irregular, or because they are in denial about their pregnancies. They often face greater difficulties in obtaining the procedure, either because of the cost (between $350 and $900 for a first-trimester abortion; a late second-trimester abortion can cost up to $3,000) or the relative dearth of abortion providers. (This is not solely a problem for adolescents, but generally for women, especially those who are financially disadvantaged.) "Eighty-seven percent of all U.S. counties lacked an abortion provider in 2005; 35% of women

185. Ibid., p. 684.

186. Planned Parenthood. 2007. "Abortion After the First Trimester," http://www.plannedparenthoodnj.org/library/topic/abortion_access/after_first_trimester. Accessed July 6, 2010.

187. Ibid., citing CDC, "Abortion Surveillance–2006," http://www.cdc.gov/mmwr/preview/mmwrhtml/ss5808a1.htm?s_cid=ss5808a1_e. Accessed July 8, 2010.

live in those counties."[188] Teenagers, however, face special difficulties in obtaining abortions. They often delay telling their parents, out of fear of their reaction, which also may delay the abortion decision. In states with parental involvement laws, minors might need more time to receive court approval or to make plans to travel to another state. "Adolescents approaching age 18 years also have been reported to wait until they are old enough to obtain an abortion without parental involvement."[189]

A second reason for late abortions is the development of health problems in the woman. These include certain types of infections, heart failure, malignant hypertension, including preeclampsia, out-of-control diabetes, serious renal disease, and severe depression. These symptoms may not appear until the second trimester, or they may become worse as the pregnancy advances.[190] A third reason is detection of fetal anomalies. Amniocentesis is usually done between the 15th to 18th week of pregnancy. It may take 2 or 3 weeks to get the results back from the laboratory. Thus, fetal diagnosis of chromosomal, biochemical, or DNA abnormalities can rarely be established prior to 18 weeks, and possibly later. In addition, if gestation is miscalculated, the fetus may be 20 weeks old.

Thirty-eight states prohibit abortion, except when necessary to protect the woman's life or health, after a specified point in pregnancy, most often fetal viability, although some prohibit abortions after 24 weeks and a few in the third trimester.[191] In *Doe v. Bolton*,[192] the companion case to *Roe*, the Court made clear that the health exception is a matter of physician discretion and must be interpreted broadly to include all the physical, emotional, psychological, and familial factors that contribute to the woman's well-being. No explicit mention of fetal deformity was made, although two states—Maryland and Utah—permit postviability abortions for this reason. In some states, an exception for fetal abnormality is interpreted as coming under the health exception. In others, late-term abortions are permitted only if there is a threat to the woman's life or health, narrowly interpreted. Although this conflicts with the Supreme Court's decisions in *Roe* and *Bolton*, such laws remain on the books. In many places, it is difficult, if not impossible, for women to obtain late-term abortions.

Nan Hunter, of the American Civil Liberties Union, argues that there should be no time limits on abortion. If the state does not have the right to impose the burdens of pregnancy on women during early gestation, why does it acquire that right later on in pregnancy? Hunter says, "The burden to a woman of continuing a pregnancy

188. Guttmacher Institute. 2010. "Facts on Induced Abortion in the United States." http://www.guttmacher.org/pubs/fb_induced_abortion.html. Accessed July 6, 2010. Citing R. K. Jones et al. 2008, "Abortion in the United States: Incidence and Access to Services, 2005," *Perspectives on Sexual and Reproductive Health* 40 (1): 6–16.

189. CDC, "Abortion Surveillance–2006" (see note 186).

190. Planned Parenthood, "Abortion After the First Trimester" (see note 185).

191. Guttmacher Institute. 2010. "State Policies on Later-Term Abortions," http://www.guttmacher.org/statecenter/spibs/spib_PLTA.pdf. Accessed October 29, 2010.

192. *Doe v. Bolton*, 410 U.S. 179 (1973).

against her will is stupefying."[193] Instead of imposing time limits on abortion, society should adopt measures that will reduce the number of late abortions, such as contraceptive education and services, restoring Medicaid funding for abortions, and repeal of parental-consent laws.

When I wrote the first edition of this book, I disagreed with Hunter, saying ". . . it does not seem unfair for society to require women to decide within a reasonable period of time whether or not they will continue the pregnancy. Twenty-four weeks should ordinarily be enough time for a woman to learn that she is pregnant and to gain access to the health-care system. . . . Imposing a time limit acknowledges the claims of the late-gestation fetus to social protection, while also recognizing the right of the woman to decide not to become a mother." A similar view was taken by the plurality in *Casey:* "The viability line also has, as a practical matter, an element of fairness. In some broad sense it might be said that a woman who fails to act before viability has consented to the State's intervention on behalf of the developing child."[194]

However, this suggests that the woman could have chosen to abort earlier in pregnancy, but simply chose not to do so. Such cases are possible, though unlikely. Imagine a mature woman who discovers she is pregnant at 6 weeks but keeps delaying the abortion decision until finally she makes up her mind and has an abortion at 24 weeks. Such dithering fails to give any consideration to the now sentient fetus, for no good reason, and is therefore irresponsible and immoral. I would not make it illegal, because I do not see how the state could determine the reason for the delay.

In any event, this does not reflect the reality of late-term abortions. Women do not have late abortions because they cannot or will not make up their minds. If a late-term abortion is chosen because of a health condition which developed or became manifest late in the pregnancy, the woman could not have chosen an earlier abortion. If the pregnant woman is a young teen, who is either ignorant about the signs of pregnancy, or in denial, the issue of choice also does not arise. Since late-term abortions are far more expensive than early abortions, but also riskier for the woman, delays are often not a matter of choice, but rather a matter of finding the money.

> The difficulties that low-income women face when making arrangements underscore the importance of financial support for such women when they seek abortion. Yet, under the Hyde Amendment, which was enacted in 1977, the use of federal funding is prohibited for most abortions, and only 17 states use state funds to cover all or most medically necessary abortions (only four do so voluntarily, while the other 13 do so pursuant to a court order). . . . Our findings suggest that gestational age at abortion in the United States could be further reduced if financial barriers faced by disadvantaged groups were removed

193. Nan Hunter. 1989. "Time Limits on Abortion," in Sherrill Cohen and Nadine Taub, eds., *Reproductive Laws for the 1990s.* Clifton, NJ: Humana Press, p. 147.

194. *Casey* (see note 171), p. 870.

and if women, especially young women, were better educated about how to recognize pregnancy.[195]

Social policy that aims at removing these barriers seems fairer and more humane than punishing women for not being able to surmount them. In addition, the situations that lead to late abortions are often heart-wrenching. One patient recounts her story of learning late in pregnancy that her fetus had a condition, posterior urethral valves, that would entail a brief life of respirators, dialysis, surgeries, and pain. She writes:

> When we arrived at the Women's Health Center, we immediately felt the compassion and understanding from the entire staff. We had a story, and they listened. The doctor instantly connected with us and assured us that although our decision was a difficult one, he knew how sick our son was and that the choice we made was because we love him so much and couldn't bear to put him through a short life full of pain and suffering.[196]

This sort of painful and personal decision is one that should be made by the prospective parents and their doctor. The guiding principle should be the motto Dr. Tiller put on buttons he had created for members of his staff: "Trust women."

Partial-Birth Abortion

The latest strategy in the anti-abortion movement has been to focus on a particular method of abortion, used in second- and third-trimester abortions, called "partial-birth abortion" by its opponents. In 2000, the Supreme Court struck down Nebraska's law prohibiting partial-birth abortion in *Stenberg v. Carhart,*[197] where this was defined as partially delivering vaginally a living unborn child for the purpose of killing it. Justice Stephen Breyer wrote that the statute was unconstitutional for two reasons: one, because it lacked an exception to preserve the health of the mother and two, by depriving a woman of a method of abortion deemed safer for her, it unduly burdened her right to choose abortion. Justice Sandra Day O'Connor was the swing vote in a 5-4 decision.

A Republican-dominated Congress then passed essentially the same law, known as the "Partial-Birth Abortion Ban Act" in 2003, which was signed into law by President George W. Bush. The law was challenged by four physicians and was held unconstitutional by a series of federal courts. *Gonzales v. Carhart*[198] reached the Supreme Court in 2006 and was decided April 18, 2007. By that time, Sandra Day O'Connor had been replaced by the Bush-appointed Samuel Alito. In another

195. L. B. Finer, L. F. Frohwirth, L. A. Dauphinee, S. Singh, and A. M. Moore. 2006. "Timing of Steps and Reasons for Delays in Obtaining Abortions in the United States," *Contraception* 74 (4): 334–344, at 344.

196. http://www.aheartbreakingchoice.com/kansasdelays.html. Accessed July 7, 2010.

197. *Stenberg v. Carhart,* 530 U.S. 914, 120 S. Ct. 2597 (2000).

198. *Gonzales v. Carhart,* 550 U.S. 124, 127 S. Ct. 1610 (2007).

5-4 decision, the Court reversed its decision in *Stenberg* and declared the Partial-Birth Abortion Ban Act to be constitutional.

Many Americans, even those who are generally pro-choice, support a ban on so-called partial-birth abortions. However, this support seems to derive from ignorance about what the law entails. Much of the support comes from revulsion at the idea of aborting a late-gestation fetus—a nearly born baby. However, as we saw earlier, *Roe v. Wade* already gave states the right to prohibit postviability abortions; no "partial-birth abortion" ban was necessary for that purpose. Another source of support for the law derives from the thought that it is a "particularly gruesome," as well as medically unnecessary, method.[199] To understand why this objection makes no sense, it is necessary to understand abortion options after the first trimester.

In the first trimester, almost all abortions are performed through suction curettage in which the cervix is dilated, and a suction device removes the contents of the uterus.[200] After 12 weeks, that method is no longer feasible and doctors use a procedure known as dilation and evacuation (D&E). Here is a description of this procedure:

> In the usual second-trimester procedure, "dilation and evacuation" (D&E), the doctor dilates the cervix and then inserts surgical instruments into the uterus and maneuvers them to grab the fetus and pull it back through the cervix and vagina. The fetus is usually ripped apart as it is removed, and the doctor may take 10 to 15 passes to remove it in its entirety.[201]

Abortion by D&E was left untouched by the Partial-Birth Abortion Ban Act. The method banned by the Act is a variation on D&E known as "intact dilation and evacuation" (or sometimes D&X—dilation and extraction). "The main difference between the two procedures is that in intact D&E a doctor extracts the fetus intact or largely intact with only a few passes, pulling out its entire body instead of ripping it apart. In order to allow the head to pass through the cervix, the doctor typically pierces or crushes the skull."[202]

While intact D&E is certainly gruesome, it is hard to see why it is more gruesome than ripping the fetus apart before removing it. Responding to this objection, Justice Kennedy wrote, "The objection that the Act accomplishes little because the standard D&E is in some respects as brutal, if not more, than intact D&E, is unpersuasive. It was reasonable for Congress to think that partial-birth abortion, more than standard D&E, undermines the public's perception of the doctor's appropriate role during delivery, and perverts the birth process."[203] Justice Kennedy gave no reason why

---

199. This is how Senator Orrin Hatch characterized the procedure in his questioning of Supreme Court nominee Elena Kagan. See Jane McGrath, "Kagan Rejects Suggestions by GOP Senators She Authored Language in Key ACOG Statement on Partial-Birth Abortion," CNSNews.com (July 7, 2010), http://www.cnsnews.com/news/article/69037. Accessed July 7, 2010.

200. American College of Obstetricians and Gynecologists (ACOG), 2008. "Induced Abortion," http://www.acog.org/publications/patient_education/bp043.cfm. Accessed October 29, 2010.

201. *Gonzales* (see note 197), p. 1614.

202. Ibid.

203. Ibid., at 1617.

he found this judgment to be reasonable. The truth is that any method of killing and removing from the uterus a fully formed fetus will be unpleasant. Whether the method is correctly characterized as brutal and inhumane depends on whether it inflicts pain; it has nothing to do with whether the fetus is removed in one piece or dismembered. Moreover, as we saw earlier, the concern about fetal pain in abortions after mid-gestation can be addressed through the use of fetal anesthesia, if this is safe for the woman. In terms of gruesomeness, the distinction between the two procedures is nonexistent, and therefore it is absurd to assume that intact D&E would, but D&E would not, undermine the public's perception of the doctor's role, perverting the birth process. Another basis for differentiating between the two procedures is that intact D&E involves removing the body of the fetus, while still alive, from the woman's body. This, it is alleged, is similar to the killing of a newborn infant.[204] However, in both methods, the fetus is killed before being removed from the woman's body. Partly removing the body of the fetus prior to killing it does not make intact D&E infanticide or akin to infanticide.

Why did the Partial-Birth Abortion Ban Act not include an exception for the woman's health, in clear contravention of *Roe v. Wade*? The reason, according to Congress, is that such an exception is unnecessary since intact D&E is never medically necessary. This was not the view of the American College of Obstetricians and Gynecologists, according to its amicus brief in *Stenberg*:

> Depending on the physician's skill and experience, the D&X procedure can be the most appropriate abortion procedure for some women in some circumstances. D&X presents a variety of potential safety advantages over other abortion procedures used during the same gestational period. Compared to D&Es involving dismemberment, D&X involves less risk of uterine perforation or cervical laceration because it requires the physician to make fewer passes into the uterus with sharp instruments and reduces the presence of sharp fetal bone fragments that can injure the uterus and cervix. There is also considerable evidence that D&X reduces the risk of retained fetal tissue, a serious abortion complication that can cause maternal death, and that D&X reduces the incidence of a "free floating" fetal head that can be difficult for a physician to grasp and remove and can thus cause maternal injury. That D&X procedures usually take less time than other abortion methods used at a comparable stage of pregnancy can also have health advantages. The shorter the procedure, the less blood loss, trauma, and exposure to anesthesia. The intuitive safety advantages of intact D&E are supported by clinical experience. Especially for women with particular health conditions, there is medical evidence that D&X may be safer than available alternatives.[205]

In striking down the Act as unconstitutional, Justice Breyer held that an abortion regulation must contain a health exception if "substantial medical authority supports the proposition that banning a particular procedure could endanger

204. Ibid.

205. *Stenberg v. Carhart*, 2000 WL 340117 (U.S.) (Appellate Brief), pp. 21–22.

women's health."[206] Justice Kennedy rejected this standard as too exacting, saying, "Marginal safety considerations, including the balance of risks, are within the legislative competence where, as here, the regulation is rational and pursues legitimate ends, and standard, safe medical options are available."[207] In a commentary on the case,[208] Ronald Dworkin notes that Justice Kennedy conceded that there might be situations in which the standard procedure did pose a real danger to a woman's health, and he said that the courts could then reexamine whether the statute was constitutional as applied to her. Dworkin writes, "But as Justice Ruth Ginsburg pointed out in her powerful dissenting opinion, women cannot wait for the result of lengthy litigation when they need an abortion, and few doctors will act on their own judgment of a demonstrable health risk when they know they face jail if a court later disagrees."[209] Kennedy's ruling would have been wrong, even if Congress had discovered impressive medical opinion on its side, Dworkin says. "Forcing a woman either to abandon abortion or to accept a procedure that distinguished medical opinion, as well as her own doctor, regards as unsafe is obviously a serious burden on her right to choose, even if other doctors disagree."[210] Even more basically, Dworkin asks, "What business does Congress or a state have in choosing among methods of abortion at all?"[211] If anything is a medical matter, surely that is. If a woman has a right to an abortion, she ought to be able to rely on her physician to choose the safest method for her. Moreover, as Dworkin points out, the state's interest in protecting fetal life, enunciated in *Casey*, is not served by a ban on a particular method of abortion. Full compliance with the Act "would not save a single fetal life, since in each case doctors could use the standard D&E method."[212]

Although abortion has occupied center stage in the debate over "fetal rights," it is only one area where the status of the fetus is an issue. Other issues include whether there can be civil or criminal liability for killing a fetus, whether fetuses are included in family insurance policies, and whether severely impaired children whose existence is the result of a physician's negligence can recover in a civil suit for "wrongful life." These and other questions are addressed in the next chapter, where I consider the legal status of the unborn beyond abortion.

206. *Stenberg* (see note 196), at 938.

207. *Gonzales* (see note 197), at 130.

208. Ronald Dworkin, 2007. "The Court and Abortion: Worse Than You Think," *New York Review of Books* 54 (9): 20–21.

209. Ibid., p. 20, footnote 3.

210. Ibid., p. 21.

211. Ibid.

212. Ibid.

3

Beyond Abortion

The Fetus in Tort and Criminal Law

As we saw in the last chapter, the U.S. Supreme Court's recognition of the right to abortion was based, in part, on the recognition that the unborn have never been recognized in the law as persons in the whole sense. Traditionally the law has been reluctant to accord legal rights to the unborn "except in narrowly defined situations and except when the rights are contingent upon live birth."[1] This reluctance to recognize the unborn as a person (outside criminal abortion statutes) meant that at common law a fetus, viable or otherwise, could not be the subject of homicide. When the first edition of this book appeared in 1992, most states continued to follow the common law. Today, however, at least 38 states have fetal homicide laws,[2] which allow for additional punishment of someone whose attack on a pregnant woman results in the death of her viable fetus. The issue of the legal status of the unborn occurs in other areas of the law, including prenatal and preconception torts, prenatal wrongful death, and wrongful life suits. Physicians and others who negligently inflict injury on a fetus may be successfully sued. In most states, there can be recovery in a wrongful-death action for the loss of a viable fetus. Since the wrongful-death acts of most states allow recovery only for the death of a "person," this suggests that a viable fetus is a person for purposes of recovery in wrongful-death suits. Some argue that this demonstrates an inconsistent attitude toward the fetus, treating it as a person in some legal contexts, but not others. Some find these discrepancies intellectually dissatisfying; others worry about the political fallout of fetal protection laws. Such laws, it is argued, are intended to subvert the right to abortion and should be opposed on that ground.

1. *Roe v. Wade*, 410 U.S. 113, 161 (1973).

2. National Conference of State Legislatures (NCSL) 2010. "Fetal Homicide Laws." http://www.ncsl.org/default.aspx?tabid=14386. Accessed April 15, 2010. States with fetal homicide statutes include Alabama, Alaska, Arizona, Arkansas, California, Colorado, Florida, Georgia, Idaho, Illinois, Indiana, Iowa, Kansas, Kentucky, Louisiana, Maine, Maryland, Massachusetts, Michigan, Minnesota, Mississippi, Nebraska, Nevada, North Carolina, North Dakota, Ohio, Oklahoma, Pennsylvania, Rhode Island, South Carolina, South Dakota, Tennessee, Texas, Utah, Virginia, Washington, West Virginia, and Wisconsin.

I maintain that a more nuanced approach, based on the interest view, can help to resolve apparent contradictions and avoid a purely ad hoc approach to the legal status of the unborn. The interest view denies moral and legal status to the early-gestation fetus, providing part of the justification for legal abortion. However, acceptance of the interest view does not preclude prenatal torts, that is, civil suits brought against physicians whose negligence causes children to be born with serious injuries. Although the harm is inflicted prenatally, when the child is a fetus, it is not the fetus, but the surviving child, who is affected and wronged by the negligence. Allowing surviving children to recover for injuries inflicted prior to birth in no way implies that preconscious fetuses have interests, rights, or moral or legal status. There is no contradiction in a legal system that both allows for abortion and allows recovery for prenatal torts.

Prenatal wrongful-death actions pose a different problem. Recovery for the wrongful death of a fetus should be seen, on the interest view, not as according personhood, interests, or rights to the unborn, but as compensating prospective parents for the loss of an expected child. Fetal homicide laws can be similarly rationalized. The aim is to protect pregnant women from physical attack and from the harm of losing a wanted pregnancy. As Dawn Johnsen notes, "Holding third parties responsible for the negligent or criminal destruction of fetuses is therefore consistent with, and even enhances, the protection of pregnant women's interests."[3] Such laws thus do not ascribe an independent status to the unborn or conflict with the Supreme Court's abortion decisions.

In the first section, I discuss recovery in torts for prenatal injury and preconception torts, against third parties and mothers, and for purposes of insurance coverage. Prenatal wrongful death is covered in the second section. The third section considers the criminal law relating to fetuses, including prenatal neglect, murder, and vehicular homicide. Wrongful life suits are the topic of the fourth section.

RECOVERY FOR PRENATAL INJURY IN TORTS

Against Third Parties

Prior to 1946, there was no recovery for prenatal injuries. Then, in the landmark case of *Bonbrest v. Kotz*,[4] the U.S. District Court for the District of Columbia allowed recovery against an attending physician for injuries inflicted in utero on a child who was subsequently born alive. Within a few years after *Bonbrest*, most American jurisdictions followed suit.[5] Today, all American jurisdictions allow tort claims for

---

3. Dawn Johnsen. 1986. "The Creation of Fetal Rights: Conflicts With Women's Constitutional Rights to Liberty, Privacy, and Equal Protection," 95 *Yale Law Journal* 599 (hereafter "Women's Rights/Fetal Rights"), p. 603.

4. *Bonbrest v. Kotz*, 65 F. Supp. 138 (1946).

5. The same result was reached earlier in Canada in *Montreal Tramways v. Leveille* (4 D.L.R. 337, 345 [S.C.C. 1933]). In England the same result was reached by statute through the Congenital Disabilities Act (1976). The act totally supersedes common law.

prenatal injuries if the child is subsequently born alive, and it generally does not matter whether the injury occurred before or after viability.[6]

What explains the refusal of American courts until the middle of the 20th century to allow a cause of action for prenatal torts? The judicial stance toward the unborn was based on a decision of the Massachusetts Supreme Court in *Dietrich v. Northampton*.[7] Justice Oliver Wendell Holmes held that no duty of care was owed to the unborn child. Until live birth, it was not a separate being, but part of the mother. Any damage to it that was not too remote to be recovered for at all was recoverable by her.

Although Holmes's decision concerned the death of a nonviable fetus, the Illinois Supreme Court appealed to *Dietrich* in its decision in *Allaire v. St. Luke's Hospital*[8] when it held that there was no cause of action for a child born seriously and permanently disabled from injuries to his mother just prior to delivery. The case was significant not only because it was relied on for the next 46 years but also because of the cogent dissent of Justice Boggs.

Acknowledging that there was no case law upholding a right of prenatal recovery, Justice Boggs argued that nevertheless the fact that the injuries were inflicted prior to birth should not operate to deny a cause of action. "The appellee corporation owed it as a duty to the plaintiff, though unborn, to bestow due and ordinary care and skill to the matter of his preservation and safety before and at the time of his birth."[9] To regard the fetus, once it is viable, as merely a part of its mother is "to deny a palpable fact . . . though within the body of the mother, it is not merely a part of her body, for her body may die in all of its parts and the child remain alive, and capable of maintaining life, when separated from the dead body of the mother."[10] If the viable fetus is a separate being, and not merely a part of its mother, then negligence that causes him to be born maimed and crippled is an injury to him, and not to his mother. Justice Boggs concluded that once the fetus had reached the stage where it could live separable from the mother, and is afterwards born, the "child has a right of action for any injuries wantonly or negligently inflicted upon his or her person at such age of viability, though then in the womb of the mother."[11]

The Irrelevance of Viability

The implicit rationale for the viability requirement, as regards a surviving child, is that, prior to viability, there is no independent being to whom the defendant owes a duty of care. In his effort to refute Justice Holmes's mistaken notion that the unborn was merely a part of the mother's body, Justice Boggs focused on viability as the basis for separate existence. It is true that, prior to viability, the fetus cannot exist separately. However, the fetus is a separate entity, biologically distinct from its mother, throughout pregnancy.

6. *Farley v. Sartin*, 195 W. Va. 671, 466 S.E.2d 522 (1995).

7. *Dietrich v. Northampton*, 138 Mass. 14 (1884).

8. *Allaire v. St. Luke's Hospital*, 184 Ill. 359, 56 N.E. 638 (1900).

9. Ibid., 56 N.E. at p. 642.

10. Ibid., 56 N.E. at p. 641.

11. Ibid., 56 N.E. at p. 642.

This led the New York Supreme Court, Appellate Division in *Kelly v. Gregory* to allow recovery by a surviving child for injuries sustained by its mother in her third month of pregnancy. The court began by noting that the Court of Appeals had previously allowed recovery by a surviving child if the injury were inflicted after viability. The question the court faced in *Kelly* is whether recovery should be allowed for injuries inflicted prior to viability. The court held that "the same rule should govern both cases" because "legal separability should begin at biological separability" and "separability begins at conception."[12] The court concluded, "If the child born after an injury sustained at any period of his prenatal life can prove the effect on him of the tort, as for the purpose of this appeal and on the face of the complaint before us we must assume plaintiff will be able to do, we hold he makes out a right to recover."[13]

This ruling reaches the right result for the wrong reason. The reason that viability at the time of the injury is not a prerequisite for recovery by a surviving child is not that separate existence begins prior to viability, at conception, as the court held. It is rather that the separate existence of the fetus *at the time of the injury* is irrelevant to the merits of the *surviving infant's* cause of action. As Justice Proctor pointed out in *Smith v. Brennan*, "whether viable or not at the time of the injury, the child sustains the same harm after birth, and therefore should be given the same opportunity for redress."[14] In other words, it is the *surviving child*, not the fetus, who has the cause of action, although the injury was sustained prior to birth. Whether the fetus is separable from the pregnant woman at the time of the injury is not relevant to the surviving child's cause of action. Indeed, once it is understood that it is the surviving child who has the cause of action, there is no philosophical or logical reason to restrict recovery to injuries incurred after conception.

Preconception Torts

Not only can there be a duty of care prior to viability, but the duty of care can exist even before the conception of the individual injured by the negligence. Wrongful acts today can harm future people who have not yet been born or conceived. Professor James puts the point well: "the improper canning of baby food today is negligent to a child born next week or next year, who consumes it to his injury. The limitation of the *Palsgraf* case contains no requirement that the interests within the range of peril be known or identified in the actor's mind, or *even in existence at the time of the negligence*."[15] One relevant factor is causation, and there is no reason to bar as a matter of principle the possibility of injury caused before birth, or even conception. The first American court to recognize this was the U.S. Court of Appeals for the Tenth Circuit in *Jorgensen v. Meade Johnson Laboratories*.[16] In that case, the father of

12. *Kelly v. Gregory*, 282 A.D. 542, 125 N.Y.S.2d 696 (1953).

13. Ibid.

14. *Smith v. Brennan*, 31 N.J. 353, 367, 157 A.2d 497, 504 (1960).

15. Harper and James. 1956. *Law of Torts*, vol. 2, p. 1030, emphasis added.

16. 483 F.2d 237 (10th Cir. 1973). Cited in David L. Runner. 1984. "The Prenatal Plaintiff and the *Feres* Doctrine: Throwing the Baby out With the Bath Water?" 20 *Willamette Law Review* 495, p. 502.

twin girls with Down syndrome alleged that, prior to the twins' conception, their mother's genetic structure had been altered through her ingestion of birth control pills. The district court found that the plaintiffs failed to state a cause of action under Oklahoma law and dismissed the suit. On appeal, the Tenth Circuit reversed, holding that the timing of the tortious conduct should not be determinative in allowing or denying the child's right of action. Assuming that causation could be established, the fact that the injury resulted from preconception conduct was no reason for denying recovery.

In addition to causation, another factor in assigning a duty of care is foreseeability, defined in *Black's Law Dictionary* as "the reasonable anticipation that harm or injury is a likely result from certain acts or omissions . . . That which is objectively reasonable to expect, not merely what might conceivably occur."[17] The question is then whether the defendant reasonably could have foreseen the harm to the infant plaintiff, who did not exist at the time of the negligent conduct. This has been a controversial point. In *Monusko v. Postle*,[18] a woman charged that the physicians who treated her during her second pregnancy negligently failed to test her for or immunize her against rubella, with the result that her third child was born with rubella syndrome and was severely mentally and physically impaired. The Court of Appeals of Michigan upheld her cause of action, saying, "It is readily foreseeable that someone not immunized may catch rubella and, if pregnant, bear a child suffering from rubella syndrome."[19] In his dissent, Presiding Judge MacKenzie rejected the majority's conception of foreseeability, saying, "the question is whether it is foreseeable that the defendant's conduct may create a risk of harm to the plaintiff, not whether it is foreseeable that the plaintiff will exist. Under the majority's logic, all persons would be deemed to foresee, and thus owe a duty to, the future children of all other persons."[20]

In *Albala v. City of New York*,[21] an infant sought recovery for congenital brain damage, allegedly due to his mother's uterus having been perforated during an abortion more than 3 years before his conception. Despite precedents from several jurisdictions,[22] the New York Court of Appeal rejected the concept of preconception negligence, primarily on policy grounds. Concluding that "foreseeability alone is not the hallmark of legal duty,"[23] Judge Wachtler, writing for the majority, held that to allow such a cause of action would stretch traditional tort concepts beyond manageable bounds. It seems likely that the court's decision was based largely on the fear that recognition of preconception torts would create limitless liability and a flood of cases. This is understandable, particularly

17. *Black's Law Dictionary*. 1990. 6th edition. St. Paul, MN: West Publishing Co., p. 649.

18. *Monusko v. Postle*, 175 Mich. App. 269, 437 N.W.2d 367.

19. Ibid., 175 Mich. App. at 275.

20. Ibid., 175 Mich. App. at 278.

21. *Albala v. City of New York*, 54 N.Y.2d 269, 429 N.E.2d 786, 445 N.Y.S.2d 108 (1981).

22. *Renslow v. Mennonite Hospital*, 67 Ill.2d 348, 367 N.E.2d 1250 (1977) [alleged that negligent blood transfusion to plaintiff's mother 8 years prior to her conception caused injuries to plaintiff's brain, nervous system, and other organs]; *Bergstresser v. Mitchell*, 577 F.2d 22 (8th Cir. 1978) [infant plaintiff alleged that due to a negligent cesarean performed 2 years before his conception, he was born with brain damage and other severe injuries].

23. *Albala* (see note 21), 54 N.Y.2d at 273.

in light of the factual situation in *Albala*. However, this is no reason to exclude preconception liability, which can be limited to cases where both causation and foreseeability can be demonstrated. Admittedly, both causation and foreseeability are often difficult to prove, but that difficulty is no reason to deny a cause of action. Moreover, in some cases, the connection between the negligent act and the future child is far from tenuous, a point stressed by the court in *Monusko*: "We emphasize the direct connection between the test and immunization procedure and the harm in this case, and the fact that the test and the preconception immunization are specifically designed to prevent rubella syndrome in children that are not yet conceived."[24] Finally, New York's rejection of preconception torts on policy grounds can be criticized on grounds of fairness. It seems grossly unfair to deny compensation to someone who has been seriously injured by another's negligence, where the harm was reasonably foreseeable, simply because there are many others in the same boat. Despite some critical comment by courts in other states,[25] *Albala* remains the law in New York today.

Preconception tort liability has arisen in connection with diethylstilbestrol (DES). "In the U.S. an estimated 5 to 10 million persons were exposed to DES from 1938 to 1971, including pregnant women prescribed DES and their children."[26] The drug, which was given to women in order to prevent miscarriage, was eventually found to be ineffective, but before that was learned, it caused some adverse effects, including a rare vaginal and cervical cancer known as clear-cell adenocarcinoma in some of the daughters of the women who took it. Research has confirmed that DES daughters are also more likely to have reproductive difficulties, including infertility, such as ectopic pregnancy and preterm delivery, and miscarriages or stillbirths.[27] In 1990, the New York Appellate Division ruled that the granddaughters of women who took DES, who were not even conceived at the time, could sue for the drug's alleged harmful effects.[28] The plaintiff was Karen Enright, who was born in 1981 with cerebral palsy. The complaint alleged that Karen's mother, Patricia, was exposed in utero to DES, resulting in certain anatomical abnormalities and deformities in her reproductive system that prevented her from carrying a baby to full term. Karen's disabilities were allegedly caused by her premature birth, which was attributed to her mother's exposure to DES. The lower court (which in New York is the Supreme Court) had dismissed all causes of action seeking to recover damages for Karen's injuries. The appellate court reversed, saying, "Although plaintiff is not a 'DES daughter'—one who was exposed to DES while *in utero*—she may be no less a victim of the devastation wrought by DES than her mother, who is a DES daughter, and we see no sound basis for denying

24. *Monusko* (see note 18), 175 Mich. App. at 277.

25. See *Yeager v. Bloomington Obstetrics and Gynecology*, Inc., 585 N.E.2d 696 (Ind.App. 1992); *Taylor v. Cutler*, 306 N.J.Super. 37, 703 A.2d 294 (1997); *Lynch v. Scheininger*, 162 N.J. 209, 744 A.2d 113 (2000); *Monusko v. Postle*, 175 Mich.App. 269, 437 N.W.2d 367 (1989); *McNulty v. McDowell*, 415 Mass. 369, 613 N.E.2d 904 (1993); *Lough v. Rolla Women's Clinic, Inc.*, 866 S.W.2d 851 (Mo. 1993).

26. CDC. 2010. DES Update Home, http://www.cdc.gov/des/index.html. Accessed May 17, 2010.

27. CDC. 2010. DED Update Consumers, http://www.cdc.gov/des/consumers/about/effects_daughters.html. Accessed May 17, 2010.

28. *Enright v. Eli Lilly & Co.*, 155 A.D.2d 64 (1990).

plaintiff her day in court along with her mother."[29] The court maintained that its decision did not conflict with the Court of Appeals' rejection of preconception torts in *Albala*, because the necessity of establishing manageable bounds for liability—the rationale for denying a cause of action in *Albala*—is "conspicuously absent" under a strict products-liability theory. Moreover, while restriction of liability is an important policy consideration, it is balanced in this case by a competing consideration—namely, the need for a remedy for those who have suffered the devastation caused by DES. The court noted that both the Court of Appeals and the New York State Legislature had made it easier for DES victims to sue the manufacturers of the drug,[30] demonstrating "deep concern for those injured by toxic substances in general and DES in particular."[31] The economic incentive of manufacturers to turn out safe products would only be diluted by creating "an arbitrary generational limitation on the legal responsibility for birth defects caused by DES."[32] The court stressed that DES is a "singular case,"[33] which does not have implications for preconception torts in general.

On February 19, 1991, the Court of Appeals, New York's highest court, decided against Karen Enright.[34] The court held in accord with their decision in *Albala* that no cause of action accrues in favor of a "third generation" plaintiff against the drug manufacturers. As in *Albala*, the reason for the decision was fear of limitless liability. The court said, "For all we know, the rippling effects of DES exposure may extend for generations. It is our duty to confine liability within manageable limits. Limiting liability to those who ingested the drug or were exposed to it in utero serves this purpose."[35] On October 7, 1991, the U.S. Supreme Court declined to hear *Enright v. Lilly*, thereby blocking the first suit to come before the Court that sought to establish preconception torts.[36]

At least 16 states have addressed the preconception tort issue: California, Colorado, Georgia, Illinois, Indiana, Louisiana, Maryland, Massachusetts, Michigan, Minnesota, Mississippi, Missouri, New York, Ohio, Oklahoma, and Pennsylvania.[37] Seven (Colorado, Illinois, Indiana, Michigan, Mississippi, Missouri, and Oklahoma) have allowed recovery, four (Maryland, Minnesota, New York, and Pennsylvania) have denied recovery, and five (California, Georgia, Louisiana, Massachusetts, and Ohio)

---

29. Ibid., p. 70.

30. In *Hymowitz v. Eli Lilly & Co.*, 73 NY2d 487 (1989), the New York Court of Appeals held that liability could be imposed on DES manufacturers in accordance with their share of the national DES market, notwithstanding the plaintiff's inability to identify the manufacturer particularly at fault for her injuries.

31. *Enright v. Eli Lilly & Co.* (see note 28), p. 69.

32. Ibid., pp. 70–71.

33. Ibid., p. 70, quoting *Hymowitz v. Eli Lilly & Co.*, 73 NY2d 487, 508 (1989).

34. *Enright v. Eli Lilly & Co.*, 77 NY2d 377, 568 N.Y.S.2d 550 (1991).

35. Ibid., 568 N.Y.S.2d at p. 555 (citations omitted).

36. *Enright v. Eli Lilly & Co.*, 502 U.S. 868, 112 S. Ct. 197 (1991).

37. Julie A. Greenberg. 1997. "Reconceptualizing Preconception Torts," 64 *Tennessee Law Review* 315, p. 320.

"have implied that a duty may be owed to the later-conceived in limited circum-stances."[38] As for third-generation DES claims (which account for most of the actions against pharmaceutical companies), it appears that no state has specifically imposed liability, although such claims might be allowed in Illinois and Oklahoma, and pos-sibly in Pennsylvania as well.[39] In other states in which such claims have been brought, courts have declined to impose liability. The reasons are all variations on the theme of opening the floodgates of liability. Yet according to one commentator, the feared tidal wave of lawsuits has not occurred.[40] Even if it did, this would not "justif[y] the adop-tion of a blanket no-duty rule or strict and arbitrary limitations."[41] I agree. The inter-mediate appellate court in *Enright* was correct: there was no sound basis for denying the plaintiff her day in court. An injured person should be given the opportunity to prove negligence, causation, and reasonable foreseeability. If these factors are proven, the plaintiff should be able to recover damages. When the negligent act (or omission) occurred, and specifically whether the victim existed at the time of the act, is irrelevant.

The right of surviving children to sue third parties for prenatal injuries is well established. Some commentators have urged the states to expand the conception of fetal rights to permit the fetus to sue its mother in tort for prenatal injuries.[42] Such an extension raises both practical questions about implementation, as well as theo-retical questions about the parent-child tort immunity doctrine and the infringement of the mother's rights to privacy and bodily self-determination.

Against the Mother

PARENTAL IMMUNITY

The doctrine of parental immunity is that a child cannot sue his or her parent in tort for personal injuries resulting from a negligent or intentional act. The doctrine is relatively new in American common law. It was created by the Mississippi Supreme Court in 1891 in *Hewellette v. George*.[43] Without citing any prior case law or statutory authority, the court simply held that a child's personal tort action against a parent would disturb the peace of society and be contrary to public policy. Within a few years, most states had adopted the doctrine of parental tort immunity, relying on three primary justifications; "that allowing a child to sue a parent for a personal tort would (1) disrupt family harmony, (2) encourage collusion, perjury and fraud between family members, and (3) impair parental authority and discipline."[44]

38. Ibid.

39. Ibid., p. 339.

40. Ibid., p. 341.

41. Ibid., p. 342.

42. See, for example, John Robertson. 1983. "Procreative Liberty and the Control of Conception, Pregnancy and Childbirth," 69 *Virginia Law Review* 405, pp. 437–442.

43. *Hewellette v. George*, 68 Miss. 703, 9 So. 885 (1891).

44. *Stallman by Stallman v. Youngquist*, 152 Ill.App.3d 683, 504 N.E.2d 920, 924 (1987).

For the next 30 years, courts continued to uphold the doctrine of parental immunity, while creating numerous exceptions to it. Then, in 1963, in the landmark case of *Goller v. White*, the Wisconsin Supreme Court abolished the general rule of nonliability, with immunity in two areas: parental authority and ordinary discretion in providing food, clothing, housing, and medical care.[45] *Goller* has been criticized for not going far enough in abolishing parental immunity, because it implies that "within certain aspects of the parent-child relationship, the parent has carte blanche to act negligently toward his child."[46] For this reason, the Supreme Court of Arizona rejected *Goller* as providing guidance, approving instead the "reasonable parent test," set out in the California case of *Gibson v. Gibson*, "in which a parent's conduct is judged by whether that parent's conduct comported with that of a reasonable and prudent parent in a similar situation."[47] Today, states that remain loyal to the parental immunity doctrine are in the minority.[48]

The ability of a surviving child to sue for prenatal injuries, combined with the abrogation of the common-law doctrine of parental immunity, has resulted in the potential for lawsuits by surviving children against their mothers. According to Ron Beal, the majority of jurisdictions should recognize a duty on the part of a woman to her fetus in order to remain "consistent with their policy justifications as set forth in their decisions abolishing parental immunity and recognizing the right of a child born alive to recover for prenatal injuries."[49] In other words, if surviving children can recover for their prenatally indicted injuries from third parties, and if parents are no longer immune from liability simply because they are parents, injured children should be able to sue their mothers for injuries negligently inflicted during pregnancy.

The Woman's Right of Privacy

In deciding whether such suits should be allowed, we cannot ignore the "geography of pregnancy."[50] The fetus is inside its mother's body. Whatever she is required to do to benefit or avoid harming the fetus will also have an impact on her own body. So the issue is not simply the extent of the duty a parent owes to a child but also what risks and costs a pregnant woman is required to bear for the sake of her not-yet-born child. Some have argued that a woman could be obligated to undergo surgery if necessary to sustain the life or health of the fetus. This imposes an obligation on pregnant women that is not imposed on anyone else, and so it violates equal protection. In addition,

45. *Goller v. White*, 20 Wis.2d 402, 122 N.W.2d 193, 198 (1963).

46. *Broadbent v. Broadbent*, 184 Ariz. 74, 81, 907 P.2d 43, 50 (1995), quoting *Gibson v. Gibson*, 3 Cal.3d 914, 479 P.2d 648, 652–653 (1971).

47. Ibid., citing *Gibson v. Gibson*, 3 Cal.3d 914, 479 P.2d 648.

48. Ron Beal. 1984. "'Can I Sue Mommy?'" An Analysis of a Woman's Tort Liability for Prenatal Injuries to Her Child Born Alive" (hereafter "Prenatal Injuries"), 21 *San Diego Law Review* 325, p. 336.

49. Ibid., p. 357.

50. See Janet Gallagher. 1987. "Prenatal Invasions & Interventions: What's Wrong With Fetal Rights?" 10 *Harvard Women's Law Journal* 9, pp. 13, 38–40.

it ignores the woman's rights to privacy and bodily self-determination, rights that do not arise in the case of third-party lawsuits.

In response, it might be said that the woman's legitimate interests could be considered in determining the duty owed to the child. A woman would not have a duty to do *whatever* was necessary to protect the not-yet-born child, but only a duty to behave reasonably during pregnancy. This was the finding of the Court of Appeals of Michigan in *Grodin v. Grodin*,[51] the first case explicitly to consider the right of a surviving child to sue its mother for injuries resulting from the mother's negligence during pregnancy. The case concerned a child born with tooth discoloration caused by his mother's taking tetracycline during pregnancy. The child, Randy Grodin, sued his mother for negligence in failing to seek proper prenatal care, for her failure to request that her doctor perform a pregnancy test, and for her failure to inform her doctor that she was taking a medication that might be contraindicated for pregnant women.

The child also sued his mother's doctor. The suit against the physician alleged that he was guilty of malpractice in not administering a pregnancy test to Mrs. Grodin after symptoms of pregnancy were brought to his attention. Indeed, the doctor allegedly assured Mrs. Grodin that it was impossible for her to become pregnant. After a different doctor told her she was 7 or 8 months pregnant, Mrs. Grodin stopped taking the medication that caused the discoloration of her son's teeth.

John Robertson provides the background to the case:

> The child originally filed suit against the physician alone for his injury. During discovery the physician claimed that he had warned the mother to stop taking tetracycline. To guard against the possibility that the jury might ascribe the child's injury to the mother and refuse to award damages, the attorney advised amending the complaint to include the mother as a defendant because a homeowner's policy insured the mother against tort liability. But for the existence of a homeowner's policy with broad coverage, the suit against the mother would not have been filed.[52]

The main issue in the case was whether the parental tort immunity doctrine protected the mother from liability. Michigan overruled the doctrine of intrafamily tort immunity in the early 1970s, using the *Goller* approach, which creates two immunity exceptions. The trial court granted Mrs. Grodin's motion for summary judgment, based on the second exception, parental discretion in the provision of ordinary care. The summary judgment precluded testimony on either the necessity of the use of tetracycline to maintain the mother's health, or the risk created for her child. The Michigan Court of Appeals reversed and remanded the case to determine whether the mother had acted *reasonably*.

Some commentators have viewed *Grodin* as alarming in that it sanctions monitoring the behavior of women during pregnancy. "Reasonable" behavior might include regular prenatal checkups, a balanced diet with vitamin supplements, judicious use of medications and caffeine, and abstention from tobacco, alcohol, and narcotics.

51. *Grodin v. Grodin*, 102 Mich. App. 396, 301 N.W.2d 869 (1980).

52. Robertson, "Procreative Liberty" (see note 42), p. 441, footnote 114.

It might require women to abstain from too much exercise, sexual intercourse, or working. Virtually every area of a woman's life could come under scrutiny, seriously threatening women's rights to privacy and bodily self-determination. As Dawn Johnsen notes, "If the current trend in fetal rights continues, pregnant women would live in constant fear that any accident or 'error' in judgment could be deemed 'unacceptable' and become the basis for a criminal prosecution by the state or a civil suit by a disenchanted husband or relative."[53]

Concern for privacy distinguishes third-party lawsuits from lawsuits against mothers, and it should make us extremely reluctant to extend civil liability to women for their behavior during pregnancy. In theory, an exception could be in the case of surrogate motherhood or contract pregnancy, in those states that recognize and uphold such contracts. Unlike regular mothers, surrogate mothers typically contractually agree to restrict their behavior during pregnancy. A typical surrogate contract specifies that the surrogate will comply with all medical instructions given to her by her physician as well as by her independent obstetrician or midwife, have regular prenatal examinations, take medications and vitamins prescribed by her treating obstetrician or midwife, not smoke cigarettes, drink alcoholic beverages, or use any illegal drugs, or take prescription or nonprescription drugs without consent from her obstetrician or midwife. The surrogate often agrees not to participate in dangerous sports or hazardous activities or knowingly allow herself to be exposed to radiation, toxic chemicals, or communicable diseases. One sample contract even specifies that the surrogate shall "comply with the instructions of the Treating Physician and the obstetrician with respect to the use of hair sprays, hair dyes, and permanent solutions, and agrees that she shall not remain in close proximity to cat litter, cleansers, oven cleaners, pesticides, second hand smoke, or other aerosol sprays during and through the end of her pregnancy."[54] Some contracts specify that the woman shall not abort the pregnancy, or they may require her to abort if prenatal testing reveals fetal deformity. Some commentators have criticized such contracts as unduly onerous, or even unconstitutional, precisely because they deprive the woman of control over her own body and behavior. However, assuming that the contract is valid, if a surrogate knowingly engages in behaviors she agreed to forego, and if these behaviors cause the child to be born with injuries that otherwise would have been avoided (something that might be extremely difficult to prove), she might reasonably be civilly liable to the contracting couple and to the child once born. I know of no such lawsuits that have been brought, undoubtedly because it is unlikely that a woman who becomes a surrogate is likely to have the "deep pockets" that would make such a suit worthwhile.

Concern for women's interests in liberty, privacy, and bodily self-determination does not apply to the circumstances in *Grodin*. Mrs. Grodin's privacy was not threatened by allowing her son to recover damages under the family's insurance coverage. Recognition of such causes of action will not make women live in fear of civil suits resulting from some accident or error of judgment, because the woman herself benefits if the insurance company compensates her child for his injuries. It is unlikely

---

53. Johnsen, "Women's Rights/Fetal Rights" (see note 3), p. 607.

54. All About Surrogacy, Sample Traditional Surrogacy Contract. http://www.allaboutsurrogacy. com/sample_contracts/TScontract1.htm. Accessed November 6, 2010.

that any suits would be filed in the absence of an insurance policy. On the other hand, having allowed a child to sue his mother where there was a family insurance policy, the Michigan courts might find it difficult to deny a cause of action where there was no insurance. In that case, fears about exposing virtually every area of a woman's life to judicial scrutiny would be justified. Imposing an open-ended duty of reasonable care in pregnancy sets a dangerous precedent and threatens women's liberty and privacy interests. However, as I will argue in the next section, the situation is different in the case of automobile liability.

Automobile Liability

Seven states have abolished the parental-immunity doctrine in the area of automobile liability, because of the prevalence of insurance coverage. This type of suit is not a truly adversarial situation, but rather one in which *both* parties are seeking to recover from the insurance carrier to provide for the child so as not to deplete the family assets.[55]

This approach has been criticized as legally weak and untidy. The mere presence of insurance without additional justification has never been the basis for recognizing a cause of action. However, the claim is not that the parent is liable because there is insurance. Liability stems from the principle that an injured party has the right to compensation for negligently inflicted injuries. It is immunity from liability that must be justified. The primary justification for parental immunity is the preservation of family harmony. The harmony of the family is not threatened when an injured child recovers damages from an insurance company. Thus, there is no justification for exempting parents from liability in this situation.

This was the reasoning of the Appellate Court of Illinois in *Stallman v. Youngquist*.[56] Bari Stallman was 5 months pregnant in 1985 when her auto collided with another, driven by Clarence Youngquist. Her subsequently born daughter, Lindsay, filed suit against both her mother and Youngquist, alleging that their negligent driving resulted in serious prenatal injuries that became apparent at birth. Because the plaintiff sought to recover damages from Mrs. Stallman's automobile insurance policy, Mrs. Stallman's insurer controlled her trial.

The trial court dismissed Lindsay's complaint against her mother on grounds of the state's parent–child tort immunity doctrine. The Illinois Appellate Court reversed, holding that Lindsay should have the opportunity to show that her mother's actions fell outside the doctrine. On remand, the trial court found that the immunity doctrine did apply to the case and granted the mother's motion for summary judgment. Once again, the Appellate Court reversed, holding that, as the Illinois Supreme Court had never adopted the parent–child tort immunity rule, it was subject to abrogation by the Appellate Court. The court announced that it was joining the many states that have abrogated the doctrine, saying, "We agree with the Massachusetts Supreme Judicial Court that '[c]hildren enjoy the same right to protection and to legal redress for wrongs done them as others enjoy. Only the strongest reasons, grounded in public

---

55. Beal, "Prenatal Injuries" (see note 48), p. 340.

56. *Stallman v. Youngquist*, 125 Ill.2d 267, 531 N.E.2d 355 (1988).

policy, can justify limitation or abolition of those rights.' "[57] The court concluded that an unemancipated minor child may recover damages against a parent for personal injuries caused by the negligence of the parent in the operation of a motor vehicle, and an infant who is born alive can maintain a tort action to recover for prenatal injuries.

The Supreme Court of Illinois reversed.[58] Declining to address the issue of parental immunity, the court held that a fetus has no cause of action against its mother for unintentional infliction of prenatal injuries. The court distinguished such suits from suits against third parties on three grounds. First, such causes of action would establish a legal duty on the part of the mother to create the best prenatal environment possible. They would make the mother and fetus legal adversaries from conception until birth, and they would require the mother to guarantee the health of that potential adversary.[59]

Second, holding a third party liable for prenatal injuries does not interfere with the defendant's right to control his or her own life, whereas imposing such liability on a mother subjects to state scrutiny all the decisions a woman must make during her pregnancy and thus infringes on her right to privacy and bodily autonomy.[60] Third, the absence of any clear, objective standard of due care during pregnancy would create the danger that prejudicial and stereotypical beliefs about the reproductive abilities of women might skew jury determinations of liability.[61] Finally, the court suggested that disparities in wealth, education, and access to health care would prevent a fair application of any legal standard of prenatal care. The best way to achieve healthy newborns, the court argued, is not "through after-the-fact civil liability in tort for individual mothers, but rather through before-the-fact education of all women and families about prenatal development."[62]

These are all good arguments against the creation of broadly construed duties of pregnant women to their not-yet-born children (see Chapter 4). But none of these arguments applies where a surviving child seeks to recover under a parent's automobile insurance policy. The duty to drive carefully and avoid injuring others is not a duty of prenatal care. It is a duty of care imposed on all drivers to everyone who might be injured by the failure to drive carefully. Allowing surviving children to sue their mothers for prenatal injuries caused by negligent driving does not imply a legal duty on the part of the mother to create the best prenatal environment possible. Nor does it subject the entire lives of pregnant women to state scrutiny or infringe on their rights to privacy. If there is automobile insurance, allowing such suits does not make the mother and fetus—or, rather, subsequently born child—genuine adversaries, since the whole family benefits by allowing the child to recover. If Mrs. Stallman had had a pregnant passenger in her car, that woman's subsequently born child would have a cause of action against Mrs. Stallman, and it would be able to collect

57. *Stallman v. Youngquist*, 152 Ill.App.3d 683, 504 N.E.2d 920, 925 (1987), quoting *Sorensen v. Sorensen*, 369 Mass. 350, 359, 339 N.E.2d 907, 912 (1975).

58. *Stallman v. Youngquist*, 125 Ill.2d 267, 531 N.E.2d 355 (1988).

59. Ibid., p. 276.

60. Ibid., p. 278.

61. Ibid.

62. Ibid., p. 280.

damages under her insurance policy. Why should Mrs. Stallman's own child be denied the benefit of insurance that would be available to a stranger? Finally, even if the best way in general to achieve healthy newborns is through prenatal education and care, this has no relevance for the compensation of infants injured in car accidents. The best prenatal care in the world would not have protected Lindsay from being injured in a car accident. Concern for women's autonomy and privacy should not lead us to deny Lindsay Stallman her right to recover for her injuries. If she is entitled to make a case against Clarence Youngquist, she should also have been permitted to make her case against Bari Stallman.

PRENATAL WRONGFUL DEATH

So far I have been discussing suits in which the fetus survives and seeks to recover damages for injuries negligently inflicted before birth. What if the negligence results in the death of the fetus? Can there be a cause of action for the wrongful death of a fetus?

To understand the special case of prenatal wrongful-death actions, it is necessary to understand the nature of wrongful-death actions in general.

Wrongful-Death Actions

Until the middle of the 19th century, there was no right of recovery for the death of a human being killed by the negligence or wrongful act of another.[63] This common-law rule left the bereaved, and often destitute, family of the victim without a remedy. This intolerable result was changed in England by the passage of the Fatal Accidents Act of 1846, otherwise known as Lord Campbell's Act. The Act provides that whenever the death of a person is caused by the wrongful act or negligence of another, in such manner as would have entitled the party injured to have sued if he or she had survived, an action may be brought in the name of his or her executor for the benefit of certain relatives, such as husband, wife, parent, or child.

In wrongful-death actions, the duty of care is to the deceased, but the damages are measured by the loss suffered by the survivors. This feature—unique (so far as I know) in tort law, means that the basis for recovery is not the loss suffered by the one who is tortiously killed, but rather the loss suffered by his or her survivors. As we will see, this has particular importance for prenatal death.

In general, common-law countries do not allow the relatives of a wrongful-death victim compensation for mental anguish. Where there is no pecuniary loss, as is likely in the death of a minor child or aged parent, there can be no recovery. Financial loss may be prospective, but it must be likely, and not merely possible. This obviously rules out recovery for the loss of an unborn child. The pecuniary-loss rule has been vigorously

63. For a more extensive treatment of wrongful-death actions, see my 1987 article, "Prenatal Wrongful Death," *Bioethics* 1 (4): 301–320.

criticized, and it has been rejected by a number of common-law jurisdictions.[64] In a number of American states, some form of mental distress damages is explicitly recognized.

Most states now permit prenatal wrongful-death actions, at least after viability. Some commentators regard this as part of the trend toward recognizing the separate existence of the fetus, which led to allowing recovery on the part of surviving children for injuries indicted prenatally. On the interest view, however, there is an important difference between prenatal torts and prenatal wrongful death. A child who is injured before her birth, and must go through life crippled or maimed, has had her most basic interests set back; she has been harmed. By contrast, when a fetus is killed before it acquires any interests, it is not harmed. Permitting recovery on the part of surviving children for injuries inflicted prenatally does not imply a right of recovery if the fetus is tortiously killed.

In Chapter 2, I argued that death can be a harm to conscious fetuses. For this reason, it might be thought that prenatal wrongful-death actions should be permitted for, but limited to, late-gestation (viable) fetuses. This seems to me to misconceive the nature and purpose of wrongful-death actions. Despite a persistent tendency on the part of some courts to view prenatal wrongful-death actions as redressing the wrong to the unborn,[65] their real function is to redress the wrong to the parents, who have suffered the loss of an expected and wanted child. The correct basis for allowing recovery for prenatal wrongful-death was expressed by the Supreme Court of Washington, when it held that damages for anguish at the loss of an 8-month-old fetus were recoverable under the state's wrongful-death statute, because a parent's mental anguish would not be dependent on whether the child survived to full term.[66] The court offered no conclusion as to whether there could be recovery for a nonviable fetus.

The Implications for Abortion

Several judges have expressed the view that recognition of prenatal wrongful-death suits conflicts with the right to abortion. One court maintained that it is "incongruous" to allow a woman the constitutional right to abort and yet hold a third party liable to the fetus for merely negligent acts.[67] Another held that "There would be an inherent conflict in giving the mother the right to terminate the pregnancy yet holding that an action may be brought on behalf of the same fetus under the wrongful death act."[68]

64. Stuart M. Speiser and Stuart S. Malawer. 1976. "An American Tragedy: Damages for Mental Anguish of Bereaved Relatives in Wrongful Death Actions," 51 *Tulane Law Review* 1.

65. See, for example, *Kwaterski v. State Farm Mutual Automobile Insurance Company*, 34 Wis. 2d 14, 20, 148 N.W.2d 107, 110 (1967), holding that barring prenatal wrongful death "would produce the absurd result that an unborn child who was badly injured by the tortious acts of another, but who was born alive, could recover while an unborn child, who was more severely injured and died as a result of the tortious acts of another, could recover nothing."

66. *Moen v. Hanson*, 85 Wn.2d 597, 537 P.2d 266 (1975).

67. *Wallace v. Wallace*, 120 N.H. 675, 679, 421 A.2d 134, 137 (1980).

68. *Toth v. Goree*, 65 Mich. App. 296, 304, 237 N.W.2d 297, 301 (1975).

The same theme is voiced by those on both sides of the abortion debate. Conservatives see hypocrisy in recognizing prenatal wrongful-death actions while also allowing abortion; liberals worry that recognition of prenatal wrongful death will threaten women's rights of reproductive choice. As a policy matter, this is a realistic concern. Nevertheless, recovery for prenatal wrongful death need not conflict with the right to abortion. Acknowledging the woman's right to have an abortion, stemming from her right to privacy, is entirely consistent with recognizing her right to be compensated when a wanted pregnancy is negligently terminated. Indeed, both prenatal wrongful-death actions and legal abortion can be seen as aspects of reproductive liberty. The perception of inconsistency stems, I think, from the error of regarding prenatal wrongful-death actions as primarily intended to protect the lives of the unborn. Why, it may be asked, should such protection be extended to some fetuses and not others? The corrective is to realize that prenatal wrongful-death suits are not premised on entitlement of the *fetus* to the protection of law, but rather on the right of its prospective parents to compensation for their loss.

The fact remains that the Supreme Court held in *Roe* that the unborn is not a person within the language and meaning of the Fourteenth Amendment, while the death statutes of most states restrict recovery to the death of a person. Some judges have regarded this as an insurmountable obstacle to prenatal wrongful-death actions. In response, it has been noted that *Roe* is a federal constitutional decision rather than a tort or death-statute decision, and so its interpretation of "person" does not compel for these decisions.[69] Does this mean that judges should be able to interpret the meaning of "person" for the purpose of wrongful-death actions, or is this a matter to be addressed by the legislature?

This was an issue in *Young v. St. Vincent's Medical Center,*[70] a case in Florida, one of the minority of states that does not allow recovery for the death of a fetus. In November 1989, Gwendolyn Young, in her 34th week of pregnancy with twins, went into premature labor and was admitted to St. Vincent's. To determine the maturity of the fetal lungs, a resident attempted to withdraw amniotic fluid. Instead, she punctured one of the fetuses, drawing blood instead of amniotic fluid. At that point, the attending physician took over and completed the amniocentesis, and Ms. Young was discharged. She returned the next day with labor pains. After it was discovered that one of the fetuses had no heart beat, an emergency cesarean section was performed. One of the babies, Jessica, survived, but the other, Willisha, was stillborn. Ms. Young sued St. Vincent's in a wrongful-death action, alleging that negligent prenatal care led to the death of her daughter. The trial court entered summary final judgment in favor of St. Vincent's on the basis that Willisha was not born alive and Florida law does not permit a cause of action for wrongful death of an unborn child.

The trial court was correct on Florida law; the Florida Supreme Court has consistently refused to allow a cause of action for the wrongful death of unborn children, based largely on its view that if the Florida legislature intended to include a fetus within the meaning of person in its wrongful-death statute, it would have explicitly

69. David Westfall. 1982. "Beyond Abortion: The Potential Reach of a Human Life Amendment," *American Journal of Law & Medicine* 8 (2): 95–135, p. 112.

70. *Young v. St. Vincent's Medical Center, Inc.,* 673 So.2d 482 (Fla. 1996).

amended the law. Nevertheless, because of the "great public importance"[71] of the issue, in April 1995, the Florida District Court of Appeal asked the Florida Supreme Court to reconsider the question of whether a stillborn fetus has a right of recovery under Florida's Wrongful Death Act. The policy arguments in favor of such a right were put forward by Judge Mickle in a specially concurring opinion. First, it seems illogical to allow a surviving child to recover for injuries that are not severe enough to cause death, but to deny recovery for worse injuries, and second, it is perverse to provide a tortfeasor with an economic motive for killing a fetus rather than merely injuring it. In response to the Supreme Court's view on legislative intent, Judge Mickle wrote, "there is no clear evidence to suggest that the Florida Legislature intended to govern exclusively the cause at issue. It appears more likely that the Legislature merely intended to provide a wrongful death action, leaving its adminis-tration and construction to the courts."[72] He concluded:

> The record in this case contains a physician's sworn statement that Willisha was capable of independent survival outside of her mother's womb, and that she would have survived delivery but for the negligence of St. Vincent's. Ms. Young requests very simply that she be granted the opportunity to prove up her claim that her daughter would be alive today were it not for negligent acts alleged in the complaint. Reflecting upon a change in the attitude of our sister states permitting these actions, and in light of the fact that the reasons formerly relied on to deny maintenance of such actions no longer are persuasive, I agree that the time has come for our supreme court to reconsider joining our sister states in recognizing that wrongful death actions lie by the estates of stillborn children for fatal injuries they received while viable children *en ventre sa mere*.[73]

The Florida Supreme Court declined the invitation to revisit the issue, citing *Hernandez* v. *Garwood*,[74] which established that there is no cause of action under Florida's wrongful-death statute for the death of a stillborn fetus. This ruling was supported the American Civil Liberties Union (ACLU) Reproductive Freedom Project and the ACLU of Florida, which filed a friend-of-the-court brief urging the Court to continue to limit wrongful-death actions to those *born alive*. In a 1996 paper, the ACLU explained its position:

> The central question posed by *Young v. St. Vincent's Medical Center* was not whether the prospective parent's loss should be compensated, but rather, *how* it should be compensated. The Project and the ACLU of Florida urged that any money damages should go to the prospective parent, who should be compensated for the loss of her child and the harm she suffered when her choice to continue a pregnancy to term was frustrated. The understandable impulse to compensate the loss of a fetus, we argued, should not lead to an award of damages to the

71. *Young v. St. Vincent's Medical Center, Inc.*, 653 So.2d 499 (Fla. Dist. Ct. App. 1995), at 499.

72. Ibid., at 505.

73. Ibid., at 507.

74. *Hernandez v. Garwood*, 390 So.2d 357 (Fla. 1980).

stillborn fetus. Instead, the prospective parent's loss could and should be compensated within the existing tort law framework, which recognizes a unified legal interest between the pregnant woman and her fetus.[75]

This analysis is consistent with the interest view, which denies that a fetus has full moral status. Moreover, recognition of the fetus as a person is not necessary to achieve the desirable aim of redressing the injury of the loss of an expected child. Prospective parents have a right that others refrain from tortiously killing their unborn children, and a right to compensation for emotional distress when this right is abridged. Recognition of prenatal wrongful-death actions admittedly serves the important purpose of compensating prospective parents, but at the cost of extending legal personhood to the unborn. The compensation-for-emotional-distress approach has the advantage of focusing on the wrong done to the parents, without implying that a person has been killed.

If parental anguish is the basis for recovery, *neither live birth nor viability at the time of the injury* should be a condition of recovery. Admittedly, the grief occasioned by losing a baby during labor or delivery is likely to be greater than the grief caused by an early miscarriage, and this might properly affect *the amount of damages*. Nevertheless, expectant parents may experience emotional distress whenever a wanted pregnancy is negligently terminated, regardless of the fetus's stage of development. The viability requirement is as unwarranted here as it is regarding prenatal injury, although for entirely different reasons. In the case of prenatal injury, it is the *born child* who is harmed by the negligence that occurred when she was a fetus. Her characteristics at the time of the injury are irrelevant. What matters is that there now exists a harmed individual whose suffering is the result of another's negligence, and who thus deserves to be compensated. In the case of prenatal death, the previable fetus is not harmed by being killed, but this is irrelevant because the wrong is not to the fetus anyway, but to its parents. They are entitled to be compensated for their grief and anguish at the loss of an expected and wanted child, when that loss is occasioned by someone else's negligence.

THE CRIMINAL LAW

In the first two sections, I have argued that there should be civil liability for tortiously injuring or killing a fetus. What about criminal liability? A journalist comments, "Laws that make killing a fetus a form of murder have been one of the most hot-button debates of the past decade."[76] Basically, there are two approaches that have been taken to the issue of fetuses killed by violent acts against pregnant women. One approach is to make the killing of a fetus by someone other than a pregnant woman or abortion provider a criminal homicide, either by amending the state's homicide statute to include fetuses or by passing a fetal homicide law. In some states, the killing of a fetus in the course of an attack on a pregnant woman is manslaughter. In others,

75. ACLU. 1996. "What's Wrong With Fetal Rights?" http://www.aclu.org/print/reproductive-freedom/whats-wrong-fetal-rights. Accessed November 6, 2010.

76. David France. 2006. "The Laci Effect," *O, The Oprah Magazine*: 224–252, p. 250.

such as California, the unlawful killing of a fetus with malice aforethought is murder. The other approach is to mandate additional criminal penalties when an attack on a pregnant woman causes her to miscarry, focusing "on the harm done to a pregnant woman and the subsequent loss of her pregnancy, but not on the rights of the fetus."[77]

A range of issues are raised in conjunction with criminal liability for injuring or killing a fetus. These include the interpretation of statutes, the evolution of the common law, and the proper functions of the judiciary and the legislature. We will need to consider the distinction between civil and criminal law, and how much consistency is possible or desirable in these two areas of law. We will also need to consider the social and political impact of treating feticide as a form of homicide.

Prenatal Neglect

A number of commentators advocate subjecting women to criminal penalties for behavior during pregnancy that harms a viable fetus.[78] In Chapter 4, I argue that such an approach is not warranted on public-policy grounds; that it is unlikely to protect any babies, while being certain to infringe women's rights to privacy and bodily self-determination. In this section, I would like to stress that such an approach is not legally warranted either.

It is sometimes claimed that the imposition of criminal liability follows from the existence of civil liability. In a Comment in the *Whittier Law Journal*, the author notes that the court in *Grodin* imposed civil liability on a woman for damage to her fetus, and concludes, "Therefore, if both a third person and a pregnant woman can be held equally culpable for negligent harm to a viable fetus, then it logically follows that the prospective mother should be subject to criminal sanctions resulting from identical conduct."[79] Nothing of the kind follows. From the fact that someone is civilly liable for injuring another, it does not follow that he or she is criminally liable. The degree of culpability for criminal liability is much higher than it is for civil liability, because the penalty imposed by the criminal law (imprisonment) is so much more serious than that imposed by the civil law (payment of damages). In general, criminal wrongs are those that merit moral condemnation by the community.[80] *Grodin*, cited in the earlier-quoted Comment as a "perfect example"[81] of maternal obligation, carries no

77. National Conference on State Legislatures (NCSL). 2010. "Fetal Homicide Laws." http://www.ncsl.org/IssuesResearch/Health/FetalHomicideLaws/tabid/14386/Default.aspx. Accessed November 6, 2010.

78. See, for example, Margery Shaw. 1984. "Conditional Prospective Rights of the Fetus," *Journal of Legal Medicine* 5; John E. B. Myers.1984. "Abuse and Neglect of the Unborn: Can the State Intervene?" 23 *Duquesne Law Review* 1; and Michael A. Shekey. 1987. Comment, "Criminal Liability of a Prospective Mother for Prenatal Neglect of a Viable Fetus," 9 *Whittier Law Review* 363 (hereafter "Prenatal Neglect").

79. "Prenatal Neglect" (see note 78), p. 387.

80. See J.C. Smith and Brian Hogan. 1978. *Criminal Law*, 4th ed. London: Butterworths, pp. 4–8, 20–21.

81. "Prenatal Neglect" (see note 78), p. 387.

implication of moral wrong. The harm to the child (discolored teeth) was hardly egregious, the mother did not act recklessly or wantonly in taking a prescribed medicine, and the "penalty" was imposed, not on the mother, but on the insurance company. It is ludicrous to imagine that criminal sanctions might be imposed against Mrs. Grodin. Even where the culpability is much greater, and the mother's actions morally condemnable, there are compelling policy reasons not to impose criminal liability on women for their behavior during pregnancy (see Chapter 4).

Homicide

THE BORN-ALIVE RULE

Since at least the 14th century, the destruction of a fetus in utero has not been held a homicide at common law.[82] Only someone who has been born alive can be the victim of a homicide. This is known as the "born-alive rule" (BAR). A number of commentators have criticized the rule,[83] calling it arbitrary and illogical because it permits a conviction for homicide if the fetus survives birth, however briefly. If the same fetus is stillborn, however, it cannot be the victim of a homicide.

Clarke Forsythe, Staff Counsel for Americans United for Life Legal Defense Fund, argues that the BAR is obsolete. He maintains that if we examine the origins of the rule, we will see that it was "entirely an evidentiary standard, mandated by the primitive medical knowledge and technology of the era"[84] Before the 20th century, it was difficult to determine whether the fetus died as the result of an attack on the mother, or from natural causes. Live birth was required to prove that the fetus was alive in the womb at the time of the attack, since obviously there can be no homicide if the "victim" was already dead. Today, medical technological advances, such as fetal heart monitoring, ultrasound examinations, and fetal autopsies, make it possible to know whether the fetus was living at the time of the material acts, what gestational stage it had attained, and the cause of its death. According to Forsythe, the problems of proof that led to the formulation of the BAR no longer exist, and therefore the rule should be dropped.

I think that Forsythe is wrong about the purely evidentiary nature of the BAR. It seems rather that there are three reasons why the common law insisted on live birth for a homicide conviction, only one of which is evidentiary. That is the reason Forsythe gives—namely, that in the past it was not possible to be sure that a miscarriage or stillbirth was the result of the attack on the pregnant woman, or whether the fetus was dead before the attack. Indeed, in the past, it was not always clear if the woman was even pregnant. However, in addition to this evidentiary reason, there are two other reasons why live birth traditionally has been considered significant.

---

82. *Commonwealth* v. *Cass*, 392 Mass. 799, 467 N.E.2d 1324, 1328 (1984).

83. See John T. Shannon. 1987–1988. Note, "A Fetus Is Not a 'Person' as the Term Is Used in the Manslaughter Statute" (hereinafter "A Fetus Is Not a 'Person'), 10 *University of Arkansas at Little Rock Law Journal* 403 and Clarke D. Forsythe. 1987. "Homicide of the Unborn Child: The Born Alive Rule and Other Legal Anachronisms," 21 *Valparaiso University Law Review* 563.

84. Forsythe, "Homicide of the Unborn Child" (see note 83), p. 564.

First, prior to live birth, the fetus was considered to be a part of the pregnant woman, and not a separate existence. As Justice Holmes said in *Dietrich*,[85] it was not *in esse* until it was born alive. Second, a fetus is not yet a fully developed human being, a person like the rest of us. This was expressed by the great common-law authority, Sir Edward Coke, who held that the killing of a fetus is a "great misprision, and no murder." But if the child is born alive and then dies from the attack on its mother, this is murder, "for in law it is accounted a reasonable creature, *in rerum natura*, when it is born alive."[86] Blackstone, in his Commentaries, closely followed Coke. "[T]he person killed must be a 'reasonable creature in being and under the king's peace,' at the time of the killing, . . ."[87]

Forsythe argues that the "reasonable creature" requirement is itself based on evidentiary considerations. He points out that in his section on the "law of persons," Blackstone says that the right to life—the most basic right of persons—begins as soon as the infant is able to stir in the mother's womb—that is, at quickening, when the fetus was considered to be alive. Yet although Blackstone ascribes a right to life to the quick fetus, he nevertheless maintains that the killing of a quick fetus is not murder. This sounds contradictory, Forsythe says, but only if the BAR is taken to be substantive. "There is no contradiction when the born alive rule is recognized to be an evidentiary principle that was required by the state of medical science of the day. Thus, Blackstone held that the unborn child was a 'person' with a right to life at quickening, but recognized that proof of the denial of that right at common law could not be obtained without live birth."[88]

Blackstone may have been influenced by evidentiary considerations. However, this explanation does not cohere with the fact that the common law did not allow recovery for prenatally inflicted wounds by a child who survived live birth. The reason for refusing to allow such suits was not the evidentiary problem of proving that the plaintiff's injuries were caused by the defendant's negligence. Rather, it was universally held that the defendant owed no duty of care to a being that was not *in esse* at the time of the negligence.

It seems, then, that neither the requirement of separate existence, nor that of being a reasonable creature, is based solely on the difficulties of proving that the attack on the pregnant woman killed the fetus. If the BAR is properly interpreted as a substantive definition of a legal person, and is not merely evidentiary, it is not made obsolete by advances in medical technology.[89]

It could be argued that even if the BAR was not formulated entirely because of problems of proof, nevertheless only such considerations support the rule. For

85. *Dietrich v. Northampton*, 138 Mass. 14 (1884).

86. Edward Coke. 1628. *The Third Part of the Institutes of the Laws of England* 50 (Garland Pub. Reprint 1979). Cited in Forsythe, "Homicide of the Unborn Child" (see note 83), p. 583.

87. W. Blackstone. 1765. Commentaries on the Laws of England 198 (University of Chicago Press Facsimile 1979). Cited in Forsythe, "Homicide of the Unborn Child" (see note 83), p. 585.

88. Forsythe, "Homicide of the Unborn Child" (see note 83), p. 586.

89. My argument that the BAR is properly interpreted as a substantial definition of a legal person was cited by the Connecticut Supreme Court in *State v. Courchesne*, 296 Conn. 622, 998 A.2d 1, June 15, 2010, fn 47. See also Kristin Savell. 2006. "Is the 'Born Alive' Rule Outdated and Indefensible?" 28 *Sydney Law Review* 625, 633.

example, it might be argued that it is simply untrue that the fetus is only a part of its mother, like a limb or an organ. From conception onward, it has its own unique genetic code, and, unlike any mere bodily part of the pregnant woman, is developing into a being capable of independent existence. As a matter of biological fact, the separate existence of the fetus throughout pregnancy must be conceded. It is not a mere body part. On the other hand, neither is the pregnant woman a mere "fetal container."[90] The geography of pregnancy—the fact that the fetus is inside the mother and capable of being affected only through her body—provides very strong reasons for refusing to treat the fetus as a separate legal entity prior to live birth.

Even if there are good reasons not to extend legal personhood to fetuses, it could be argued that the similarities between a newly born infant and a nearly born infant are sufficiently great that late-gestation fetuses deserve some legal protection, especially since punishing individuals who attack pregnant women, killing their fetuses, does not raise the issues of privacy and bodily self-determination that are central to the abortion debate. Moreover, sometimes the behavior is so egregious that prosecution for murder seems not only warranted, but called for.

MURDER

During the 1980s, many state courts used the BAR to prohibit homicide convictions for the deaths of viable fetuses, even in cases where the attacks were vicious and deliberate.[91] For example, Robert Lee Hollis told his estranged wife that he did not want a baby, then forced his hand up her vagina, manually aborting her fetus, alleged to be 28 to 30 weeks old. "In separate indictments, Hollis was charged with murder 'of the unborn infant child' and assault in the first degree on his estranged wife."[92] The Kentucky Supreme Court held that until the fetus was born alive, it was not a "person," as that word is used in the context of criminal-homicide statutes, and could not be the victim of criminal homicide.[93] Another defendant repeatedly struck and kicked his 8 ½ months pregnant girlfriend, killing both her and the fetus.[94] The Illinois Supreme Court held that, although the killing of the woman was murder, the killing of the fetus was not. In *Keeler v. Superior Court of Amador County*,[95] an estranged husband, upon learning that his former wife was pregnant by another man, told her, "I'm going to stomp it out of you," and shoved his knee into her abdomen. She later delivered a stillborn fetus of up to 36 weeks gestation. The California Supreme Court held that an unborn but viable fetus is not a human being within the meaning of the statute defining murder.[96] Its ruling was based partly on the fact that the California legislature had declined to create a crime of feticide. Nor had the California Code Commission, which was supposed to revise all statutes, correct errors and omissions,

90. George J. Annas. 1986. "Pregnant Women as Fetal Containers," *Hastings Center Report* 16 (6): 3–4.

91. Shannon, "A Fetus Is Not a 'Person'" (see note 83), p. 407.

92. *Hollis v. Commonwealth*, 652 S.W.2d 61 (Kentucky 1983), p. 62.

93. Ibid.

94. *People v. Greer*, 79 Ill.2d 103, 402 N.E. 2d 203 (1980).

95. *Keeler v. Superior Court of Amador County*, 2 Cal.3d 619, 470 P.2d 617 (1970).

96. Ibid., 2 Cal.3d at 631.

and recommend enactments to remedy defects, proposed any feticide laws for California. Thus, the *Keeler* court was persuaded that the legislative intent was to exclude fetuses from the homicide statute (much as the Supreme Court of Florida concluded from "legislative silence" that the Florida legislature did not intend to include fetuses under its wrongful-death statute). To include fetuses as subjects of murder would be rewriting the murder statute, not interpreting it. To create a new common-law crime would violate the due-process rights of the defendant.[97]

Not all courts have agreed. In South Carolina, a man stabbed his former wife, who was pregnant with a full-term fetus. The South Carolina Supreme Court stated that it would prospectively apply the state homicide statute to fetuses that could be proved viable at the time of the injury to the mother.[98] The court declared that it had a right and a duty to develop the common law to better serve a changing society, and that it would be grossly inconsistent to classify a fetus as a human being for the purpose of imposing civil liability, but as a nonhuman for the imposition of criminal liability.

When the first edition of this book appeared in 1992, most states followed the common law and held that a fetus, viable or not, could not be the subject of homicide. Since then, at least 38 states have passed fetal homicide laws,[99] and in 21 of these states they apply to the earliest stages of pregnancy.[100] Passage of a fetal homicide law often follows a high-profile case that causes public outrage; the California legislature amended its homicide statute to apply fetuses in reaction to *Keeler*.[101] California courts have interpreted the statute as applying only to the intentional killing (murder) of a fetus.[102] *People v. Smith*[103] held that the statute applied only to viable fetuses, but *Smith* was overruled by *People v. Davis*,[104] in which the court said that, to the extent *Smith* required a fetus to be viable for its murder to be prosecuted, it misconstrued the statute. Another California case, *People v. Apodaca*,[105] concerned the killing of a 22- to 24-week fetus, that is, one on the border of viability. The defendant told his former

97. Ibid., 2 Cal.3d at 633–634.

98. *State v. Horne*, 282 S.C. 444, 319 S.E.2d 703 (1984).

99. They are Alabama, Alaska, Arizona, Arkansas, California, Colorado, Florida, Georgia, Idaho, Illinois, Indiana, Iowa, Kansas, Kentucky, Louisiana, Maine, Maryland, Massachusetts, Michigan, Minnesota, Mississippi, Nebraska, Nevada, North Carolina, North Dakota, Ohio, Oklahoma, Pennsylvania, Rhode Island, South Carolina, South Dakota, Tennessee, Texas, Utah, Virginia, Washington, West Virginia, and Wisconsin (National Conference of State Legislatures. 2010. "Fetal Homicide Laws." http://www.ncsl.org/default.aspx?tabid=14386, Accessed November 6, 2010).

100. They are Alabama, Arizona, Arkansas, Georgia, Idaho, Illinois, Kansas, Kentucky, Louisiana, Minnesota, Nebraska, North Dakota, Ohio, Oklahoma, Pennsylvania, South Carolina, South Dakota, Texas, Utah, West Virginia, and Wisconsin (National Conference of State Legislatures. 2010. "Fetal Homicide Laws." http://www.ncsl.org/default.aspx?tabid=14386, Accessed November 6, 2010.)

101. California Penal Code, sect. 187(a).

102. *People v. Carlson*, 37 Cal. App.3d 349, 358 (1974) ("[T]here is no crime constituting manslaughter of a fetus.").

103. *People v. Smith*, 59 Cal.App.3d 751 (1976).

104. *People v. Davis*, 7 Cal. 4th 797, 872 P.2d 591 (1994).

105. *People v. Apodaca*, 76 Cal. App.3d 479 (1978).

wife, Caroline Apodaca, that he intended to kill her fetus because he was not the father, and she was not going to have anyone else's baby. He tied her up, repeatedly struck her in the stomach, and raped her. "Afterwards, he went to the closet, got a dirty towel from the laundry basket and used it to wipe between Caroline's legs. He showed the towel, which was red with blood, to his former wife and said, 'I've done it. I've killed it.'"[106] As a result of this attack, she gave birth to a dead fetus. The defendant argued that his conviction for murder violated his right to due process of law because section 187 did not notify him as to exactly what stage of development the term "fetus" was intended to cover. The court rejected this argument, saying that the statute, as written, was sufficient to give "all persons of common intelligence ample warning that an assault on a pregnant woman without her consent for the purpose of unlawfully killing her unborn child can constitute the crime of murder."[107] *Apodaca* was not dispositive for the killing of a nonviable fetus being murder since the defendant had no evidence that the fetus was not viable, and that all medical evidence pointed toward viability. However, the subsequent ruling in *Davis* makes it clear that viability is not required for a murder conviction in California. In *People v. Dennis*,[108] the California Supreme Court upheld inclusion of fetal homicide under Penal Code 190.2(3), which makes a defendant eligible for capital punishment if convicted of more than one murder.

This was the fate of Scott Peterson, who murdered his wife, Laci Peterson, who was 8 months pregnant with her first child when she went missing on Christmas Eve, 2002. About one-third of all female murder victims are killed by a past or present intimate partner,[109] and police usually look first at the husband or boyfriend. However, the police did not suspect her husband during the first month after Laci's disappearance, especially because Laci's family and friends strongly defended his innocence. Then in January 2003 it was discovered that Scott had had numerous affairs, including one with a massage therapist, Amber Frey. She went to the police when she learned that Scott was married to a missing woman. Frey told the police that 2 weeks before Laci's disappearance, Peterson had implied that he was a widower by telling her that he had "lost" his wife. This convinced Laci's family that Scott had planned to kill Laci long before her disappearance. On April 14, 2003, the body of a dead male fetus was washed ashore in the San Francisco Bay in a park north of Berkeley, where Peterson had been boating the day of Laci's disappearance. A day later, a partial female torso missing its hands, feet, and head was found in the same area. The body was identified as Laci Peterson; the fetus was confirmed to be hers.

Peterson was arrested on April 18, 2003, on a golf course. At the time, he had on his person "approximately $15,000 in cash; four cell phones; multiple credit cards belonging to various members of his family; an array of camping equipment, including knives, implements for warming food, tents and tarpaulins and also a water purifier; a dozen pairs of shoes; several changes of clothing; a t-handled double-edged dagger; a MapQuest map to Frey's workplace (printed the previous day); a shovel; rope;

106. Ibid., p. 484.

107. Ibid., 76 Cal. App.3d at 486.

108. *People v. Dennis*, 17 Cal. 4th 468, 950 P.2d 1035 (1994).

109. National Center for Injury Prevention and Control. 2003. *Costs of Intimate Partner Violence Against Women in the United States*. Atlanta, GA: Centers for Disease Control and Prevention.

24 blister packs of sleeping pills; Viagra; and his brother's driver's license."[110] Prosecutors alleged that the motive for the murder was the affair with Frey, as well as concerns about money and having to support a family. The defense based its case on the lack of direct evidence and suggested that Laci had been kidnapped by a Satanic cult, held until she gave birth, and then both bodies were dumped in the bay. "However, the prosecution's medical experts were able to prove that the baby had never grown to full term, and died at the same time as his mother."[111] The jury, convinced that Peterson planned Laci's murder, convicted Peterson of murder in the first degree for Laci. For the fetus, he was convicted of murder in the second degree, which does not require premeditation. At this writing, Scott Peterson is on death row in San Quentin State Prison while he appeals to the California Supreme Court. He continues to maintain his innocence.

The deaths of Laci and her unborn son, whom the couple had planned to call "Conner," led to the passage of the federal Unborn Victims of Violence Act, widely known as "Laci and Conner's law."[112] It was signed into law on April 1, 2004, by President George W. Bush. The President's action culminated a 5-year campaign by the National Right to Life Committee (NRLC) to win enactment of the legislation. The law recognizes a "child in utero" as a legal victim if he or she is injured or killed during any of over 60 federal crimes of violence. As a federal law, the law applies only to certain offenses over which the federal government has jurisdiction, such as crimes committed on federal property. In addition, it applies to certain crimes defined by statute as federal offenses, such as certain crimes of terrorism. Federal criminal law does not apply to crimes prosecuted by the states. However, courts have given fairly expansive interpretations of federal jurisdiction. If a defendant used anything that traveled across state lines, he probably could be charged federally. I have not been able to find any prosecutions under the Unborn Victims of Violence Act, and it is unlikely that the federal government would become involved, unless there was no state law permitting prosecution. Undoubtedly, the passage of the Act was motivated more by political concerns than by a real interest in prosecuting cases, and its significance may be more symbolic than actual.

The sheer viciousness of the attacks in *Greer, Apodoca, Keeler,* and *Hollis* led many people to support convictions for murder. A different approach treats the fact that the attack causes the death of a fetus as an aggravating factor, making the assault a more serious crime.[113] This seems particularly appropriate when the woman survives the attack that kills her fetus. The loss of her expected child compounds the suffering the attack has caused her. By focusing on the assault on the pregnant woman, laws of this kind do not imply fetal personhood and do not conflict, even in theory, with the right to abortion. The convicted person is punished for what he did to her—namely, forcibly and violently causing her to miscarry. This approach is supported by

110. Wikipedia. 2010. "Scott Peterson." http://en.wikipedia.org/wiki/Scott_Peterson. Accessed November 7, 2010.

111. Ibid.

112. Pub. L. No. 108–212, 118 Stat. 568.

113. Technically, assault is an act by which a person, intentionally or recklessly, causes another to apprehend immediate and unlawful personal violence. The actual infliction of such violence is a battery. In ordinary usage, the term "assault" is used to cover both assault and battery.

Lynn Paltrow, executive director of National Advocates for Pregnant Women, who says, "The assault is first and foremost on the woman, and to create laws that separate the woman from the fetus distracts from the violence women face and from solutions that would truly protect both mothers and babies."[114] Pregnant women are particularly vulnerable to assault and murder. Homicide is the second most common cause of injury-related death among pregnant women and new mothers, according to a 2005 CDC study.[115]

On an aggravated assault approach, fetal viability should not be a condition for conviction, since losing a pregnancy at any stage would be an additional trauma, aggravating the seriousness of the assault. However, the punishment for causing a woman to lose a baby late in her pregnancy should be more severe, as her suffering will undoubtedly be greater the closer she is to giving birth. Similarly, a specific intent to kill the fetus should not be necessary to convict someone of aggravated assault (although it might affect the severity of the sentence). It would be enough that the defendant knew, or should have known, that the woman was pregnant when he attacked her.

A few states have adopted the aggravated assault approach, although the trend appears to be toward fetal homicide laws. Which approach is dictated by the interest view? The interest view maintains that early-gestation fetuses are not harmed by being killed, and so the wrong is a wrong to the expectant parent or parents, not the fetus. However, the interest view acknowledges that late-gestation fetuses, capable of experiencing and valuing their lives in at least a rudimentary way, have some interest in continued existence, albeit a fairly weak time-relative interest (see Chapter 2). There is therefore no conceptual bar to ascribing to them a right to life for the purpose of acknowledging them as homicide victims. When a pregnant woman in late pregnancy is murdered, as in the Laci Peterson case, the aggravated assault approach, which focuses on the loss to the pregnant woman, seems inadequate: a dead woman cannot grieve for the loss of her expected child. The aggravated assault approach seems to leave out an essential element—namely, that an innocent victim has been deprived of his or her life. According to the National Right to Life Committee, polls have shown that 56%–84% of Americans believe that two murder charges, not one, are merited when a pregnant woman is killed. Douglas Johnson, its legislative director, says that in his experience, the families of murdered pregnant women do not say, "My daughter was deprived of her reproductive rights." They say, "He killed the baby." This is irrespective of their position on abortion.[116]

Everyone agrees that crimes of violence against pregnant women should be punished severely. The question is whether changing the common law to allow fetuses to be homicide victims threatens the rights of women. It seems clear that many of those who advocate this change have a larger agenda: the ultimate abolition of abortion and the coercion of pregnant women to protect the fetus.

114. France, "The Laci Effect" (see note 76), p. 250.

115. Jeani Chang et al. 2005. "Homicide: A Leading Cause of Injury Deaths Among Pregnant and Post-Partum Women in the United States, 1991–1999," *American Journal of Public Health* 95:471–477.

116. France, "The Laci Effect" (see note 76), p. 250.

This was made clear in the case of Sean Patrick Merrill, who was charged in Minnesota with murder for killing his girlfriend and the 28-day-old embryo she was carrying at the time of her death. Mr. Merrill is widely believed to be the first person charged with homicide of a fetus in such an early stage of development. His lawyers say there is no evidence that either the defendant or the woman, Gail Anderson, knew she was pregnant when Mr. Merrill was alleged to have killed her with a shotgun blast to the chest in November 1988. Arguing that the law has "profound implications" that go beyond the arena of criminal homicide, the Minnesota Civil Liberties Union wrote in a brief that "if fetuses are persons within the meaning of the 14th Amendment, it is difficult to imagine how a state could constitutionally permit abortion." Pro-life advocates agree. Laurie Anne Ramsey, director of public affairs for Americans United for Life, said fetal-homicide statutes "sensitize the public to the fact that the unborn child—at any stage of his or her development—deserves protection and does have rights." Ms. Ramsey went on to say, "Such laws will make people think about the humanity of the unborn child; to understand that abortion—like murder—is violence against a member of our society."[117]

We need to keep the threat to abortion rights in mind when considering the merits of the born alive rule. The aggravated-assault approach does not threaten women's rights to privacy and autonomy. As long as assaults against pregnant women that cause them to miscarry can be punished sufficiently severely, the aggravated-assault approach, despite its limitations when both mother and fetus are killed, may be preferable to abrogating the BAR.

Vehicular Homicide

Most vehicular-homicide statutes make it a felony to cause the death of "another person" by driving recklessly or driving while intoxicated. In recent years, a number of courts have considered the question of whether a fetus should be considered a "person" for the purposes of vehicular homicide. The highest court in at least one state has refused to uphold vehicular-homicide convictions involving the demise of a fetus.[118]

A notable exception is the Supreme Judicial Court of Massachusetts in *Commonwealth v. Cass*.[119] The case involved a female pedestrian, 8½ months pregnant, who was struck by a car. The fetus died in the womb and was delivered by cesarean section. The autopsy revealed that the fetus was viable at the time of the incident and that it died of internal injuries caused by the impact of the vehicle operated by the defendant. The court had to decide whether a viable fetus is a "person" within the meaning of the vehicular-homicide statute. The court ruled that it was, although it applied this prospectively. On due-process grounds, its decision was not applied to the instant case, saying that the decision may not have been foreseeable.

The court's decision was based on two arguments. The first concerned legislative intent. The court held that it was reasonable to assume that the legislature intended the statute to include viable fetuses. This assumption was based in part on the "ordinary"

---

117. William E. Schmidt. 1990. "Murder Trial Now Focus of Abortion Debate," *The New York Times*, Friday, June 15, B5.

118. *State v. Trudell*, 243 Kan. 29, 755 P.2d 511 (1988).

119. *Commonwealth v. Cass*, 392 Mass. 799, 467 N.E.2d 1324 (1984).

meaning of the word *person*, which the court took to be synonymous with "human being": "An offspring of human parents cannot reasonably be considered to be other than a human being, and therefore a person, first within, and then in normal course outside, the womb."[120] In addition, the Supreme Judicial Court had already ruled, in *Mone v. Greyhound Lines, Inc.*,[121] that a viable fetus would be considered a person for purposes of the state's wrongful-death statute: "Despite the fact that *Mone* was a civil case, we can reasonably infer that, in enacting [Mass. Gen. Laws tit. XIV, ch. 90] § 24G, the Legislature contemplated that the term 'person' would be construed to include viable fetuses."[122]

The court's second argument was that the BAR was based on evidentiary considerations that have been made obsolete by advances in medical technology. It decided to formulate a "better rule": "that infliction of prenatal injuries resulting in the death of a viable fetus, before or after it is born, is homicide."[123]

Justice Wilkins dissented, joined by Justices Liacos and Abrams. The dissenters dismissed as totally implausible the majority's claim that the legislature intended to include fetuses in the vehicular-homicide statute. "Nowhere does the court explain why the Legislature should be assumed to have disregarded hundreds of years of the criminal common law nor why this court should ignore the commendable judicial restraint of every other court that has considered the point."[124] Justice Wilkins characterized the decision as "an inappropriate exercise of raw judicial power."[125]

Cass has been widely criticized as a usurpation of legislative power, both by scholars[126] and judges, who have held that the matter "must be left to the good judgment of the legislature, which has the primary authority to create crimes."[127] Several states have done just this. For example, in 1999, Florida enacted a vehicular-homicide law that makes it a crime to kill a viable fetus in a car accident.[128] Its law was enacted in response to vigorous lobbying on behalf of a woman whose daughter and grandson were killed in a car accident along with the daughter's unborn child.[129]

120. Ibid., 467 N.E.2d at 1325.

121. *Mone v. Greyhound Lines, Inc.*, 368 Mass. 354, 331 N.E.2d 916 (1975).

122. *Cass* (see note 118), 467 N.E.2d at 1326.

123. Ibid., at 1329.

124. Ibid., at 1330.

125. Ibid (quotation omitted).

126. See, for example, Bruce Palmer. 1986. Note, "State Protection of Future Persons: *Commonwealth v. Cass*," 18 *Connecticut Law Review* 429; J. H. Henn. 1986. Comment, "Vehicular Homicide of a Viable Fetus–Judicial Statutory Amendment," 70 *Massachusetts Law Review* 201.

127. *State* ex rel. *Atkinson v. Wilson*, 175 W. Va. 352, 332 S.E.2d 807, 813 (1984).

128. Fla. Stat. Ann. § 782.071.

129. Sandra L. Smith. 2000. Note, "Fetal Homicide: Woman or Fetus as Victim? A Survey of Current State Approaches and Recommendations for Future State Application," 41 *William & Mary Law Review* 1845, p. 1857.

Arkansas originally subscribed to the BAR, as evidenced in its 1987 ruling in *Meadows v. State*.[130] In *Meadows*, a drunk driver killed the driver of an oncoming car, as well as the viable fetus of a pregnant passenger, and the defendant was convicted of two counts of manslaughter. The Supreme Court of Arkansas held that the fetus was not a "person" for purposes of the manslaughter statute. The court determined that such a decision should be made by the legislature; to do otherwise would create a new common-law crime.[131] The Arkansas legislature responded to *Meadows* by enacting a statute enlarging the crime of battery to include injuries to pregnant women resulting in miscarriage. "As a further reaction to the *Meadows* decision, the Arkansas legislature recently enacted a comprehensive fetal protection act and amended the Arkansas Code to expand the definition of 'person' to include fetuses at twelve weeks of development.[132] Accordingly, Arkansas is unique because it has laws protecting both women and fetuses."[133]

Kansas is another state with an inconsistent approach to fetal vehicular homicide. In *State v. Burrell*,[134] the defendant was charged with two counts of involuntary manslaughter after running a stop sign, striking another car, and killing a passenger and her viable fetus. "The [Kansas Supreme C]ourt, without comment, appeared to abandon the born alive rule by reversing, on other grounds, the trial court's dismissal of the two charges, and remanding the case."[135] But 3 years later, in *State v. Trudell*,[136] the Kansas Supreme Court upheld the BAR when it held that the district court properly ruled that a viable fetus was not a "human being" within the meaning of the aggravated vehicular-homicide statute. In 1995, the Kansas legislature responded to these cases with two new laws providing penalties for injuries that cause pregnant women to miscarry. One statute relates to injuries causing miscarriage inflicted in the commission of a felony or misdemeanor, the other to miscarriage-producing injuries caused by a vehicle. Originally, the bill was drafted to define a " 'preborn human being' as 'a human being in existence from fertilization until birth.' "[137] Abortion-rights advocates protested that this could make abortion first-degree murder. "The legislature revised the proposal and modeled it after New Mexico's laws penalizing those who cause miscarriages by injury to the woman. Additionally, like the New Mexico statutes, the Kansas statute does not specify the fetus's gestational age. Pro-choice and pro-life activists were pleased with the final result."[138]

Statutes that treat fetuses as persons, even for a rather narrow and desirable purpose, might serve as a wedge, opening the door to legislation that protects fetuses at the expense of women's rights of privacy and self-determination. A legislative

130. *Meadows v. State*, 291 Ark. 105, 722 S.W.2d 584 (1987).

131. Ibid.

132. See Ark. Code Ann. § 5–1–102(13)(B). Cited in Smith (see note 128), p. 1859.

133. Smith, Fetal Homicide (see note 128), p. 1859.

134. *State v. Burell*, 237 Kan. 303, 699 P.2d 499 (1985).

135. Smith, Fetal Homicide (see note 128), p. 1866.

136. *State v. Trudell*, 243 Kan. 29, 755 P.2d 511 (1988).

137. Smith, Fetal Homicide (see note 128), p. 1868.

138. Smith, Fetal Homicide (see note 128), pp. 1868–1869.

approach that focuses on the harm to the pregnant woman, and does not make the fetus a separate victim, seems the preferable approach. In the words of one commentator:

> Proposals using this alternative focus have received less opposition from pro-choice advocates, and, if the statutes are crafted carefully, will likely enjoy support from both pro-choice and antiabortion advocates, as well as groups concerned about the effects of domestic violence. Although these laws would not result in separate prosecutions for fetal deaths or injuries, they would provide a greater level of comfort for victims' families than laws in states that do not punish third-party harms to fetuses.[139]

A novel twist in the debate over the protection of fetuses by vehicular-homicide statutes occurred when the driver who was charged with killing the fetus was also its mother.[140] On the evening of July 14, 1989, Beth Levey, 8½ months pregnant, stopped at a bar in Waltham, Massachusetts. Authorities say that she drank five gin-and-tonics and then drove away, hitting first a parked car and then a utility pole.[141] She was found slumped over the wheel. Her fetus was stillborn, the imprint of the steering wheel in its head. Ms. Levey was indicted for several charges, including operating a motor vehicle under the influence of alcohol, but she was also charged with felony motor-vehicle homicide. It was the first time anyone had been prosecuted in a comparable situation anywhere in the United States.

Middlesex County District Attorney Scott Harshbarger brought the homicide charge against Ms. Levey for two reasons. First, he considered this to be an egregious drunk-driving case, because her blood alcohol content was very high and she had a previous conviction for drunk driving.[142] As it happened, she hurt herself and lost her own baby, but she could very well have injured someone else. Second, Mr. Harshbarger said that he had "no option," given the decision by the Massachusetts Supreme Court in *Cass*, which held that the vehicular-homicide statute includes viable fetuses. In a public statement he issued, defending his decision to prosecute, Mr. Harshbarger wrote, "Until that decision is overruled or limited, or until the legislature acts, I feel obliged to proceed."[143] If another pregnant woman had been in Ms. Levey's car, and she lost her viable unborn child as a result of the accident, Ms. Levey would undoubtedly have been charged with vehicular homicide. So why should the fact that the dead fetus was her own be a reason not to charge her? It would not be a reason if the victim was Ms. Levey's own born child. Drunk drivers often kill the people they love most. Sympathy for their loss may be relevant at the sentencing stage, on the ground that the person has already suffered enough, but it is not considered a reason for not prosecuting.

139. Smith, Fetal Homicide (see note 128), p. 1884.

140. *Commonwealth v. Levey*, Nos. 89–2725-2729 (Mass. Superior Court, 1989).

141. Christopher B. Daly. 1989. "Woman Charged in Death of Own Fetus in Accident," *Washington Post*, November 25, A4.

142. Ibid.

143. Ibid.

The defense argued that *Cass* was not a relevant precedent, because it addressed only the case in which a pregnant woman was herself the victim of violence. The cases cited by the Court in *Cass* were exclusively cases in which a third party intentionally and brutally harmed a woman. "The Court did not—nor could it—cite a single civil case in which a mother was held liable for wrongful death, much less a single criminal case in which a mother was prosecuted for vehicular homicide."[144] The defense called the application of the vehicular-homicide statute to this case "a grotesque extension of the criminal law."[145]

The defense acknowledged that the common law of torts has evolved to allow recovery for prenatal injuries; however, with very few exceptions, this has been limited to third parties. The defense argued that the rationale for the extension of liability was not to protect the fetus, but "to vindicate the mother's interest in having a live, uninjured child."[146] It interpreted *Bonbrest* v. *Kotz*,[147] the first case allowing a surviving child to recover for injuries indicted in utero, as vindicating the interests of the parents, not the child, nor the fetus.

In my view, this reading of *Bombrest* is mistaken. While permitting recovery for prenatal torts is not aimed at vindicating the interests of the *fetus*, neither is it aimed at vindicating the interests of the *parents*. Rather, it is the *surviving child* who has been injured and who deserves compensation. This interpretation not only gives the most plausible explanation of the law but also vindicates the interest view, which is the foundation of this book. The interest view enables the important distinction between actions brought by surviving children for prenatally inflicted injuries from prenatal wrongful-death suits. The interests of the parents are vindicated in prenatal wrongful-death suits, but it is the interests of the surviving child that are vindicated in prenatal-injury cases. It may be wise social policy not to allow children to sue their mothers for prenatally caused injuries, but we should not pretend that the justification is that the only interests involved are those of the mother.

The fundamental question raised by *Levey* is the rationale for punishing someone whose negligent or reckless driving causes the death of a fetus. If the rationale focuses on the harm done to the pregnant woman, as the defense argued, then it is absurd to press charges when the pregnant woman herself is the driver. On the other hand, if the rationale is that a viable fetus is entitled to the protection of the state or commonwealth, then it is irrelevant that the person responsible for causing the death is the mother.

This issue was never resolved because the prosecution entered a *nolle prosequi*. This is an entry on the record of a legal action denoting that the prosecutor will proceed no further with the action. The district attorney decided not to prosecute further for several reasons. First, Ms. Levey had already pleaded guilty to several lesser charges, including operating under the influence of alcohol. As part of her sentence, she was ordered to complete a 14-day residential alcoholism-treatment program, after which the charges were dropped, and she was prohibited from driving

144. *Commonwealth v. Levey*, Nos. 89–2725-2729, *Memorandum in Support of Motion to Dismiss*, p. 9.

145. Ibid., p. 3.

146. Ibid., p. 9.

147. *Bonbrest v. Kotz* (see note 4).

during her period of 5 years probation. Finally, a review of confidential medical records regarding the diagnosis and treatment of the defendant and her fetus indicated that the fetus was alive for a long time after Ms. Levey was hospitalized. Certain standard medical procedures had not been performed; for example, she was not put on a fetal monitor and her placenta was not checked for damage. If these procedures had been done, the fetus's death (which the autopsy indicated was due to placental abruption, not the trauma to the head) could have been prevented.

The entry of a *nolle prosequi* in the *Levey* case left open the question of whether other pregnant women could be prosecuted for vehicular homicide in Massachusetts. The defense lawyers argued that the implications of such prosecutions would be ominous:

> . . . if it is appropriate for the courts to interpret "personhood" for the vehicular homicide statutes, then it could be no less appropriate for the courts to reinterpret "personhood" for all offenses under the criminal law. If *Cass* is seen as announcing the principle that a viable fetus is a person for purposes of the criminal law, then pregnant women will be at risk of prosecution for a host of offenses deriving from what they did or did not do during pregnancy—from negligent driving to delivering alcohol or controlled substances to a minor."[148]

To my knowledge, after *Levey*, no other woman in Massachusetts—or anywhere else in the United States—has ever been prosecuted for vehicular homicide for the death of her own fetus. Nevertheless, as we will see in the next chapter, prosecutions against women for behavior during pregnancy that was held to harm, or risk harming, their unborn children have taken place. While they are not ruled out by the interest view, I will argue in Chapter 4 that there are substantial policy reasons not to use the criminal law against pregnant women as a means for protecting "not-yet-born" children.

WRONGFUL LIFE

"Wrongful-life" suits are suits in which infants with birth defects seek to recover damages from allegedly negligent physicians.[149]

These suits differ in important ways from ordinary medical malpractice suits, and they raise special legal and philosophical questions. While most jurisdictions allow "wrongful-birth" suits (distinguished from wrongful-life suits in the following discussion), only California, New Jersey, and Washington recognize wrongfullife as stating a legally cognizable cause of action.

148. *Memorandum in Support of Motion to Dismiss* (see note 143), p. 19.

149. I have drawn on my previous writings on wrongful life for this section, including "The Logical Case for 'Wrongful Life,'" *Hastings Center Report* 16:2 (April 1986), pp. 15–20; a report prepared under contract for the Office of Technology Assessment, U.S. Congress, Washington, D.C., "Ethical Implications of Population Screening for Cystic Fibrosis: The Concept of Harm and Claims of Wrongful Life"; and "When Is Birth Unfair to the Child?" co-authored with Ronald McClamrock, *Hastings Center Report* 24:6 (November-December 1994), pp. 15–21.

The claim in a wrongful-life suit is not that the negligence of the physician was the cause of the child's impairment. It is, rather, that the physician, by failing to inform the parents adequately, is responsible for the birth of an impaired child who otherwise would not have been born and therefore would not have experienced the suffering caused by the impairment. The plaintiff in a wrongful-life suit is the child; typically, such suits are brought by the parents on behalf of the infant plaintiff. By contrast, in "wrongful-birth" suits, the plaintiffs are the parents, who claim that because of negligence on the part of health care providers or laboratories (either in performing failed sterilizations or abortions, often referred to as "wrongful conception" suits, or in giving improper advice about the risk of having children with serious birth defects), the parents were wrongfully deprived of the option to abort. The distinction between wrongful-birth and wrongful-life suits is critical, because the legal basis for each is quite distinct. Nevertheless, the two kinds of suits are frequently confused in the mind of the public and in the media. For example, a newspaper story about *DeChico v. Northern Westchester Hospital Center*[150] reported that "New York provides for 'wrongful life' actions where 'malpractice by a physician deprived the parent of the opportunity to terminate the pregnancy within the legally permissible time period.'"[151] In fact, New York courts have never accepted wrongful life as a cause of action. *DeChico* acknowledged a cause of action on behalf of the parents, that is, a wrongful-birth suit.[152] As the result of a growing recognition of the responsibilities of medical workers to meet ordinary standards of care in advising parents about the risk of genetic abnormalities, and a corresponding recognition of the rights of parents to collect damages when these standards are not met, wrongful-birth suits have met with increasing success in the courts.[153] There has been considerably more resistance to wrongful-life suits.

The infant plaintiffs in wrongful-life cases typically have severe and often multiple disabilities, both mental and physical. They may suffer from such crippling and sometimes fatal ailments as cystic fibrosis, neurofibromatosis, polycystic kidney disease, or Tay-Sachs disease. They typically require expensive medical care and often need special education and training. It seems only fair that such children, whose impaired existence is allegedly due to the negligence of others, should have a legal remedy. At the same time, it is acknowledged that the negligent parties are not responsible for the children's handicaps. Nothing the physician did, or failed to do, caused the child to be born blind or severely developmentally disabled or sick. Had the physician acted properly and nonnegligently, the child would not have been born

150. *DeChico v. Northern Westchester Hospital Center*, 73 A.D.3d 838, 900 N.Y.S.2d 743 [2010].

151. Mark Fass. 2010. "N.Y. Court Throws Out 'Wrongful Life' Suit Over Birth of Brain-Damaged Child," New York Law Journal, May 17. http://www.law.com/jsp/article.jsp?id=1202458273287. Accessed November 6, 2010.

152. *DeChico* (see note 149), 73 AD3d at 840 ("Although a child may not maintain a wrongful life cause of action, a parent may, under some circumstances, maintain a cause of action on his or her own behalf for the extraordinary costs incurred in raising a child with a disability.")

153. See, for example, *Berman v. Allan*, 80 N.J. 421, 404 A.2d 8 (1979); *Speck v. Finegold*, 497 Pa. 77, 439 A.2d 110 (1981); *Karlsons v. Guerinot*, 57 A.D.2d 73, 394 N.Y.S.2d 933 (1977); *Harbeson v. Parke-Davis, Inc.*, 98 Wash.2d 460, 656 P.2d. 483 (1983).

healthy—the usual claim in a tort action. Rather, he or she would not have been born at all. In essence, these suits allege that the infants (and not merely their parents) would be better off if they had never been born, that the children themselves have been harmed or wronged by being born. As one commentator expresses it, the decision of prospective parents to avoid birth or conception upon learning that their unborn child is likely to be severely disabled "stems primarily from a genuine concern for the welfare of their potential offspring. Most prospective parents are likely to opt for not burdening their would-be children with an awful existence, intuitively believing that such a devastated life would be worse than no life at all."[154] Some find this claim morally offensive; others regard it as metaphysically puzzling.

The term "wrongful life" was used first in 1963 in *Zepeda v. Zepeda*,[155] in which a healthy infant plaintiff claimed that his father had injured him by causing him to be born illegitimately. The Illinois appellate court declined to permit recovery, fearing that it would be flooded with suits for wrongful life brought by parties born under adverse conditions. Subsequent courts have distinguished between being born under adverse conditions and being born with a severe handicap or fatal disease. Presiding Justice Jefferson wrote for the majority in *Curlender v. Bio-Science Laboratories* (1980):

[A] cause of action based upon impairment of status—illegitimacy contrasted with legitimacy—should not be recognizable at law because a necessary element for the establishment of any cause of action in tort is missing, injury and damages consequential to that injury. A child born with severe impairment, however, presents an entirely different situation because the necessary element of injury is present.[156]

Nevertheless, even if wrongful-life suits are limited to cases involving severe impairment, they pose difficult problems. To see why, let us examine the reasons why courts have rejected wrongful-life suits.

Gleitman v. Cosgrove[157] was an early wrongful-life suit, decided by the New Jersey Supreme Court on March 6, 1967. The Gleitmans contended that the defendant doctors had erroneously assured Mrs. Gleitman that the rubella she had contracted early in her pregnancy posed no risk to her unborn child, who was born deaf, mute, probably developmentally disabled, and nearly blind. The Gleitmans claimed that they would have chosen abortion had they been accurately advised. The New Jersey Supreme Court barred recovery by either the parents or the infant, Jeffrey, holding that there were no damages cognizable at law and also, in the case of his parents, that public policy precluded recovery.

The court rejected Jeffrey's suit on the ground that it was "logically impossible" to measure the infant's alleged damages. The *Gleitman* court asserted that since nonexistence is beyond the experience of juries, there is no reasoned way to calculate

154. Amos Shapira. 1998. "'Wrongful Life' Lawsuits for Faulty Genetic Counselling: Should the Impaired Newborn Be Entitled to Sue?" *Journal of Medical Ethics* 24: 369–375, p. 370.

155. *Zepeda v. Zepeda*, 41 Ill. App.2d 240, 190 N.E.2d 849 (1963).

156. *Curlender v. Bio-Science Laboratories*, 106 Cal.App.3d 811, 825 (1980).

157. *Gleitman v. Cosgrove*, 49 N.J. 22, 227 A.2d 689 (1967).

the difference in value between nonexistence and the child's impaired life. It is an established principle of tort law that damages that are uncertain, contingent, or speculative in nature cannot be made the basis of a recovery. However, the comparison of existence and nonexistence is not unique to wrongful-life cases. In wrongful-death suits, juries must measure damages by comparing the value of the deceased's existence, healthy or impaired, with the value of nonexistence. As one commentator has noted, "If the jury is capable of making this comparison in wrongful-death suits, there is no reason to doubt their ability to make the same comparison in wrongful-life suits."[158]

A related point regarding the assessment of damages was made by the New York Court of Appeals in *Becker v. Schwartz*.[159] The amount paid by a negligent defendant to the successful plaintiff is supposed to be what is needed to restore the injured plaintiff to the position that he or she would have occupied but for the defendant's negligence. But in wrongful-life cases, had the defendant not been negligent, the infant plaintiff would never have existed. "Simply put, a cause of action brought on behalf of an infant seeking recovery for wrongful life demands a calculation of damages dependent upon a comparison between the Hobson's choice of life in an impaired state and nonexistence. This comparison the law is not equipped to make."[160] However, as one commentator notes, "it is frequently the case that tort damages will not put the plaintiff in her original position or make her whole. Money damages are often a poor substitute but, of course, are better than no damage award at all."[161]

A different argument against wrongful-life suits is based on the value of human life. In *Berman v. Allen*,[162] the New Jersey Supreme Court explicitly rejected its earlier rationale offered in *Gleitman* for dismissing the infant plaintiff's cause of action—namely, the difficulty of ascertaining damages. Instead, it based its dismissal on the premise that life, however handicapped, cannot be an injury. The court held that the infant, Sharon Berman, who was born with Down syndrome, would be able to love and be loved and to experience happiness and pleasure, and therefore it could not be said that she would be better off had she never been born.

The *Berman* court was no doubt right that Sharon's life was not an injury to her. Views about Down syndrome have changed dramatically over the last 50 years. Parents who had children with Down syndrome in the 1950s were discouraged from keeping their children at home. Today it is recognized that the symptoms of the disorder can vary from mild to severe. No longer are children routinely consigned to institutions; they live at home and attend school. They are also living longer than in previous generations. "Although many children have physical and mental limitations,

158. Dawn Currier. 1983. Note, "The Judicial System's Wrongful Conception of Wrongful Life," 6 *Western New England Law Review* 493.

159. *Becker v. Schwartz*, 46 N.Y.2d 401 (1978).

160. Ibid., at 412.

161. Mark Strasser. 1999. "Wrongful Life, Wrongful Birth, Wrongful Death, and the Right to Refuse Treatment: Can Reasonable Jurisdictions Recognize All But One?" 64 *Missouri Law Review* 29, p. 74.

162. *Berman v. Allan*, 80 N.J. 421, 404 A.2d 8 (1979).

they can live independent and productive lives well into adulthood."[163] It is increasingly recognized that the lives of children with Down syndrome can be happy, even if they cannot be completely normal. However, this decision provides no guidance with respect to the lives of more seriously impaired children. One of the most serious genetic diseases is Tay-Sachs disease, "a rare inherited disorder that progressively destroys nerve cells (neurons) in the brain and spinal cord."[164] The Tay-Sachs child is doomed to a short and increasingly handicapped existence, with death occurring in early childhood. The child appears well at birth and develops normally for 3–6 months, when progressive psychomotor degeneration slowly begins. "As the disease progresses, [the child] experiences seizures, vision and hearing loss, intellectual disability, and paralysis."[165] "Ultimately, the patient will progress to an unresponsive vegetative state with death resulting from bronchopneumonia resulting from aspiration in conjunction with a depressed cough."[166]

There is no comparison between the life of a child with Down syndrome and the life of a child with severe infantile Tay-Sachs disease. The child with Down syndrome can have relationships with other people, learn, and enjoy life, even though his or her life will be limited compared with an unaffected child. By contrast, the life of a baby with Tay-Sachs cannot be seen as a good to that child. The infant cannot see, eat, sit up, or even hold up his or her head, much less crawl around. What possible pleasure can there be in such an existence? The best that can be said is that once the child enters a vegetative state, he or she no longer suffers. But the mere absence of suffering is not sufficient to make life a good.

There are two variations on the argument based on the value of human life. One version, often called "sanctity of life," maintains that life is sacred, a gift from God, and something that it would be wrong to reject. Although its origin is clearly religious, in its secular formulation, it is the view that life, whatever its condition or quality, is of intrinsic value. On this view, there is no such thing as a life not worth living. Those who accept this maintain that life, with whatever disabling conditions and no matter how filled with suffering or devoid of pleasure, must be a good. This seems simply false. A life devoid of any of the things that give meaning to human life—pleasure, the ability to love, to learn, to have relationships—is not a life worth living.

The other version, sometimes referred to as "the disability critique," does not insist that life is sacred or that life is always worth living, whatever its condition. The disability critique can acknowledge that the life of a child with severe infantile Tay-Sachs disease is probably not worth living. However, disability advocates emphasize that this disease is unusually severe, and not indicative of most disabling conditions. (Indeed, one participant, Marsha Saxton, in a Hastings Center working group

163. Google Health–Down Syndrome. https://health.google.com/health/ref/Down+syndrome. Accessed November 6, 2010.

164. Genetics Home Reference–Tay Sachs Disease. Reviewed September 2008. http://ghr.nlm.nih.gov/condition=tay-sachs-disease. Accessed November 6, 2010.

165. Ibid.

166. Tay-Sachs Disease. http://themedicalbiochemistrypage.org/taysachsdisease.html. Accessed November 6, 2010.

on disability and prenatal testing[167] often repeated the mantra, "Tay-Sachs is off the table!") The disability critique emphasizes that the lives of people with disabilities, including extremely severe disabilities, are usually well worth living. It maintains that the common belief that disability is incompatible with life satisfaction is due largely to prejudice and ignorance about the lives of people with disabling conditions. A prominent bioethicist and disability advocate, Adrienne Asch, points to research showing that people with disabilities generally find their lives satisfying. When they do not, it is often not because of the disability itself, but rather because of "societal arrangements that exclude some people from participating in school, work, civic, or social life."[168] It is these social arrangements that need to be fixed, according to disability advocates, rather than preventing the existence of people with disabilities. Because wrongful-life suits maintain that life is a wrong to the child, and indeed, that the child should never have been born, disability advocates typically oppose such suits.

A third argument against wrongful-life suits is that they are logically incoherent. This argument maintains that it is impossible for a person to be better off never having been born. For if I had never been born, then I never was; if I never was, then I cannot be said to have been better off. The problem can be put another way. To be harmed is to be made worse off; but no individual is made worse off by coming to exist, for that suggests that we can compare the person before he existed with the person after he existed, which is absurd. Therefore, it is logically impossible that anyone is harmed by coming to exist and wrongful-life suits are both illogical and unfair in that they require the defendant to compensate someone he has not harmed. As Justice Schreiber noted in his dissent in *Procanik v. Cillo*, "sympathy for a handicapped child and his parents should not lead us to ignore the notions of responsibility, causation and damage that underlie the entire philosophy of our system of justice. It would be unwise—and, what is more, unjust—to permit the plaintiff to recover damages from persons who caused him no injury."[169] The challenge, then, for the advocates of the infant plaintiff is to express precisely the nature of the injury or wrong done to the infant.

One formulation was given by the New York Supreme Court, Appellate Division (an intermediate appellate court) when it upheld a claim for wrongful life in *Park v. Chessin*[170] in 1977. That case concerned an infant born with polycystic kidney disease. The parents already had one child with the condition, who had lived only a few hours after birth. Their obstetrician falsely informed them that polycystic kidney disease was not genetic and therefore the chances were "practically nil" that any subsequent child would be affected. Relying on this advice, Mrs. Park gave birth to a second child, Lara, who lived for 2½ years before succumbing to the fatal disease. In holding that the infant could recover for injuries and conscious pain and suffering, the court cited "the fundamental right of a child to be born as a whole, functioning

167. The final report of this two-year project, "The Disability Rights Critique of Prenatal Genetic Testing," appeared in the *Hastings Center Report* (September-October 1999): S1–S22.

168. Adrienne Asch. 1999. "Prenatal Diagnosis and Selective Abortion: A Challenge to Practice and Policy," *American Journal of Public Health* 89 (11): 1649–1657.

169. *Procanik v. Cillo*, 97 N.J. 339, 371–372, 478 A.2d 755 (1984).

170. *Park v. Chessin*, 60 A.D.2d 80, 400 N.Y.S.2d 110 (1977).

human being."[171] This sweeping claim has been universally rejected by other courts and commentators, and it was overruled the following year when the New York Court of Appeals (New York's highest court) considered *Park v. Chessin* as a companion case to *Becker v. Schwartz*.[172] The court denied that the infants suffered any legally cognizable injury and held that there was no precedent for recognition of a fundamental right to be born as a whole, functional human being.

Another approach is to express the injury to the child in terms of the wrong done to the parents.[173] Alexander Capron argues that the impaired infant has the right to have his or her parents determine whether birth would be in the infant's best interests.[174] Thus, the deprivation of the parents' right to choose abortion is not only a wrong to the parents (as is claimed in a wrongful-birth suit) but also a direct wrong to the infant.

The interpretation is ingenious because it neatly avoids the logical puzzles associated with claiming that the infant was harmed by being born, while it strengthens the infant's cause of action by basing it on the increasingly accepted right of the parents to choose not to have a child with severe impairments. Despite these advantages, I reject Capron's interpretation, because it suggests, implausibly, that the *child* has been wronged whenever; because of the negligence of health care providers, the *parents* are deprived of the choice of abortion.

The implausibility of this view is revealed if we think of an infant born with a relatively minor impairment, something that can be corrected, but not completely, such as a club foot. There may be individuals who would choose abortion rather than have a child with a clubfoot, because they consider life with even a minor disability, such as a limp, to be not worth living. If the doctor negligently fails to inform the parents that the child will have a club foot, he or she wrongs the parents, since they were deprived of the chance to terminate the pregnancy. Yet, according to Capron, the infant has the right to have his parents decide whether birth would be in his or her best interests. It follows that, by depriving the parents of the chance to decide whether life with a club foot is in the child's best interests, the doctor wrongs both the parents and the child. This seems implausible; surely a child born with a minor and fixable defect is not wronged by birth. This suggests that the wrong done to the infant cannot be understood solely in terms of violating the parents' right to decide whether to terminate a pregnancy. The notion of wrongful life cannot be divorced from the welfare of the infant plaintiff.

We cannot either ignore the logical puzzles in wrongful-life suits or sidestep them by construing the infant plaintiff's right as a right to have their parents decide whether birth is in their best interests. The infant plaintiff's claim makes sense only if we recognize that existence itself can sometimes be an injury and that a child who will be forced to live under such conditions has a right not to be born.

171. Ibid., 60 A.D.2d at 88.

172. *Becker v. Schwartz* (see note 158).

173. Alexander M. Capron. 1979. "Tort Liability in Genetic Counseling," 79 *Columbia Law Review* 618; K. J. Jankowski. 1989. "Wrongful Birth and Wrongful Life Actions Arising From Negligent Genetic Counseling: The Need for Legislation Supporting Reproductive Choice," 17 *Fordham Urban Law Journal* 27.

174. Capron, "Tort Liability in Genetic Counseling" (see note 172).

To understand the claim that there can be a right not to be born, we must explain how someone can have an interest in not being born. Fetuses, for most of gestation, do not have interests. So if there is an interest in not being born, it must belong to the born child. A child can be said to have an interest in not being born if his or her existence is inexorably and irreparably such that life is not worth living. Joel Feinberg explains the right not to be born this way: "Talk of a 'right not to be born' is a compendious way of referring to the plausible moral requirement that no child be brought into the world unless certain very minimal conditions of wellbeing are assured. When a child is brought into existence even though those requirements have not been observed, he has been wronged thereby . . . "[175] The crucial idea is that the condition of the infant at birth can doom the child's future interests to total defeat. Feinberg argues that the advance dooming of a child's most basic interests—that is, those that are essential to the existence and advancement of any ulterior interests—deprives the child of what can be called his or her birthrights. And if you cannot have that to which you have a birthright, you are wronged if you are brought to birth.

In *Harm to Others*, Feinberg concedes that the infant plaintiff in a wrongful-life suit has not been, strictly speaking, harmed. For to harm someone is to make that person "worse off"; coming into existence cannot make someone worse off than he or she would otherwise have been. If the physician in these cases had acted properly, the parents would have chosen abortion, and the child would never have existed. Nonexistence is not a *better* condition to be in; *it is no condition at all*. Therefore, Feinberg concludes that the negligent physician in a wrongful-life case cannot be said to have *harmed* the child, because the physician's negligence did not make the child worse off than he or she was. However, the physician can be said to have *wronged* the child by depriving the child of his or her birthright: the right not to be brought into the world if all of one's most basic interests are doomed. In a subsequent article,[176] Feinberg came to the conclusion that it is possible to harm someone by being responsible for his being brought into existence, and that his failure to see this in *Harm to Others* stemmed from the failure to clarify what it means to say that someone has been made "worse off." This phrase is ambiguous. It could be interpreted to mean "worse off than he was before the wrongdoer acted." Feinberg dubs this interpretation "the worsening condition." Clearly, the worsening condition cannot be satisfied in the wrongful-life situation. That is, no one can be worse off than he was before he existed, since this suggests comparing the individual before he existed with the individual after he existed, which is absurd. In some cases, however, the individual who has been harmed is not worse off than he was; rather, he is worse off than he *would have been* had the wrongdoer not acted in he did. This expresses a *counterfactual condition*. Expressed intuitively, the counterfactual claim is that the individual would have been better off not coming into existence, or "better off unborn." Once we distinguish the counterfactual test from the worsening test, Feinberg suggests, the logical problem posed by coming into existence disappears. For although, as we have seen, the worsening condition cannot be satisfied in wrongful-life suits, the possibility

175. Joel Feinberg. 1984. *Harm to Others*. New York: Oxford University Press, p. 101.

176. Joel Feinberg. 1987. "Wrongful Life and the Counterfactual Element in Harming" (hereafter "Wrongful Life"), *Social Philosophy & Policy* 4 (1): 145–178.

remains that the counterfactual condition can be satisfied. And if the counterfactual condition is satisfied, and the plaintiff is "worse off" because of something the defendant did, then the defendant can be said to have harmed the plaintiff. This enables us to place wrongful-life suits squarely within traditional tort concepts. The challenge is to explain what it means to say that someone is "worse off" for coming into existence, or "better off unborn."

It may help to start with the expression "better off dead," a common expression that is not logically odd. To say that someone is better off dead is not to compare her condition while alive with her condition after she is dead. That would be absurd, since after someone ceases to exist, she is in no condition at all. Instead, the phrase "better off dead" simply means that life is so terrible that it is no longer a benefit or a good to the one who lives. In the case of a competent adult, the criterion by which we judge whether a person is better off dead is ordinarily whether the person himself considers life not worth living.[177] This test, however, cannot be applied in the case of infants. It is not just that infants cannot *express* their preferences; they do not yet have the intellectual equipment necessary for *having* the relevant preferences. Infants cannot understand the choice between severely handicapped existence and no existence at all. They cannot weigh up benefits and harms to reach a decision as to whether life is, on balance, worth living. Therefore, it does not make any sense to ask what the infant would want, if he could only tell us. The test of "substituted judgment" is simply inapplicable in the case of never-competent individuals.[178]

What sense, then, can be given to the judgment that the infant would be better off not existing? It might be thought that if we cannot consult the infant's own preferences, then life is necessarily a benefit and a good to the child. The implausibility of this is seen if we consider the example of an infant whose medical condition will dooms the baby to unremitting and unrelievable pain, followed by an early death. An example would be dystrophic epidermolysis bullosa (EB),[179] discussed in Chapter 2. Even if we cannot ascribe a *preference* for nonexistence to the child, for the reasons given earlier, surely we can say that this is a life so awful that no one could possibly wish it for the child. In saying this, we are not making a "substituted judgment," since this is not possible in the case of infants, but rather offering the judgment of a "proxy chooser," someone who acts as the infant's advocate, concerned to promote his or her welfare.

Parents occasionally play this role in deciding whether to continue invasive and painful, treatment on their extremely premature or severely impaired newborns. Sometimes they decide that saving or prolonging the baby's life is not in the baby's

177. I say "ordinarily" to leave open the possibility that someone irrationally prefers death when, objectively speaking, he has, as we say, "everything to live for." Such a person would not be "better off dead," although he might, contrary to reason, believe that he would be. Similarly, someone might really be "better off dead," but irrationally prefer not to die. This would be the case when the only options are a relatively painless death now and a far more terrible death in the future, and out of sheer fear, the person opts for the later and worse death. See Philippa Foot. 1977. "Euthanasia," *Philosophy & Public Affairs* 6: 85–112.

178. This point is made by Allen Buchanan. 1981. "The Limits of Proxy Decisionmaking for Incompetents," 29 *UCLA Law Review* 386.

179. Jonathan Glover uses this example in "Future People, Disability, and Screening," in Peter Laslett and James Fishkin, eds., *Justice Between Age Groups and Generations* (New Haven, CT: Yale University Press, 1992): 127–143.

own best interest (see Chapter 2). If such a decision can be made regarding treatment, it would seem that it can be made regarding wrongful life. The danger in both situations is that the proxy chooser will be biased against the sort of life available to a person with severe disabilities. It should be remembered that being deaf, blind, unable to walk, or severely mentally impaired is not necessarily incompatible with having a life worth living. A life that a normal individual might find intolerable might not be so awful for an infant who has known nothing else. Disabilities, even severe ones, do not necessarily make a child better off dead, or better off unborn.

The proxy chooser is therefore neither to express the child's own preferences, nor to ascribe his or her own values, goals, ideals, or aspirations to the child. Rather, the proxy is to represent the child's best interests. Feinberg explains his choice as follows:

> [The proxy chooser] exercises his judgment that whatever interests the impaired party might have, or come to have, they would already be doomed to defeat by his present incurable condition. Thus, it would be irrational—contrary to what reason decrees—for a representative and protector of those interests to prefer the continuance of that condition to non-existence. The proxy might also express the retroactive preference, on the incompetent's behalf, not to have been born at all.[180]

There are two important features of the proxy's choice. First, the choice of nonexistence is not merely rational in the weak sense of being in accordance with reason, but in the strong sense of being required by reason. Second, his or her nonexistence is rationally preferable in the strong sense only if all of his or her interests, present and future, are "doomed to defeat."

The "doomed-to-defeat" test works best where there is chronic pain, combined with either an early death or such severe developmental disabilities that the child will not be able to develop any compensating interests. This was the prognosis given to the parents of "Baby Jane Doe," when their first child was born with a severe case of spina bifida in 1983. They were told that she would never know happiness, only pain. Her mental disability would be so severe that she would never talk, never learn, never even recognize her parents. In addition, she would be bedridden, paralyzed, and subject to constant bladder and urinary-tract infections. Her parents decided that such a life would not be in her best interest, and so they decided against surgery to close her spine, having been told that her death would soon follow.[181] As it turned out, she did not die, and the hole in her spine closed naturally. The prognosis given

---

180. Feinberg, "Wrongful Life" (see note 175), p. 164.

181. The parents' judgment was challenged by a right-to-life Vermont lawyer, Lawrence Washburn, but ultimately the parents prevailed when New York's Court of Appeals held that the trial judge had abused his authority by hearing the case, since Washburn had no relationship to the child or her parents, and reports of abuse must go through child protective services. *Weber v. Stony Brook Hospital*, 60 NY2d 208, 456 N.E.2 1186, 469 N.Y.S.2d 63 (1983). For discussions of the case, see my 1984 article, "Baby Jane Doe in the Courts," *Hastings Center Report* 14 (1): 13–19, and George J. Annas. 1984. "The Case of Baby Jane Doe: Child Abuse or Unlawful Federal Intervention?" *American Journal of Public Health* 74 (7): 727–729.

her parents turned out to be unduly pessimistic. She became a self-aware little girl who "not only experienced and returned the love of her parents"[182] but also attended a school for the physically and neurologically handicapped, where she took classes in speech, and physical and occupational therapy. An article in *Newsday* in 2003, when she was 20 years old, was entitled, "A Fighter's Spirit: Keri-Lynn–Baby Jane Doe–Beat Stiff Odds."[183]

Relatively few impaired newborns, even those with the severest anomalies, have lives that are filled with severe, chronic, and intractable pain. Far more common are cases in which the infant's condition precludes the ability to develop or to do any of the things that human beings characteristically develop, and which make lives subjectively worth living. This would include children like Jeffrey Gleitman and Peter Procanik, who, because of congenital rubella syndrome, were born deaf, blind, and severely mentally retarded. Is nonexistence clearly preferable for such infants?

John Robertson argues that life-prolonging treatment is almost always in the best interest of even severely handicapped babies. In an article about euthanasia and withholding treatment from infants with severe disabilities, Robertson considers the case of a profoundly retarded, nonambulatory, blind, and deaf infant who will spend his few years in a crib in the back wards of a state institution.[184] He writes:

> One who has never known the pleasures of mental operation, ambulation, and social interaction surely does not suffer from the loss as much as one who has. While one who has known these capacities may prefer death to a life without them, we have no assurance that the handicapped person, with no point of comparison, would agree. Life and life alone, whatever its limitations, might be of sufficient worth to him.[185]

John Arras agrees.[186] Such a child suffers no pain. He is neither horrified by his plight nor depressed by his neglect in the state institution. He just lies there. We may consider such a life totally miserable, but can we be sure it appears so to the infant? If we confine ourselves to the infant's own perspective, it does not seem that we can

182. B. D. Colen. 1994. "Whatever Happened to Baby Jane Doe?" *Hastings Center Report* 24 (3): 2.

183. Jamie Talan. 2003. "A Fighter's Spirit: Keri-Lynn–Baby Jane Doe–Beat Stiff Odds," *Newsday*, October 12. http://www.newsday.com/news/a-fighter-s-spirit-20-year-old-keri-lynn-baby-jane-doe-beat-steep-odds-1.365134. Accessed November 7, 2010.

184. John A. Robertson. 1974–1975. "Involuntary Euthanasia of Defective Newborns: A Legal Analysis," 27 *Stanford Law Review* 213. Robertson includes the child's being ignored on a back ward to emphasize that a life that seems dreadful from our perspective might still have value for the infant. Of course, the child's being neglected is not inherent to his disability. This is a social condition that could be ameliorated to make the life of the infant as worthwhile as possible.

185. Ibid., p. 254.

186. John D. Arras. 1985. "Ethical Principles for the Care of Imperiled Newborns: Toward an Ethic of Ambiguity" (hereafter "Ethic of Ambiguity") in Thomas Murray and Arthur Caplan, eds., *Which Babies Shall Live?* Clifton, NJ: Humana Press, pp. 83–135.

say with confidence that the child is "better off dead" or "better off unborn." It is not even clear that the most radically impaired infant suffers from or has interests of his own that are defeated by his impaired condition.

We are left with two possibilities. We can restrict ourselves to the child's own interests (a "best-interests" standard) and acknowledge that an infant is clearly "better off dead" and thus a candidate for wrongful life only in cases that combine severe physical and mental handicaps with chronic, severe, and intractable pain. (A child who dies after a very brief life of pain might also have a wrongful life, but there would be little case for damages in such a short life. Wrongful-life suits are most compelling in the case of children who survive and have extraordinary medical expenses.) Alternately, we can broaden the criteria for wrongful life to encompass a more objective, or intersubjective, notion, that of a "minimally decent existence." As regards withdrawal of treatment, Arras says that if we are honest with ourselves, we will acknowledge that in most cases where it is thought best to stop life-prolonging treatment, death is not necessarily in the child's "best interest." (Indeed, in some of these cases, the infants barely have any interests.) Rather, we support letting the child die because we do not believe that a life of little more than biological existence constitutes a minimally decent existence. We do not think that such a life is worth sustaining, even if it does not impose undue suffering on the child. A paradigm case would be anencephaly, where most or all of the forebrain is missing. Without a cerebellum, it is believed that children with anencephaly are unable to feel or think or experience anything.[187] For this reason, life cannot be a good to them, but neither do they suffer. Most anencephalic babies are stillborn or die within hours or days of birth, although with aggressive treatment, their lives can be prolonged. Few parents opt for life-prolonging treatment, believing that it makes no sense to prolong the life of an infant who cannot experience his or her life.

The intuitive idea is that mere biological existence is not a good or a benefit. It is the ability to experience life, to partake in human experience, that makes life worthwhile, including such capacities as conscious awareness, the ability to experience pleasure, to give and receive love, to think, to learn. If all or most of these capacities are missing, then the child does not have a minimally decent existence. The suggestion here is that a child who does not have even a minimally decent existence is "better off unborn"—that is, worse off for having been brought into existence. And if

187. This is somewhat controversial. Most scientists and doctors believe that babies with anencephaly do not experience anything, or have an inner life. On the other hand, parents of such babies do not agree that this is true of all such infants. According to one Web site, "Some children are able to swallow, eat, cry, hear, feel vibrations (loud sounds), react to touch and even to light. But most of all, they respond to our love: you don't need a complete brain to give and receive love—all you need is a heart!" http://www.anencephalie-info.org/e/faq.php. Accessed November 6, 2010. Some doctors and researchers agree. See, for example, Van Assche, F.A. 1990. "Anencephalics as Organ Donors," *American Journal of Obstetrics and Gynecology* 163 (2): 599–600. "Anencephalics can be divided into a large group without a functional hypothalamohypophysial system and a smaller group with a functional hypothalamohypophysial system. Those with a functional hypothalamohypophysial system have shown pain reaction."

the child can be said to be "worse off" for having been born, then the child can be said to have been harmed by being brought to birth.[188]

I have suggested that we will have a more plausible analysis of both "better off dead" and "better off unborn" if we allow the proxy chooser to apply either the "doomed-to-defeat" or the "minimally decent existence" criterion. However, even if we broaden the criteria in this way, "wrongful life" may still be a null—or virtually null—set, on Feinberg's analysis. The reason is that Feinberg insists that the choice for nonexistence must be rational, not merely in the weak sense of consistent with reason, where this means that the choice is one that a rational person could make, but in the strong sense of required by reason, where this means that the choice is one that a rational person would have to make. According to Feinberg, a child can be said to have been harmed by being brought into existence only if it would be irrational for a proxy chooser, acting out of concern for the child's best interest, to choose existence for that child. It is unlikely that this extremely restrictive standard could be met in most cases. Perhaps it could be met in the case of Tay-Sachs disease or EB or Lesch-Nyhan syndrome. (This is an X-linked recessive condition that involves a process of neurological and physiological deterioration from approximately the sixth month of life; the most striking feature of the syndrome is compulsive self-mutilation.) However, in the majority of cases, there seems room for rational people to disagree about whether life is worth living. In relatively few cases, if any, can a proxy chooser who opts for the child's existence be said to be acting "contrary to reason."

It seems to me that Feinberg sets too stringent a standard of rationality for his proxy chooser. It is a much more stringent standard than is required of parents deciding on life-prolonging care for their severely impaired newborns. No one demands that their decision be one that could not be rejected by a rational decision maker. It is acknowledged that different parents, with different values, may arrive at different decisions. So long as their decision is not clearly contrary to the child's best interests, parents are allowed to make medical decisions for their children, including decisions to stop life-prolonging treatment. Moreover, much less is at stake in the wrongful-life context than in the medical decision-making context. If a mistake is made in the medical context, a child who could have had a life worth living may be denied care and die. If a comparable mistake is made in the wrongful-life context, a negligent physician may be required to compensate a child with serious disabling conditions who was not in fact "better off unborn." That is hardly a tragedy, and for that reason, it is hard to understand why so stringent a standard of rationality should

188. An idea similar to the "minimally decent existence" standard is Richard McCormick's "relational potential" standard, according to which life is to be preserved only insofar as it contains some potential for human relationships. See "To Save or Let Die: The Dilemma of Modern Medicine," *Journal of the American Medical Association* 229: 2 (1974), pp. 172–176. As the story of Baby Jane Doe reveals, it is often extremely difficult to know at birth which babies have relational potential or will have a minimally decent existence. This epistemological problem complicates medical decision making, especially the withholding or withdrawing of treatment, although it is less relevant to wrongful-life cases, since it should be easier to determine the likely medical expenses needed than to determine the future quality of the child's life.

be required in the wrongful-life context, when it is not required in the medical decision-making context.

I conclude that Feinberg's analysis of wrongful life could be improved in two ways; first, broaden the criterion for determining that an infant is "better off unborn" to include a "minimally decent existence" test. Second, weaken the rationality criterion; that is, permit the proxy chooser to make choices that are rational in the weak sense of "consistent with reason," or reasonable, instead of insisting that the choice for nonexistence be one that a rational person would perforce make. So long as the choice for nonexistence is a reasonable one, the child can be said to have been harmed by being brought into existence. It should be pointed out that, even if we modify Feinberg's analysis in this way, relatively few wrongful-life suits would succeed. Someone playing the role of advocate for the infant could not reasonably choose nonexistence over life with such impairments as deafness, blindness, confinement to a wheelchair, mild mental retardation, or albinism.[189] These conditions do not entail a life that falls below a decent minimum. Many people with comparable disabilities have lives that are well worth living. The irony is that it is just these children who would be most able to benefit from recovery in a wrongful-life suit. There is not a lot that can be done for children so severely impaired that their lives can be plausibly said to be "not worth living." By contrast, money awarded to a child with Down syndrome or spina bifida, to a child born deaf or blind, can be used for medical treatment and education, to improve the child's life.

A solution might be to suspend traditional tort rules, Feinberg suggests this, saying:

> This would be a "victimless tort," that is, not a tort at all in the traditional sense, but perhaps justice would support it anyway, as it supports various kinds of strict and vicarious liability. It might not be fair to make a person pay damages to another whom she has not directly wronged, but it may be more unfair still to make the miserable impaired party pay, or do without the aid he needs.[190]

Something like this reasoning appears to have motivated the New Jersey Supreme Court in its ruling in *Procanik v. Cillo*,[191] the 1984 case that overturned *Gleitman*. Wrongful-birth damages could not be awarded because the statute of limitations had expired. The court recognized a wrongful-life action, saying:

> Whatever logic inheres in permitting parents to recover for the cost of extraordinary medical care incurred by a birth-defective child, but in denying the child's

189. In *Pitre v. Oupelousas General Hospital*, 530 So.2d 1151 (La. 1988), a couple sued the hospital after the doctor negligently performed a tubal ligation and failed to inform the couple of the fact. She later gave birth to their third child who was afflicted with albinism, which causes vision problems and a need for life-long medical care. The Supreme Court of Louisiana dismissed the action for wrongful life, but not on the ground that life with albinism is worth living. Rather, the court held that the physician could not have been expected to foresee the birth of a child with albinism. Because the physician had a duty to warn the parents that the tubal ligation had failed, they could recover damages relating to the pregnancy and the husband's lack of consortium, but they were not entitled to special damages arising from the child's disability.

190. Feinberg, "Wrongful Life" (see note 175), p. 174.

191. *Procanik v. Cillo* (see note 168).

own right to recover those expenses, must yield to the inherent injustice of that result. The right to recover the often crushing burden of extraordinary expenses visited by an act of medical malpractice should not depend on the "wholly fortuituous circumstance of whether the parents are available to sue."[192]

Thus, as one commentator explains, "the court's decision 'to allow the recovery of extraordinary medical expenses (was) not premised on the concept that non-life is preferable to an impaired life, but (was) predicated on the needs of the living.'"[193]

A separate issue is whether wrongful-life suits are the best way to ensure that the needs of disabled people for medical treatment and special education are met. This seems unlikely. Ideally, all people with disabilities should receive the treatment they need, regardless of whether their disability or their existence is someone's fault.[194] However, denying recovery to wrongful-life plaintiffs is not going to improve the situation of other impaired children. Until the interests of all disabled people are met through universal access to health care, litigation may be the only way for some infants to get the services they need.

Finally, there is the question of whether wrongful-life suits are contrary to the interests of people with disabilities as a class, because they suggest (or even state) that the lives of some people with disabling conditions are not worth living. Many disability advocates find this notion so offensive that they would prefer that the parents who bring such suits forego monetary damages that could be used to improve the child's life. In my view, this boils down to an empirical question: have wrongful-life suits adversely affected the lives of people with serious disabilities? If they have, that is a strong argument against them. I do not know if this is the case, although I doubt it. Activism on the part of people with disabilities has resulted in a real change in societal attitudes, as well as in the law: witness the Americans With Disabilities Act of 1990, which prohibits discrimination against individuals with disabilities. I suspect that the disability-rights objection to wrongful-life suits stems from its symbolic message, and not any real disadvantage imposed on people with disabilities by such suits. If this is the case, then it seems to me that the medical and educational needs of actual children should take precedence. Where severe disabilities are due to medical negligence, and parents cannot recover damages on their own behalf, justice requires the recognition of wrongful-life suits.

In the next chapter, I consider the problem of behavior during pregnancy that exposes the fetus to serious health risks. In contrast to wrongful-life cases, these are situations in which a child is born with defects that could have been avoided. But for the mother's behavior during pregnancy, the child would have been born "healthy and whole." Increasingly, there have been calls for coercive measures to

---

192. Ibid., 97 N.J. 339, at 351–352, 478 A.2d 755, at 762, quoting *Turpin v. Sortini*, 31 Cal.3d 320, 328, 643P.2d 954, 965 (1982).

193. Strasser (see note 160), p. 66, quoting *Procanik*, 97 N.J. at 353, 478 A.2d at 763.

194. John Harris (1990) makes this point in "The Wrong of Wrongful Life," *Journal of Law and Society* 17 (1): 1–16.

protect the "not-yet-born" child. The interest view does not rule out such measures. Whether they are wise public policy is a separate matter. Feminists and civil libertarians caution against the threat of a "pregnancy police" that would intrude into every aspect of a woman's life and decision making. These are valid concerns. Coercive measures against pregnant women are neither necessary nor likely to safeguard the health of future children, but they seriously threaten women's rights to privacy and self-determination.

4

Maternal–Fetal Conflict

Women who use illegal drugs during pregnancy have been subjected to various criminal charges, from child abuse to murder in cases of stillbirth or neonatal death. In 2001, a South Carolina woman who used cocaine while pregnant and had a stillbirth was found guilty of homicide by child abuse. She was sentenced to 20 years in prison and served 8 years before the State Supreme Court overturned her conviction in 2008. In 2004, a Hawaiian woman, addicted to crystal methamphetamine, whose son died shortly after birth, was convicted of manslaughter and sentenced to 10 years probation. The Supreme Court of Hawaii overturned her conviction, ruling unanimously that state law does not allow the prosecution of women who engage in risky behavior during pregnancy that leads to the death of a newborn. Also in 2004, a Utah woman was charged with capital murder after she delayed having a cesarean section, and one of the twins she was carrying died as a result. The murder charge was dropped after she pled guilty to a lesser charge, child endangerment, for using illegal drugs while pregnant. She was sentenced to 18 months probation and ordered into a drug treatment program.

Drug use during pregnancy in some states is sufficient to classify the child after birth as neglected, and it is grounds for removing the infant from its mother. This has been done even in cases where the baby was born healthy and there were no other indications that the woman would neglect or abuse the child. Pregnant addicts who commit minor crimes, and would ordinarily be free on probation, have been jailed in order to protect the fetus from prenatal exposure to drugs. Jailing the mother to protect the baby is one of the clearest examples of what has become known in the literature as "maternal–fetal conflict."

Some commentators regard the phrase "maternal–fetal conflict" as unnecessarily adversarial, because it suggests that the interests of the pregnant woman are opposed to the interests of the unborn. They argue that while behaviors such as drinking alcohol or smoking tobacco or using illegal drugs pose risks to the developing fetus, such behaviors also endanger maternal health. These commentators suggest that the interests of pregnant women and their fetuses are not pitted against each other, as is suggested by the expression "maternal–fetal conflict." Instead, women and the fetuses they gestate are, and should be treated by health care professionals as, a unit with common interests.

I understand and respect this criticism. All too often, the public has been willing to demonize and punish women whose behavior during pregnancy is deemed risky or irresponsible. At the same time, it must be recognized that a pregnant woman can have interests, including entirely legitimate interests, which may conflict with what will protect the life or health of her fetus. For example, cancer treatments that give a pregnant woman the best chance of survival may kill or deform her fetus. Fetal surgery that is the fetus's only chance of survival may impose considerable risks on the pregnant woman. It is wishful thinking to pretend that what is best for the pregnant woman is necessarily best for the fetus or future child, or that what is best for the fetus always promotes the pregnant woman's interests. Moreover, it is possible that some pregnant women choose to engage in behaviors that are risky both for themselves and their future children. Even if we, as a society, allow competent adults to make such choices for themselves, there is still the question of whether, and in what ways, society may intervene to protect the welfare of children from prenatally inflicted harm.

Not all cases of maternal–fetal conflict involve drug use. In the landmark case of *Automobile Workers v. Johnson Controls*,[1] workers sued the company for its "fetal protection policy," which prevented women of childbearing age from working on its battery production line, unless they could prove that they were infertile. The U.S. Supreme Court ruled in favor of the worker plaintiffs, saying that women have a constitutional right to make their own decisions about how to balance potential risks to fetuses against their own economic needs and those of their families. (This case, discussed in detail in the first edition of *Life Before Birth*, has been left out of this edition because the Supreme Court's ruling has ended the legal battle over corporate fetal protection policies.)

The potential for maternal–fetal conflicts also exists in obstetrics. Doctors who think a cesarean delivery is necessary to prevent fetal death or serious injury have sometimes sought, and been given, court orders to perform the surgery when women have refused. In some cases, the refusal has resulted in the woman's facing criminal charges.

In Chapter 2, I used the interest view to defend abortion. I argued that, before becoming conscious and sentient, the fetus has no interests at all, and so no interest in continued existence. Without an interest in continued existence, the preconscious fetus is not harmed or wronged by being killed. Since abortion is not a wrong to the preconscious fetus, and the preconscious fetus has no right to life, the state should stay out of abortion decisions, at least throughout most of gestation.

MORAL OBLIGATIONS TO THE NOT-YET-BORN

The moral situation changes when a woman decides not to abort, but to carry her baby to term. Once this decision is made, the fetus is not simply a *potential* child. It will be a child who, once born, has interests, including an interest in a healthy life. That interest can be adversely affected by his or her mother's behavior during pregnancy. If she neglects her own health, if she has an inferior diet, if she smokes or drinks too much or uses illegal drugs, she takes risks with the health of her future child. Insofar as these risks are avoidable and unreasonable, taking them is morally wrong, a violation of parental duty. That the child is, at the time of the infliction of

1. Automobile Workers v. Johnson Controls. 1991. 499 U.S. 187.

the harm, a fetus, without interests of its own, is irrelevant to the moral obligation, because the duty of the mother-to-be is to the future expected child, not to the presentient fetus. So there are things that pregnant women who plan to give birth ought to do, or refrain from doing, not only for their own health, but for the sake of the baby. As the sign in the obstetrician's office says, "Now you have two reasons to quit smoking."

For the vast majority of women, the decision not to abort, but to carry to term, is made early in the pregnancy. As we saw in Chapter 2, 90% of all abortions in the United States take place in the first trimester. Most women know very quickly whether the pregnancy is welcome. In the case of a planned pregnancy, the decision to become a mother is made even before conception. Changes in lifestyle, then, may be required as soon as pregnancy is determined, or even earlier. Women who are trying to become pregnant are told that they should improve their diets, as well as those of their husbands (the better his nutrition, the healthier his sperm). They may be advised to take vitamin-mineral supplements that have been shown to prevent certain birth defects. They are told to lose excessive weight and get into shape. It is recommended that they cut down on caffeine and alcohol, to quit smoking, to avoid marijuana and other "recreational" drugs, and to take only those medicines that their doctors prescribe. Having been told to do all these things, they are told that, above all, they should relax![2] These recommendations are aimed at giving the baby the best possible odds of being born alive and well. They reflect the idea that the decision to have a baby brings with it moral obligations to the child who will be born. At the same time, it is important to remember that women are not, in George Annas's trenchant phrase, "fetal containers."[3] They have needs and interests of their own, which may compete with, and sometimes trump, the needs and interests of their future offspring.

The idea that mothers-to-be have prima facie moral obligations to act responsibly during pregnancy, so as to avoid harming their future children, is relatively uncontroversial. Disagreement occurs when we try to say precisely what these moral obligations are. Behavior that is protective of the fetus may impose sacrifices or even risks on the pregnant woman. How much sacrifice or risk is an expectant mother morally required to undergo? And even if we could agree on that, it would be a further and much more complex question, whether these moral obligations should be made into legal ones.

The interest view does not by itself provide a resolution to these complex questions. Rather, it provides a framework for thinking about them. It maintains that, once born, children have interests in healthy existence, and that these interests can be damaged before the children are born, or even conceived. Thus, the interest view differentiates between the issue of abortion, which, crudely speaking, concerns the right to be born, and the issue of maternal–fetal conflict, which concerns the right of children to be born free of preventable injury. The interest view explains how women can have both the right to terminate their pregnancies and the obligation, if they

2. Arlene Eisenberg, Heidi Eisenberg Murkoff, and Sandee Eisenberg. 1984. *What to Expect When You're Expecting*. New York: Workman Publishing, pp. 331–333.

3. George J. Annas. 1986. "Pregnant Women as Fetal Containers," *Hastings Center Report* 16 (6): 3–4.

choose not to abort, to refrain from harming the children they will bear. However, the nature and scope of this obligation requires a richer moral debate than is provided by the interest view alone.

The interest view imposes on pregnant women a prima facie obligation not to inflict harm on the children they intend to bear. A more difficult question is whether the interest view can explain, or even acknowledge, an obligation on the part of the pregnant woman to avoid fetal *death*, as opposed to postnatal injury. This is trickier, because, on the interest view, the early-gestation, presentient fetus is not harmed or wronged by being killed. But if death is not a harm to the fetus, then it would seem that there is nothing wrong with prenatal behavior that causes the death of the fetus. It is hard to see why it should be morally acceptable for a woman deliberately to cause the death of the fetus through abortion, but morally wrong for her accidentally to cause its death by her behavior during pregnancy. In either case, she does not harm or wrong the fetus.[4] Of course, a woman who wants to have a child has strong *prudential* reasons to avoid behaviors likely to cause a miscarriage, but she has no *moral* obligations to the early fetus to avoid causing its death. After the fetus becomes sentient, sometime in mid- to late-gestation, it has an interest in avoiding pain, and also a weak time-relative interest in continued existence, as I argued in the last chapter. Thus, on the interest view, a woman has a prima facie obligation to the late-gestation fetus to avoid causing its death. The nature of this obligation—that is, what she is actually required to do—depends on the risks and burdens she would have to undergo. For example, she is not required to sacrifice her own life or health to preserve the life of a sentient fetus.

Because a woman has a prima facie obligation to the late-gestation fetus to avoid causing its death, and no obligation at all to the early-gestation fetus to avoid causing its death, it appears that, on the interest view, the stage of gestation is relevant to the obligations of the pregnant woman, with regard to the preservation of fetal life. However, because virtually all the behaviors that risk *killing* the fetus also risk *harming* the future child, a pregnant woman has moral obligations not to engage in certain behaviors even in early pregnancy, when abortion is permissible. For example, binge-drinking in early pregnancy might cause a miscarriage (no moral wrong done), but it might instead cause fetal alcohol syndrome (FAS) in the child after birth (a wrong to the child). On the interest view, the pregnant woman is morally responsible for the damage her behavior during pregnancy causes to her child. Therefore, once a woman has decided not to terminate the pregnancy, but to carry the fetus to term, her obligation to the future child to avoid harming it makes it wrong for her to engage in behavior likely to be lethal to the early-gestation fetus, even though she does not have a moral obligation to the early-gestation fetus to avoid causing its death.

Some people find this analysis puzzling for two reasons. One is that a woman might change her mind about having an abortion. But, the objection goes, how can the fact that she might change her mind affect the morality of her behavior during gestation? Imagine a woman, Alice, who does not use contraception because she wants to have a baby, and believes that her partner, with whom she is very much in love, also wants to have a child with her. She takes a pregnancy test on Wednesday, which confirms the joyous news. On Thursday, she learns that her boyfriend is

4. I am grateful to my students in my Philosophy and Public Affairs seminar in fall 2009, especially Leahanna Pelish, for pressing me on this point.

cheating on her and has been doing so for the past year, with her best friend. This changes everything. She throws the bum out and schedules an abortion for Monday. On Friday night, miserable and depressed, she goes to a bar and has six bourbons.

Has Alice done anything wrong? Surely not, on the interest view. Binge-drinking would be wrong if she were going to continue the pregnancy, since she would be risking inflicting neurological damage on her future child. However, as she is planning to abort, there is no future child to whom she has an obligation. So Alice does nothing wrong. But suppose she meets her old high school boyfriend, Zack, at the bar, where she is drowning her sorrows. He is kind and sympathetic, and they realize that they have never stopped loving each other. They spend the weekend together, and on Sunday night, Zack pleads with Alice not to have the abortion, but to marry him. He loves her and will raise the child, as if it were his own. Alice, who really did want to have a baby from the start, is delighted. On Monday morning, she calls the clinic and cancels the appointment.

Earlier I said that, on the interest view, it was not wrong (or at least not a wrong to the fetus) for Alice to binge-drink on Friday night. Now, however, it seems that it *was* wrong for her to drink those bourbons, and not only wrong, but a wrong to her future child. If the baby is born with FAS (an unlikely but possible outcome), it will be Alice's fault. She could have prevented the harm by not drinking to excess. So if the child is born with FAS, Alice has harmed and wronged the child. Thus, the interest view commits us to regarding Alice's binge-drinking as not wrong on Friday, but wrong on Monday, which seems paradoxical. How can the day of the week make a moral difference?

However, there is no paradox. The relevant difference is that on Friday, Alice planned to terminate the pregnancy. She reasonably believed that she would be harming no one by drinking to excess. And if she had terminated the pregnancy on Monday, this would have been true. But she did not have the abortion. Once she decided to have the baby, she had an obligation not to engage in binge-drinking, but that obligation is not retroactive. If it were, then all sexually active women of childbearing age would have a moral obligation not to binge-drink (or even drink at all, since even one drink could inflict harm on the developing fetus), since they *might* become pregnant, and if they do, they might decide to keep the child. That is clearly absurd.

However, Alice was already pregnant when she downed the six bourbons. Perhaps she ought to have considered the risk that she *might change her mind* and put off the binge-drinking until after she had the abortion. That way, she could be sure there would be no future person who could be harmed by her behavior. I agree that this would be the safest course. Had Alice abstained from drinking on Friday, she would have no regrets once she decided to have the baby. So perhaps we should say that pregnant women, even those who intend to abort, have some obligation not to engage in risky behavior, since it is possible they will change their minds. However, surely their obligation to avoid potentially risky behaviors is nowhere near as strong as that of women who intend to go to term.

On the interest view, the only moral objection to risky behavior during early to mid-gestation is that it might cause harm to the future child. However, this means that a pregnant woman can escape blame for her risky behavior during pregnancy by having an abortion, which seems counterintuitive to some people. They ask, how can it be right to avoid blame for harming the child by killing the fetus? If one takes the view that the fetus has the same moral standing as the born child, then of course it is wrong to avoid harming the child by doing something worse, namely, killing it in utero. On the interest view, however, killing the early fetus in utero is not wrong, and therefore it is not worse than inflicting harm on the future child. However, while early abortion is not in itself wrong, it may be seen as callous or unfeeling if done for a callous or unfeeling motive, and simply wishing to escape being blamed may seem such a motive. Here it seems the right thing to say is that the act is not wrong, but the motive casts doubt on the character of the person who does the act. Perhaps the motive for having an abortion after engaging in risky behavior is not to escape blame, but to protect the child from being born in a harmed condition. This would not be a callous motive, but it would be, in most cases, misguided. Despite the woman's risky behavior, the chances are good that the child will be fine, and even if there is damage, the child probably can have a perfectly good life (see Chapter 3, section on "Wrongful Life"). This suggests that there are very few cases, if any, in which risky behavior during pregnancy would make abortion morally obligatory for the sake of the child. If the woman *wants* to have the baby, the fact that she has engaged in potentially risky behavior during pregnancy in no way imposes an obligation on her to abort.

The interest view maintains that the early-gestation fetus has no interest or stake in survival because it has no interests at all. It has no interests at all because interests are compounded out of desires and goals, which themselves require (at least) sentience. David DeGrazia disagrees.[5] He maintains that even the early fetus, which is not sentient, has a weak interest in continued existence, because the early fetus is identical to (that is, an earlier stage of) the future born person. However, he also thinks that this interest in survival is discounted because the psychological unity between the future child and the presentient fetus is so weak. Thus, DeGrazia is able to adhere to a pro-choice position on early abortion, holding that virtually any interest of the pregnant woman in terminating the pregnancy would override the fetus's weak time-relative interest in continued existence.

Let us suppose that DeGrazia is right on the identity question. That is, I, Bonnie Steinbock, was once an early-gestation fetus. I came into existence at the start of the pregnancy that resulted in my birth. This sounds quite plausible, biologically speaking. Does this mean that I then had an interest or stake in my survival? I do not see that it does. In the early stages of my existence, it did not matter to me whether I continued to exist. Of course, now I am very glad that I exist, and therefore glad that my mother did not abort me. It is in my interest that a whole range of things happened, some of them before I was born (e.g., that my mother did not have an abortion), and some even before I was conceived (e.g., that my mother and father had sex at the particular time that led to my conception). For that matter, it is now in my interest that my parents went to the same high school, where they met. My existence is probably contingent on Hitler's having invaded Poland, because without that, World War II might not have occurred, and if that had not happened, my father would not have served overseas, and it is unlikely that my parents would have waited until 1946 to conceive a second child. If this is correct, then but for World War II, *I* never would have been born. It follows that it was in my interest that World War II occurred, although it seems a bit odd, and certainly egocentric, to say that I am glad

5. David DeGrazia. 2007. "The Harm of Death, Time-Relative Interests, and Abortion," *Philosophical Forum* 38 (1): 57–80.

that it did. But even if it is in my interest that the conditions that led to my birth were fulfilled, it does not follow that when I was an early-gestation fetus, I had an interest in continuing to live. At that stage of my existence, it did not matter at all to me what happened to me. Moreover, if the pregnancy had been terminated, there would have been no one who is glad that it was not. My point is this: even if we accept a biological account of identity, it does not follow that the interests of the born person accrue to the stage of nonsentient existence. The nonsentient fetus has only hypothetical interests: *if* it becomes a being with a stake in its own existence, it will have an interest in the fulfillment of all the conditions necessary for its existence to have occurred. Mere identity does not endow a being with actual interests, but actual interests can be set back or thwarted before the interested being comes into existence.

This means that there is a sense in which the interest view can accommodate "fetal rights": women can have obligations to their future children, and the fulfillment of these obligations occurs during pregnancy, when the child is still a fetus. But it is one thing to say that the notion of fetal rights is conceptually possible, quite another to say that our legal system ought to recognize fetal rights. That is a complex substantive normative issue, not merely a conceptual one. In this chapter, I argue that there are compelling policy reasons not to recognize fetal rights, as such laws do little to protect the not-yet-born, are likely to (and often intended to) restrict women's rights to abortion, and impose punishment where education and help would be more appropriate. Consider the story of a 17-year-old Utah girl who in 2009 paid a man $150 to beat her up, in an attempt to cause her to miscarry in her seventh month of pregnancy. Apparently, her boyfriend threatened to break up with her if she did not get rid of the child.[6] The girl, who was not identified because she was a juvenile, pleaded no contest to a second-degree felony count of criminal solicitation to commit murder. However, she was released because under Utah law, a woman is not criminally liable for seeking an abortion. Utah lawmakers then introduced a bill, HB 462, that would allow sentences of up to life in prison for a woman who experiences a miscarriage or stillbirth as a result of "knowing" or "reckless" behavior. Although the bill was sparked by anger at the fact that there was no law that could imprison the girl in question, the bill's reach was potentially much greater than deliberate termination of a pregnancy. Opponents said that it would open the door to a witch hunt in which every miscarriage or stillbirth would be suspect. The bill set off a firestorm of opposition, and as a result, was withdrawn by its sponsor, Representative Carl D. Wimmer. It was "revised to exempt women who commit reckless acts but permit the prosecution of women who commit 'knowing' acts that may result in stillbirths and miscarriages from the earliest stages of pregnancy."[7] This revision did not satisfy opponents who suggested that the bill would expose to criminal liability pregnant women who "know" that their cancer medications could cause pregnancy loss, or who "knowingly" stay with abusive partners, or who smoke cigarettes, "knowing" the risks to the fetus. Representative Wimmer assured critics that the bill would be applied in only

6. "Abortion Beating: Aaron Harrison Sentenced for Trying to Cause Miscarriage With Fists." 2009. http://www.cbsnews.com/8301–504083_162–5147231-504083.html. March 28. Accessed March 9, 2010.

7. Lynn Paltrow. 2010. "Utah Continues Reckless Efforts to Lock Up Pregnant Women." *The Huffinton Post*, March 6. http://www.huffingtonpost.com/lynn-m-paltrow/utah-continues-reckless-e_b_488673.html. Accessed March 9, 2010.

the most glaring cases. In response, Lynn Paltrow, founder and executive director of National Advocates for Pregnant Women, said that imprisonment of a 17-year-old girl, desperate enough to risk her own life, is not the right response, and that non-judgmental counseling would be a better approach.

A public health approach to the problem of substance abuse and other risky behaviors during pregnancy is much more likely to be successful than a criminal justice approach to achieve the obstetrician's goal of "a healthy mother and a healthy baby." In addition, punitive approaches tend to target low-income and minority women, and so are unfair as well as ineffective. Jailing women after they have given birth to a damaged child, even assuming it can be proven that the damage was due to the woman's behavior during pregnancy, also deprives the newborn of its mother, something that is rarely in the best interest of the child.

Risks to the Fetus

It used to be thought that the womb provided a shielded environment, which protected the fetus from external factors. It was not until the 1940s that experiments using animals demonstrated that maternal dietary deficiency and X-ray exposure could adversely affect intrauterine mammalian development. About the same time, the association between rubella infection and abnormal fetal development was recognized.[8] The thalidomide tragedy in the 1960s, which resulted in the births of thousands of severely malformed infants, demonstrated the potential danger to the fetus of an apparently innocuous tranquilizer.

Drugs, both legal and illegal, taken by the woman during pregnancy, pose risks to the developing fetus and born child. In terms of harmfulness, the distinction between legal and illegal drugs makes little sense. Alcohol use and cigarette smoking during pregnancy can have just as dangerous, if not more dangerous, long-term effects on the future child as heroin or cocaine. Moreover, because more pregnant women smoke cigarettes than use illegal drugs, tobacco use during pregnancy has a much greater public health impact, that is, affects more babies, than all illegal drugs put together. However, for purposes of state intervention, the distinction between legal and illegal drugs is pertinent. People who use illegal drugs are subject to criminal penalties. Since the behavior is already illegal, adding additional criminal penalties for harming a child through the behavior is a lot easier to justify than imposing criminal penalties for harm caused by the use of legal drugs.

LEGAL DRUGS

Tobacco
Tobacco can cause serious damage to the unborn, something of which the general public was not aware until the 1970s. Smokers' offspring are at higher risk for miscarriage, stillbirth, prematurity, and low birth weight.[6] The best-documented adverse effect of smoking during pregnancy is fetal growth retardation. "Infants born to women who smoke during pregnancy have a lower average birth weight and are

---

8. Sherman Elias and George J. Annas. 1987. *Reproductive Genetics and the Law.* Chicago, IL: Yearbook Medical Publishers, Inc., p. 196.

more likely to be small for gestational age than infants born to women who do not smoke. Low birth weight is associated with increased risk for neonatal, perinatal, and infant morbidity and mortality. The longer the mother smokes during pregnancy, the greater the effect on the infant's birth weight."[9]

Alcohol

In the late 1960s and early 1970s, FAS, characteristic of offspring of chronic alcoholic mothers, was first described. Full-blown FAS exists when the patient has signs in each of three categories: prenatal or postnatal growth retardation, central nervous system damage (neurological abnormality, developmental delay, or learning disabilities), and characteristic facial dysmorphology, such as microcephaly and a flattened nose.[4] "Studies by the Centers for Disease Control and Prevention (CDC) suggest that between 1,000 and 6,000 babies in the United States are born yearly with FAS."[10] Some children do not show the full FAS but have some manifestations of the syndrome. In such cases, the term "fetal alcohol spectrum disorders" (FASD) is used. Each year in the United States, up to 40,000 babies are born with FASDs,[11] with effects that range from mild to severe. "These effects include mental retardation; learning, emotional and behavioral problems; and defects involving the heart, face and other organs."[12]

According to some researchers, a clear relationship between alcohol use and adverse pregnancy outcome has been demonstrated only for heavy and prolonged maternal alcohol abuse of at least 5.0 ounces of absolute alcohol per day.[15] Other researchers claim that maternal consumption of over three drinks per day (1.5 oz. of alcohol) triples the risk of subnormal IQ.[16] They report that children born to women who had as little as one to two drinks a day in the first months of pregnancy had a slower reaction time in their early school years and difficulty in paying attention.[17] There is no known minimum "safe" level of alcohol consumption. It is possible that any consumption of alcohol produces some risk to the fetus.[13]

In light of this information, what are the moral obligations of pregnant women regarding alcohol consumption? The answer is complicated by two factors: the degree of risk and the degree of moral culpability. Let us consider risk first. Heavy and prolonged alcohol use throughout pregnancy is likely to cause FAS or FAE in the born child. This imposes on the pregnant woman a moral obligation not to engage in binge-drinking. What about moderate to light consumption of alcohol? The safest course is complete abstinence. As expressed by the March of Dimes, "Because no

9. Centers for Disease Control (CDC). 2000. "Tobacco Use and Reproductive Outcomes." http://www.cdc.gov/tobacco/data_statistics/sgr/2001/highlights/outcomes/index.htm. Accessed August 6, 2009.

10. March of Dimes. 2008. "Drinking Alcohol During Pregnancy." http://www.marchofdimes. com/professionals/14332_1170.asp. Accessed August 6, 2009. Citing Bertrand, J., et al., National Task Force on FAS/FAE. *Fetal Alcohol Syndrome: Guidelines for Referral and Diagnosis.* Atlanta, GA: Centers for Disease Control and Prevention, July 2004.

11. Ibid., citing Substance Abuse and Mental Health Services Administration, U.S. Department of Health and Human Services. Fetal Alcohol Spectrum Disorders. 2007.

12. March of Dimes. 2008 (see note 10)

13. Ibid.

amount of alcohol has been proven safe during pregnancy, a woman should stop drinking immediately if she even suspects she could be pregnant, and she should not drink alcohol if she is trying to become pregnant."[14] (Some studies have found decreased fertility among women who have five drinks or less per week.[15])

However, it does not follow that every pregnant woman who takes a drink is acting irresponsibly. In March 1991, a bartender and a waitress attempted to dissuade a pregnant woman in Seattle from ordering a rum daiquiri. First, they asked her whether she wouldn't prefer a nonalcoholic drink. When she said she would not, the bartender removed the warning label from a bottle of beer, which says that the Surgeon General has determined that pregnant women should not drink alcohol because of the risk of birth defects, and placed it before her. She complained to the management, and the waitress and bartender were fired for harassing a customer.[16]

In my view, the waitress and the bartender, though well meaning, were out of line (although firing them seems unwarranted, since a simple warning would have sufficed). It is one thing to require restaurants and bars to inform pregnant women of the risks posed by alcohol, through warning labels posted in the establishments. It is quite another for bartenders and waitresses to take on the role of enforcers by ensuring that women heed the posted warnings. Ironically, the greatest risk to the unborn occurs during the first trimester, when the pregnancy is unlikely to be evident and outside intervention therefore impractical. In this case, as it turned out, the woman was past her due date and had been very careful to avoid liquor throughout her pregnancy. She had decided that one drink was unlikely to do any harm, a perfectly reasonable assessment of the available evidence, and in fact, she later gave birth to a healthy boy.[17]

Admittedly, total abstinence is the safest course for the not-yet-born child, but are people morally obligated to follow the *safest* course? We do not require this standard of parents regarding their already-born children. If we did, we could not justify leaving children with baby-sitters to go out to dinner. What if something should happen? It seems to me that having a single drink occasionally in pregnancy falls into the area of individual discretion, because the risk of causing harm is very low (perhaps nonexistent).

Moreover, a woman may have a good reason for wishing to consume an occasional glass of wine, even during pregnancy. Although heavy use of alcohol is not good for anyone, pregnant or not, light to moderate alcohol consumption has been connected to a reduced risk of heart disease. The moderate use of alcohol may therefore be a healthful habit for the woman, which can conceivably outweigh the small risk it imposes on the future child. By contrast, smoking has nothing at all

14. Ibid.

15. Tina Kold Jensen, Niels Henrik I Hjollund, Tine Brink Henriksen, Thomas Scheike, Henrik Kolstad, Aleksander Giwercman, Erik Ernst, Jens Peter Bonde, Niels E. Skakkebæk, and Jørn Olsen. 1998. "Does Moderate Alcohol Consumption Affect Fertility? Follow-up Study Among Couples Planning First Pregnancy," *British Medical Journal* 317(7157): 505–510.

16. Janet Lynne Golden. 2000. "'A Tempest in a Cocktail Glass': Mothers, Alcohol, and Television, 1977–1996." *Journal of Health Politics, Policy and Law* 25: 473–498.

17. Janet Lynne Golden. 2005. *Message in a Bottle: The Making of Fetal Alcohol Syndrome*. Cambridge, MA: Harvard University Press, p. 95.

to recommend it from a health perspective. The risk it poses to the baby imposes on the expectant mother an obligation to make a good-faith effort to stop, or at least cut down on, smoking. However, we now know that nicotine is an addictive drug. A woman who is addicted to cigarettes may be unable to do what she ought to do for the sake of her baby.

This brings us to the second factor, namely, the culpability of the pregnant woman. It is the heavy and chronic drinker, whose drinking is most detrimental to the unborn, who is least likely to be able to modify her behavior to protect her baby. Is she nevertheless obligated to stop drinking during pregnancy? On the one hand, people cannot have obligations they cannot fulfill. I cannot have an obligation to save your life if it is literally impossible for me to save you. The "ought implies can" principle may incline some people to say that pregnant drug addicts and alcoholics are not under a moral obligation to stop using drugs and alcohol. However, the fact that they cannot stop *at will* does not mean that they are literally incapable of stopping. We can recognize that it may be very difficult for some women to fulfill their moral obligations to the babies they plan to bear, and will need help to do so, without denying that they have such obligations. However, the obligation to protect future children extends beyond their mothers (and fathers). Blaming and punishing pregnant women is unlikely to do much, if anything, to protect future children. Treatment centers must be available to all people, including pregnant women, to enable them to break their addictions. (The 2008 March of Dimes fact sheet on "Drinking Alcohol During Pregnancy" includes a section on where a woman can get help to stop drinking alcohol.[18])

ILLEGAL DRUGS
A study published in 2006 estimated that between 15% to 18% (between 625,000 to 729,000) of infants born every year in the United States are exposed to one or more illegal drugs.[19]

Cocaine
Cocaine—once popularly believed relatively harmless—can pose dangers both to fetal health and to the health of born children. These effects include retarded growth in the womb and subtle neurological abnormalities, leading to extraordinary irritability during infancy and learning disorders later. In more extreme cases, there may be loss of the small intestine and brain-damaging strokes.

Although the risks are real, it is also true that they have been exaggerated both by researchers and the media, which portrayed "crack cocaine"—cocaine that is smoked, as opposed to cocaine hydrochloride, which is snorted or injected—as especially dangerous. The crack high is reputedly more immediate and intensely euphoric than snorted cocaine, but the real differences between the two forms of cocaine have more to do with social class than psychopharmacology. "Crack, unlike cocaine hydrochloride, tends to be purchased and used by poor, working-class people.

18. March of Dimes, "Drinking Alcohol During Pregnancy" (see note 10).

19. National Institute for Drug Abuse. 2006. "The Economic Costs of Alcohol and Drug Abuse in the United States." http://www.nida.nih.gov/EconomicCosts/Chapter4b.html. Accessed September 28, 2009.

Snorting remains the mode of ingestion preferred by middle-class and wealthy cocaine users."[20] Myths about "crack babies," perpetuated throughout the 1980s, only began to be dispelled in the late 1990s. As one researcher explains:

> Political rhetoric has sometimes demonized pregnant crack cocaine users, casting them as immoral and corrupt. Instead of addressing the perceived crack baby epidemic as a public health issue, cocaine-exposed babies were represented as uneducable and worthless drains upon scant public school resources. In turn, the popular media further alarmed the general public with dire predictions for cocaine-exposed infants. However, researchers have countered that there had been a rush to judgment regarding the long-term consequences of prenatal cocaine exposure.[21]

A Case Western study done in 2004 found that 4-year-old children who were exposed to cocaine before birth scored just as well on intelligence tests as unexposed children.[22]

Methamphetamines

The use of methamphetamines, including crystal meth (also known as speed, ice, or crank) and Ecstasy, has increased dramatically in recent years.[23] There have been few studies of the effects of Ecstasy on pregnancy, but in general, methamphetamines can retard growth in utero. Even full-term babies of women who used meth during their pregnancies tend to be low birth weight for term, that is, under 5½ pounds, and have smaller than normal head circumference. Premature birth and placental problems have also been reported with prenatal use of methamphetamines. The long-term outlook for such babies is not known, although low-birth-weight babies are at risk for learning and other problems. The risk is greater for babies with small head circumference than for low-birth-weight babies who have a normal head size.

Heroin

"Women who use heroin during pregnancy greatly increase their risk of serious pregnancy complications. These risks include poor fetal growth, premature rupture of the membranes (the bag of waters that holds the fetus breaks too soon), premature birth and stillbirth."[24] Other risks include low birth weight, prematurity, and breathing problems. The babies are at risk of lifelong disability. Most babies of heroin users

20. Janet Dolgin. 1991. "The Law's Response to Parental Alcohol and 'Crack' Abuse." *Brooklyn Law Review* 56 (4): 1213–1268, p. 1224.

21. Harvey J. Ginsburg, Paul Raffeld, Kelly L. Alanis, and Angela S. Boyce. 2006. "Comparing Attitudes About Legal Sanctions and Teratogenic Effects for Cocaine, Alcohol, Tobacco and Caffeine: A Randomized, Independent Samples Design," *Substance Abuse, Treatment, Prevention and Policy* 1 (4). Published online February 1, 2006. http://www.pubmedcentral.nih.gov/articlerender.fcgi?artid=1435999. Accessed August 30, 2009.

22. March of Dimes, "Drinking Alcohol During Pregnancy" (see note 10).

23. March of Dimes. 2008. "Illicit Drug Use During Pregnancy." http://www.marchofdimes.com/professionals/14332_1169.asp Accessed October 29, 2010.

24. Ibid.

show withdrawal symptoms after birth, including continual crying, fever, diarrhea, vomiting, and even seizures. The severity depends on how long the baby was exposed to heroin in the womb. These symptoms usually disappear by 1 week of age. "The longer the baby's exposure in the womb and the greater the dose, the more severe the withdrawal. Babies exposed to heroin before birth also face an increased risk of sudden infant death syndrome (SIDS)."[25]

A study published in 2000 found that there were correlations between maternal drinking, smoking, and marijuana use during pregnancy and behaviors in the child at age 3:

> Higher activity level, greater difficulty of management, tantrums, eating problems, and eating nonfood were related to maternal drinking during pregnancy. Increased fearfulness, poorer motor skills, and shorter length of play were associated with maternal marijuana use during pregnancy. Less well developed language, higher activity level, greater difficulty of management, fearfulness, decreased ability to get along with peers, and increased tantrums were associated with maternal cigarette smoking during pregnancy.

The authors concluded that, "It may be that the effects of substance use during pregnancy, especially more subtle ones, show up in behavior before they can be measured by developmental scales."[26]

The good news is that growing awareness of the risks to infants has led to a decrease in the rate of pregnant women using illicit drugs, binge-drinking alcohol, and smoking tobacco, at least in the third trimester of pregnancy, according to the 2009 National Survey on Drug Use and Health (NSDUH) Report. "Still, a sizeable proportion of women in the first trimester of pregnancy were past month users of alcohol, cigarettes, or marijuana, and one in seven women used cigarettes in the second or third trimester."[27] Moreover, many women who stopped during pregnancy resumed drug use, smoking, or binge-drinking within 3 months of giving birth. The Report concludes, "Effective interventions for women to further reduce substance use during pregnancy and to prevent postpartum resumption of use could improve the overall health and well-being of mothers and infants."[28]

Many women who use illegal drugs, such as marijuana, methamphetamine, cocaine, heroin, or ecstasy, often also smoke tobacco or drink alcohol, making it very difficult to know whether damage to the infant was due to illegal substances, which can lead to prosecution, or legal substances, which generally do not. (There are a few cases of pregnant women who were charged with child abuse or child endangerment

25. Ibid.

26. V. B. Faden and B. I. Graubard. 2000. "Maternal Substance Use During Pregnancy and Developmental Outcome at Age Three," *Journal of Substance Abuse* 12 (4): 329–340.

27. National Survey on Drug Use and Health (NSDUH). 2009. "Substance Abuse Among Women During Pregnancy and Following Childbirth." http://www.oas.samhsa.gov/2k9/135/PregWoSubUse.htm.

28. Ibid.

for drinking during pregnancy.[29]) Finally, the harmful effects may be due not to substance abuse at all, but to the poverty that often accompanies substance abuse, which leads to poor nutrition, poor maternal health, and little or no prenatal care.

The argument so far recognizes that women do have moral obligations to the children they plan to bear, obligations to consider the impact of their behavior on the developing fetus and to avoid taking unreasonable risks with their health and well-being. These obligations can be balanced against other moral considerations, including obligations to other, already born children. The degree to which a pregnant woman can be blamed for failing to meet her obligation to her not-yet-born child depends in part on the options open to her, for example, whether there are available and affordable treatment centers that accept pregnant women. (Getting pregnant women off drugs is tricky, because going "cold turkey" can itself harm the fetus.)

A separate issue is whether the moral obligation to consider the welfare of the future child should also be a legal one. It may seem as if once moral responsibility has been established, criminal liability follows. After all, we criminally punish people who inflict injury on their born children; why not those who inflict the injury prior to birth? In the next section, I demonstrate the defects of a criminal law approach to the problem of addiction and pregnancy.

PREGNANT WOMEN AND THE LAW

The argument in favor of various kinds of legal interventions into the lives of pregnant women rests on several factors: the ability of children to be harmed prenatally (which obviates the question of the moral or legal standing of the fetus), the general obligation of individuals not to harm others or cause their deaths, and the special obligations of parents (in this case, women who have decided to become mothers) to protect and provide care for their children. The impulse to protect late-gestation fetuses and newly born babies is extremely strong, and the impulse to punish women whose behavior is regarded as selfish and irresponsible is equally strong.

Delivering Drugs Through the Umbilical Cord

In July 1989, Jennifer Johnson of Florida became the first woman to be convicted of delivering cocaine to her newborn children through the umbilical cord.[40] She was charged with drug delivery on the basis of tests performed after the births of two of her children, a son born in 1987 and a daughter born in 1989. In both cases, Ms. Johnson told doctors that she had used cocaine the day before the deliveries.

29. The Center for Reproductive Law & Policy 1996. Part I. Punishing Women for Their Behavior During Pregnancy: An Approach That Undermines Women's Health and Children's Interests. New York: Center for Reproductive Law & Policy. http://www.drugpolicy.org/library/womrepro.cfm. Citing State v. Pfannenstiel, No. 1-90-8CR (Wyo. Cty. Ct. Albany Cty. Jan. 5, 1990) (pregnant woman charged with child abuse for drinking alcohol); Joan Little, "Woman Jailed After Baby Is Born Intoxicated," St. Louis Post-Dispatch, November 26, 1991, at 3A (woman was charged with second-degree assault and child endangerment after her son was allegedly born with signs of fetal alcohol syndrome).

Both children were born healthy and full term.[30] Ms. Johnson was sentenced to 1 year in a rehabilitation program and 14 years probation. Her conviction was upheld by a Florida appeals court, but it was overturned by the state supreme court in July 1992.

By charging Ms. Johnson with delivering a drug to her newborn children, not a fetus, the prosecution avoided the issue of the legal status of the unborn. Even so, the legal basis for these prosecutions is shaky. Applying existing drug laws to the prenatal cases ignores very real differences between the two situations. For one thing, the intent ordinarily necessary for a criminal charge is missing. A woman who uses drugs during pregnancy does not intend to give her child drugs. It is absurd to treat her like a pusher in a schoolyard.

Moreover, charging her with drug delivery after the babies are born does nothing to protect those children before they are born. The way to protect them is by making drug treatment available to people who want it, including pregnant women. "The important thing to remember about the Jennifer Johnson case is that this is a woman who tried to get treatment and was turned away," says Dr. Wendy Chavkin, who did a survey of drug treatment programs in New York City.[41] She found that 54% of treatment programs categorically excluded the pregnant. Sixty-seven percent rejected pregnant Medicaid patients and only 13% accepted pregnant Medicaid patients addicted to crack.[42] And even in areas where there are treatment programs for pregnant addicts, there are not enough spaces for everyone who wants help. For example, in 1988 the waiting list for a bed in L.A. County's rehabilitation program for pregnant women was 7 months long, according to a study by the county.[43]

Have things changed substantially since 1988? It seems not. According to an article published in 2009, although there has been an increase in drug treatment services for pregnant women over the last 20 years, there are still not enough programs for pregnant women and mothers who want to get off drugs. Moreover, for a variety of reasons, many substance-abusing women are unable to access the programs that do exist, due to lack of money, difficulties with transportation, or access to child care. And even if these hurdles are overcome, substance-abusing women experience many obstacles to getting the treatment they need. They fear losing custody of their children, if they seek treatment; they are often afraid of abusive partners who do not want them to expose their own use by seeking treatment; they typically lack healthy support systems necessary for successful treatment; they feel guilty and ashamed of being addicted and do not want to face this issue; and they have a lack of knowledge about addiction and a lack of knowledge about how to access health care in general.[31] These are serious problems that will not be addressed by a simple-minded criminal justice approach.

The ruling in the Jennifer Johnson case seems to have put an end to the "delivery of drugs through the umbilical cord" approach. Instead, most states that prosecute pregnant women for prenatal drug use have turned to child abuse statutes. Since 1985,

30. Tamar Lewin. 1992. "Mother Cleared of Passing Drug to Babies," *New York Times*, July 24. http://www.nytimes.com/1992/07/24/news/mother-cleared-of-passing-drug-to-babies.html?pagewanted=1. Accessed January 31, 2010.

31. Janet W. Steverson and Traci Rieckmann. 2009. "Legislating for the Provision of Comprehensive Substance Abuse Treatment Programs for Pregnant and Mothering Women," *Duke Journal of Gender Law and Policy* 16: 315–346.

there have been prosecutions of pregnant women for drug use in many states, including Alabama, Alaska, Arizona, California, Connecticut, Florida, Georgia, Hawaii, Idaho, Illinois, Indiana, Kentucky, Maryland, Massachusetts, Michigan, Mississippi, Missouri, Nebraska, Nevada, New York, North Carolina, North Dakota, Ohio, Oklahoma, Oregon, Pennsylvania, South Carolina, South Dakota, Tennessee, Texas, Utah, Virginia, Washington, Wisconsin, and Wyoming.[32] In the lead of states prosecuting pregnant women for prenatal drug use is the state of South Carolina.

Criminal Prosecution for Child Abuse or Endangerment

THE CASE OF CORNELIA WHITNER

Cornelia Whitner, an African American woman from South Carolina, was 14 years old when her mother suddenly died at the age of 42 from heart failure. Ms. Whitner then turned to drinking beer and using drugs. She became addicted to crack cocaine, dropped out of school in the 10th grade, and had her first child at the age of 15. Her youngest was born in 1992. When a toxicology screen revealed traces of cocaine in his system, she was arrested for child abuse, even though the baby was born healthy.[33] She pled guilty. "At her sentencing, she admitted having a drug problem and said, 'I need some help, Your Honor.' The court responded, 'I think I'll just let her go to jail.' She was sentenced to 8 years in prison."[34]

After serving more than a year of her sentence, Ms. Whitner filed an application for postconviction relief, arguing that she had been convicted of a nonexistent crime. There was no crime of fetal abuse in South Carolina, but rather a crime of child abuse, which does not apply to the unborn fetus. Her application was granted and, having spent 19 months in jail, she was released in 1993.[35] However, in October 1997, the South Carolina Supreme Court reversed the lower court's decision, construing the word *child* to include viable fetuses.[36] The court held that it would be absurd to

32. Jean Reith Schroedel and Pamela Fiber, P. 2001. "Punitive Versus Public Health Oriented Responses to Drug Use by Pregnant Women," *Yale Journal of Health Policy Law Ethics* 1: 217–235, at 218.

33. A similar case is *Cochran v. Kentucky*. In 2005, Ina Cochran was charged with "wanton endangerment" after she gave birth to a healthy girl, Cheyenne, and both mother and baby tested positive for cocaine. The trial court dismissed the case, but the appellate court said that state's child endangerment statute can apply to the pregnant woman herself in light of feticide laws and unborn victims of violence laws, which were meant to punish a third party's acts against a pregnant woman. On June 17, 2010, the Supreme Court of Kentucky reversed the decision of the Court of Appeals and reinstated the trial court's dismissal of the indictment.—S.W.3d—2010 WL 2470870 (Ky.)

34. Lynn Paltrow, 1999. "Pregnant Drug Users, Fetal Persons, and the Threat to *Roe v. Wade*," 62 *Albany Law Review* 999 at 1031.

35. National Advocates for Pregnant Women. 1999. "Cornelia Whitner's Letter to the Governor of South Carolina." http://www.advocatesforpregnantwomen.org/issues/cornelialtr. htm. Accessed November 1, 2009.

36. *Whitner v. State*, 492 S.E.2d 777 (S.C. 1997), at 779.

recognize a fetus as a person for purposes of homicide laws and wrongful-death statutes, but not for child abuse.[37] Ms. Whitner was sent back to jail. Her lawyers appealed to the U.S. Supreme Court, but on May 26, 1998, the Court declined to hear the case. The Attorney General of South Carolina, Charles Condon, took the denial of review as confirmation of the personhood of viable fetuses, justifying his policy of arresting pregnant women and the prosecution of doctors who perform partial-birth abortions[38] (see Chapter 2).

THE CASE OF MALISSA CRAWLEY

One of the worst effects of the jailing of women for drug use during pregnancy is the separation of children from their mothers. This may not be unreasonable in the case of a woman with a severe crack addiction, since the focus on obtaining and using drugs may result in neglect of one's children. But not all addicts are necessarily bad parents.[39] Moreover, sometimes the punitive approach sweeps up women who have overcome their addictions and are good parents. In 1991, Malissa Crawley, an African American woman living in South Carolina, gave birth to a healthy baby boy who tested positive for cocaine. She was indicted for violating the state's child endangerment statute, and on the advice of her court-appointed attorney, she pled guilty. She was sentenced to 5 years in jail but was given a suspended sentence. She remained free on probation, where she completed an outpatient drug treatment program, and remained drug-free. She was working and taking care of her three young children. Then in 1994, she and her boyfriend got into a fight, and both were arrested for domestic violence. That charge carried only a 30-day sentence, but the conviction constituted a violation of her parole, something she did not understand when she pled guilty. She was ordered to begin serving the 5-year sentence for child endangerment. Her children were described as healthy, doing well in school, lively, and polite. Nevertheless, as a result of the *Whitner* decision, Malissa Crawley was forced back to jail on March 2, 1998, leaving behind her children, ages 6, 5, and 2.

Who benefits from such a law? Surely not the Crawley children, left without their mother at such young ages. Surely not the people of South Carolina, if the children are taken into foster care at state expense. Even Charles Condon acknowledged that putting in jail a mother who had successfully gotten off drugs was not ideal. "In fact, because she is doing well, he considered exempting Crawley from prison. But other factors forced him to put that notion aside. According to state law once a sentence is imposed, it can't be modified, Condon said. 'Her situation made a sympathetic case,' Condon said. 'But who am I to change the law?'"[40] Lynn Paltrow notes drily that

---

37. Ibid., at 780.

38. Paltrow (see note 34) at 1035.

39. Studies on the effect of drug use on parenting agree that drug addicts are more likely to neglect than to abuse their children. However, there is significant disagreement among experts about the degree to which drug use correlates with neglect. One study found that many alcoholics and opiate addicts neither abuse nor seriously neglect their children. While addiction is often one factor in neglect, it is not the only factor, nor can neglect be predicted from drug use alone. See Dolgin, note 20 at 1225.

40. Michelle R. Davis. 1998. "Mom's Past Haunts Her Future," *The State* (Columbia, SC), February 22, B1.

shortly after making this statement, Condon reduced the sentence of a white law professor who took $5,000 from a man for a lawsuit he never filed.[41]

When a baby is born healthy, despite the mother's drug use in pregnancy, the child abuse charge is based on her taking an unwarranted risk with the health of her child, just as a parent might be guilty of child neglect by leaving a young child unattended, even if nothing happens. If, however, the drug use results in the death of a child, this can lead to a charge of homicide.

Criminal Prosecution for Homicide

THE CASE OF REGINA McKNIGHT

There are some similarities between the stories of Regina McKnight and Cornelia Whitner. Both are African American, both are residents of South Carolina, and both lost their mothers at an early age. (Ms. McKnight's mother was killed by a hit-and-run driver.) Ms. McKnight was below normal in intelligence, with an IQ of 72. Deprived of her mother's care, she turned to drugs, becoming addicted to both marijuana and cocaine. Unable to cope, she became homeless and pregnant. But whereas Cornelia Whitner gave birth to a healthy boy, Regina McKnight gave birth to a stillborn girl on May 15, 1999. After a urine sample showed that cocaine was present in her body, she was arrested—her first arrest—on a charge of homicide.

At trial in 2001, prosecutors agreed that she had no intention of harming the fetus or losing the pregnancy. "Doctors who testified at the trial did not agree on whether Ms. McKnight's addiction was the cause of death. Nevertheless, a jury deliberated only 15 minutes before finding her guilty of homicide by child abuse."[42] The first woman in South Carolina to be convicted under the statute, she was given a 20-year sentence, suspended to 12 years in prison with no chance for parole.

During the trial the state never attempted to prove that her drug use in fact caused the stillbirth, which would have been difficult to prove, since rarely can a stillbirth be tied to one single cause. Nor did the state attempt to prove that Ms. McKnight was aware of the risk of stillbirth from cocaine use, nor that the risk was a substantial one.[43] All of this was simply assumed to be true, an assumption characterized by Ms. McKnight's supporters as "junk science," which would not be tolerated in a civil case, involving corporate liability. In 2002, lawyers for Ms. McKnight, lawyers, joined by 27 other medical and drug policy groups, including the American Public Health Association, the American Nurses Association, and the American Society of Addiction Medicine, sought to overturn the conviction. Their appeal to the state supreme court was unsuccessful. "The Court held that a pregnant woman who unintentionally heightens the risk of a stillbirth could be found guilty of 'extreme indifference to human life' homicide. Under this decision a conviction for homicide is

41. Paltrow, (see note 34). at 1041.

42. Bob Herbert. 2001. "In America; Stillborn Justice." http://www.nytimes.com/2001/05/24/opinion/in-america-stillborn-justice.html?scp=2&sq=Bob+Herbert+Stillborn+Justice&st=nyt. Accessed January 13, 2010.

43. Ibid.

permitted on any evidence that a pregnant woman engaged in activity 'public[ly] know[n]' to be 'potentially fatal' to a fetus. The U.S. Supreme Court refused to review the decision."[44]

Then in 2008, the state supreme court overturned her conviction, saying that there was not enough proof that the baby died because of her cocaine use. Ms. McKnight had other medical conditions, hyperthyroidism and syphilis, that could have caused the stillbirth. In addition, the court ruled that Ms. McKnight did not receive a fair trial, because her lawyer was ineffective in cross-examination and in failing to call medical experts as witnesses who could have challenged the link between cocaine use and stillbirth. The decision also indicated that the conviction was based on outdated and inaccurate medical information on the effects of cocaine on stillbirth.

"Significantly, the opinion acknowledges that current research simply does not support the assumption that prenatal exposure to cocaine results in harm to the fetus, and the opinion makes clear that it is certainly 'no more harmful to a fetus than nicotine use, poor nutrition, lack of prenatal care, or other conditions commonly associated with the urban poor.'" said Susan K. Dunn, counsel for *amici*. "This decision puts solicitors [prosecutors] across the state on notice that they must actually prove that an illegal drug has risked or caused harm—not simply rely on prejudice and medical misinformation."[45]

The court ordered a new trial, but instead Ms. McKnight pleaded guilty to involuntary manslaughter, and the court decided to release her for time already served. On June 19, 2008, she was released from prison, to go home to her three children, having served more than 8 years in jail.[46]

The McKnight decision was based largely on the facts, specifically, the absence of evidence showing that her cocaine use caused her stillbirth. In other cases, judges have determined that child abuse statutes were not intended to cover behavior in pregnancy.

THE CASE OF TAYSHEA AIWOHI

Tayshea Aiwohi, a resident of Hawaii, used crystal meth during pregnancy and while breast-feeding. When her son, Treyson, died 2 days after he was born, she was charged with manslaughter. Her lawyer, Public Defender Todd Eddins, asked to have the case dismissed, on the ground that the methamphetamine alleged to have caused his death was delivered prior to Treyson's birth, before he was legally a person. The prosecutor refused to drop charges, saying that this was the reckless killing of another human being, as deserving of prosecution as cases in which the death is caused by an attack on a pregnant woman. Hawaii Circuit Judge Michael Town sentenced Ms. Aiwohi in August 2004 to 10 years probation. However, in December 2005,

44. Drug Policy Alliance Network. 2008. "South Carolina Supreme Court Reverses 20-Year Homicide Conviction of Regina McKnight." http://www.drugpolicy.org/news/pressroom/pressrelease/pr051208.cfm. Accessed November 1, 2009.

45. Ibid.

46. Sharon Green. 2008. "Regina McKnight Released From Prison." http://www.carolinalive.com/news/news_story.aspx?id=149364. Accessed January 13, 2010.

the state supreme court overturned the conviction, ruling unanimously that state law does not permit the prosecution of women who engage in risky behavior during pregnancy that leads to the death of a newborn.

From a legal standpoint, it is crucial to determine whether the statute under which a woman has been charged applies to her behavior. From a public policy standpoint, the question is whether to create laws that allow for the prosecution and incarceration of pregnant addicts.

So far, I have been arguing against a punitive approach on the ground that sending women to jail for having used drugs in pregnancy does not protect children, and indeed, punishes them by depriving them of their mothers. It may be objected that the same considerations against "fetal abuse" laws could be used against postnatal child abuse statutes. Arguably, laws against child abuse do little to protect children. It is unlikely that such laws have much deterrent effect, because most abuse is not deliberate or planned, but stems from inability to control frustration and anger. So why punish anyone who harms a child through abuse and neglect? And if we do think that some abusers *deserve* to be punished, regardless of whether punishing them has a deterrent effect, why can't we say that *some* women who inflict prenatal harm deserve to be punished? It could be argued that criminal sanctions are, in some cases, justified, namely, when a woman is aware that her *voluntary* and *noncompulsive* behavior poses serious risks to the health of her not-yet-born child, yet she disregards these risks, causing the baby to be born seriously damaged.[47] Perhaps a yuppie weekend recreational cocaine user would come into this category. Surely we would all agree that her behavior is immoral. Why shouldn't she be prosecuted?

In response, I would concede that prosecution in such a case could be justified. My fear is that it is unlikely that prosecution would be confined to such cases—if they exist at all. That is why a bill like Utah's HB 462 is so dangerous. As Lynn Paltrow points out, whatever the intention of the law's creators, " . . . once law enforcement officials have the discretion to arrest, and judges have the opportunity to interpret the law, legislators no longer have control. In fact there have already been cases where government officials seeking to protect the 'unborn' have sought to keep pregnant women from obtaining cancer treatment . . . . The real purpose of the Utah bill, however, is to make it possible to police pregnant women and to imprison them as murderers. That deserves a firestorm of opposition as well."[48]

Experience has shown that states that punish women for drug use during pregnancy primarily prosecute uneducated, low-income addicts—women who are likely to be less than fully responsible for their harmful behavior. In addition, prosecution is aimed almost entirely at minority women (about 70%–80% of prosecutions), even though drug use is roughly comparable.[49] In other words, it is race and class that

47. I am grateful to Lawrence Nelson for pushing me on this point.

48. Lynn Paltrow. 2010. "Utah Continues Reckless Efforts to Lock Up Pregnant Women," The Huffington Post, http://www.huffingtonpost.com/lynn-m-paltrow/utah-continues-reckless-e_b_488673.html. Accessed January 25, 2011.

49. In 2004, a National Survey on Drug Use and Health found that the rate of illicit drug use for whites was 8.1%; for blacks, 8.7%. http://www.oas.samhsa.gov/nsduh/2k4nsduh/2k4results/2k4results.pdf

primarily drives such prosecutions, not degree of blameworthiness. This undercuts the argument that such prosecutions are justified because deserved.

As a matter of public policy, it makes more sense to fund drug-treatment programs than to incarcerate pregnant drug addicts. Protection of the unborn will be best accomplished not by jailing pregnant offenders, but by attacking drug addiction directly, and by securing adequate prenatal care for all women:

> Drug use during pregnancy is a health issue that should be addressed by health professionals, not law enforcement and criminal justice agents. Every major medical and public health organization in the country opposes the arrest and jailing of pregnant women for drug and alcohol use—a response that endangers rather than promotes fetal and maternal health.[50]

However, while most medical and public health organizations support a public health, rather than punitive, approach to the problem of addiction and the treatment of substance-abusing pregnant women, many physicians support legal interventions into the lives of pregnant women. According to a study published in 2002, a majority of physicians agree that existing laws regarding child abuse and neglect need to be redefined to include alcohol (54%) and drug abuse (61%) during pregnancy, and this in spite of the fact that 61% believe that fear of prosecution would deter pregnant substance abusers from seeking prenatal care. Moreover:

> . . . 52% were in favor of enacting a statute that includes drug or alcohol use during pregnancy as "child abuse" for purposes of removing that child from maternal custody. Physicians were highly in favor of compulsory treatment for illicit drug use and alcohol abuse for women already in the criminal justice system (82%–83%), neutral with respect to court-ordered contraception for alcohol- (50%) and drug-abusing women (47%), and opposed to criminal prosecution for either alcohol abuse (18%–31% depending on subspecialty) or illicit drug use (23%–34%) during pregnancy.[51]

What this shows, I think, is that physicians are no different from the rest of us. Frustrated by what appears to be feckless and irresponsible behavior on the part of pregnant women that can result in serious harm to their babies, they want the law to intervene. Experts in the field, however, tell us repeatedly that compulsory treatment and punitive strategies are unlikely to be successful in getting women off drugs or protecting their future children. Such approaches do not address the underlying issues that drive the addiction, including poverty, limited education, and trauma resulting from sexual abuse and rape. One commentator argues that when the focus is solely on the behavior (getting the woman off drugs), the woman herself is ignored

50. Drug Policy Alliance Network. 2004. "Drugs, Police & the Law: Women & Pregnancy." http://www.drugpolicy.org/law/womenpregnan/index.cfm. Accessed August 10, 2009.

51. E. L. Abel and M. Kruger. 2002. "Physician Attitudes Concerning Legal Coercion of Pregnant Alcohol and Drug Abusers," *American Journal of Obstetrics and Gynecology* 186 (4): 768–772.

and marginalized. "Strategies to control the behavior using coercive means result in continued oppression by increasing the level of shame and guilt, and by reinforcing the isolation of the addicted woman."[52] Coercive and punitive approaches have an undeniable appeal, but they do not work.

What about jailing addicts to prevent them from taking drugs while they are pregnant? The rationale here is neither retributive nor based on deterrence. Rather, the aim is to protect specific not-yet-born babies. How successful is it likely to be, and how should we balance the protection gained against the infringement of privacy and liberty?

Jailing the Pregnant Addict

In the spring of 1988, Brenda Vaughan, a 29-year-old Washington, D.C., woman, pleaded guilty to forging about $700 worth of checks. It was her first offense and one that normally would have brought probation. But because Ms. Vaughan was pregnant, and tests showed she had used cocaine, the judge sent her to jail until the date her baby was due. There were no treatment programs available, and he wanted to protect the fetus from cocaine addiction. In defending his decision, Judge Peter H. Wolf said many of his judicial colleagues have told him they incarcerate pregnant drug abusers for the same reason.[53]

In January 2005, Amber Lovill, a Texas woman, pled guilty to two counts of forgery and was given a suspended sentence of 2 years in jail.[54] She was placed on "community supervision" (probation) for 3 years. Among the terms of her probation were that she avoid the use of narcotics, meet with her probation officer at least once a month, pay fines and restitution, participate in a drug treatment program, and submit to drug testing within a Treatment Alternative to Incarceration Program (TAIP).

The state filed its first motion to revoke her supervision in September 2005, when it was discovered that she had not attended the drug treatment program. The judge did not revoke her supervision, but sanctioned her and amended the terms and conditions of her supervision. "The judge specifically ordered Lovill to serve a term of confinement in the county Substance Abuse Treatment Facility (SATF)."[55]

In 2007, the State filed a second motion to revoke her community supervision, because she had tested positive for amphetamines, failed to report to her caseworker for several months, failed to attend the SATF aftercare program, and failed to pay the fines, restitution, costs, and fees that were ordered as part of her probation. Probationers who experience a relapse are often given another chance and the ability to continue treatment. However, the recommendation of the Probation Department to the judge was that, because of her drug use and pregnancy, Lovill should be confined in Substance Abuse Felony Punishment Facility (SAFPF). Sandra Garza,

52. Robert G. Madden. 1996. "Civil Commitment for Substance Abuse by Pregnant Women? A View From the Front Lines," *Politics and the Life Sciences*, March: 56–59.

53. Rorie Sherman. 1988. "Keeping Baby Safe From Mom," The National Law Journal, October 3, p. 25.

54. Lovill v.State. No. PD-0401-09. (December 16, 2009)

55. Ibid.

her community-supervision officer, acknowledged that Lovill's use of drugs and pregnancy "drove this violation report," and that her pregnancy was a high concern of theirs. When Garza was asked about alternative to incarceration programs, she said that she thought Lovill would benefit more from incarceration.

> As a result, Ms. Lovill was imprisoned at the Nueces County Jail, where she received no drugtreatment, inadequate prenatal care, was subject to shackling during her hospital stay and during transport to and from the hospital and was separated from her child only days after giving birth.

Was sending Ms. Lovill to jail justified on grounds of protecting the health of her future child? It might be thought that at least in prison Ms. Lovill could not use drugs. However, in many prisons inmates are able to obtain illegal drugs, so sending pregnant addicts to jail to protect their fetuses from maternal drug use is not intelligent policy. More important, the protection argument is based on the assumption that her fetus and future child would be harmed by her use of amphetamines, an assumption about which many experts are skeptical. "There is no credible scientific evidence linking methamphetamine to adverse pregnancy outcomes," said Barry Lester, Ph.D., professor of psychiatry and human behavior and pediatrics at the Warren Alpert Medical School of Brown University and the director of the Brown Center for the Study of Children at Risk at Women and Infants Hospital of Rhode Island. "Pregnant women with drug addictions need treatment—not jail."[56] Even if drug use does pose a threat to the unborn child, and even if the woman has no access to drugs in jail, conditions in jail, including no drug treatment and inadequate to nonexistent prenatal care, may be far more harmful to the health of both mother and child.

In the first edition of this book, I illustrated this harm by noting a class-action lawsuit filed by Legal Services for Prisoners with Children in 1985 on behalf of pregnant and postpartum women prisoners.[57] I wrote:

> One woman suffered severe abdominal cramping and bleeding for seventeen days without being allowed to receive treatment from an obstetrician. Her son was born in the ambulance on the way to an outside hospital, and lived only two hours. Another woman was seated upright and shackled while she was in active labor, as she was being transported to an outside hospital. By the time she arrived at the hospital, the baby was in severe distress and required more than thirty days in neonatal intensive care, with some degree of permanent disability a likely result. A third woman had gained over a hundred pounds by her eighth month of pregnancy and had protein in her urine. Despite these critical high-risk factors, she was seen only twice at the high-risk OB/GYN clinic in an outside hospital. Prison officials flatly refused to issue her the special diet recommended by the clinic. It is clear that jailing women cannot ensure medical

---

56. National Advocates for Pregnant Women. 2008. "NAPW and ACLU File Amicus Brief in Lovill v. Texas." January 18. http://advocatesforpregnantwomen.org/whats_new/napwaclu_file_amicus_brief_in_lovill_v_texas.php. Accessed January 25, 2011.

57. *Harris v. McCarthy* (85-6002) (C.D. California) (1985).

screening, regular monitoring, and other such minimum-care requirements to protect the fetus.[58]

In researching the second edition, I was horrified to learn that 20 years later some of the worst practices, including shackling pregnant women in labor, still occur.

NELSON V. NORRIS

Shawanna Nelson, an African American woman, was convicted of credit card fraud and passing bad checks and sentenced to 6 years in jail in Arkansas. When she went to prison in June 2003, she was 6 months pregnant with her second child. On September 20, she went into labor. The nurses at the prison infirmary determined that she needed to go to a contracting civilian hospital to deliver the baby, and they called for a guard to escort her. Because her contractions were coming every 5–6 minutes, and Ms. Nelson was in so much pain she was unable to walk, the guard, Patricia Turesky, was instructed to rush her to the hospital, and not to put handcuffs on her. Officer Turesky handcuffed her anyway. Moreover, in spite of the fact that this was a nonviolent prisoner, who in no way threatened the officer or anyone else, Officer Turensky shackled her legs to the hospital bed at the hospital.

A nurse at the hospital questioned the need for shackling Ms. Nelson, but to no avail. Every time a nurse had to examine Ms. Nelson to determine how dilated her cervix was, she had to ask Officer Turensky to remove the shackles, and when the examination was over, the shackles were replaced. This caused enormous discomfort for Ms. Nelson, who was unable to move or stretch or shift position. In addition, many midwives recommend that the laboring woman walk, not only to relieve pain but also to speed labor and to use gravity to help the baby down the birth canal. By shackling Nelson to the hospital bed, she was not only subjected to intense unnecessary pain during labor but also lasting physical problems, including permanent hip injury, causing lifelong pain, torn stomach muscles, damage to her sciatica nerve, and an umbilical hernia requiring surgical repair. As the result of the shackling, she cannot engage in ordinary activities, such as playing with her children. She is unable to sleep, or sit or stand for extended periods, and she has been advised not to have any more children.

Ms. Nelson sued Officer Turensky and the Director of Arkansas Department of Corrections, Larry Norris, for violating her Eighth Amendment rights against cruel and unusual punishment. Director Norris and Officer Turensky moved for summary judgment based on qualified immunity, arguing that their actions did not violate any of Nelson's clearly established constitutional rights. The district court denied the defendants qualified immunity, but a three-judge panel of the U.S. Court of Appeals for the Eighth Circuit (a very conservative court) reversed and granted summary judgment for the defendants. Ms. Nelson then petitioned for *en banc* rehearing.

In a six to five decision handed down on October 2, 2009, the Eighth Circuit found in favor of the district court's denial of qualified immunity to Officer Turensky, although it held that Director Norris, who was not present and had no knowledge of the shackling, could not be held liable. The case was remanded to the district court for trial of the Eighth Amendment issues raised by Ms. Nelson against

58. Steinbock. 1996. *Life Before Birth* (New York: Oxford University Press), pp. 141–142.

Officer Turensky. However, the Eighth Circuit determined there is a constitutional right not to be shackled during labor, and that this right was clearly established in September 2003:

> Existing constitutional protections, as developed by the Supreme Court and the lower federal courts and evidenced in ADC regulations, would have made it sufficiently clear to a reasonable officer in September 2003 that an inmate in the final stages of labor cannot be shackled absent clear evidence that she is a security or flight risk.[59]

Katherine Jack, staff attorney for National Advocates for Pregnant Women, calls the decision "a major victory for the growing movement to end the inhumane practice of shackling incarcerated pregnant women."[60]

In this particular case, no harm came to Ms. Nelson's baby from the shackling, although in other cases shackling has resulted in prolonging labor and deprivation of oxygen to the fetus. The case is instructive because the practice of shackling pregnant women in labor has continued in prison despite Supreme Court decisions ruling it unconstitutional.[61] And even if this horrific practice is ended, prison remains an unhealthy environment for women and their babies. What I wrote in the first edition remains true: "Incarcerating pregnant women to ensure healthy children is an improbable venture."

Termination of Parental Rights

Parents have legal obligations to care for their children, and not to inflict harm on them. Failure to meet these obligations can result in having their children taken away, temporarily or even permanently. Some states regard the fact that a woman used illegal drugs during pregnancy, confirmed by a positive toxicology screen on the newborn, as child abuse, and sufficient grounds for removing the child from the mother's custody.

THE CASE OF BABY BOY BLACKSHEAR
On July 14, 1998, Tonya Kimbrough gave birth to a baby boy, Lorenzo Blackshear, in Canton, Ohio.[62]

---

59. *Nelson v. Correctional Medical Services*, US Court of Appeals for the Eighth Circuit, No. 07-2481, October 2, 2009.

60. Katherine Jack, " Shackling Pregnant Inmates During Labor Cruel and Unusual." American Constitution Society, ACSblog. http://www.acslaw.org/taxonomy/term/901. Accessed February 11, 2010.

61. ACLU Attorney Diana Kasdan Answers Questions about the Shackling of Women During Labor. http://www.youtube.com/watch?v=Kz6zSk88Er0&feature=related. Accessed February 11, 2010.

62. In re *Baby Boy Blackshear*, 90 Ohio St 3d 197, 2000–Ohio -173.

Some members of the hospital staff noted that the baby was "jittery." A toxicology screen was performed on the baby's urine, and he was found to have cocaine in his system. The mother also tested positive for cocaine. Stark County Department of Human Services was notified, and when the mother and baby left the hospital on July 17, the baby was taken into temporary custody. On September 30, a magistrate of the court held an evidentiary hearing and on October 6 filed a decision finding Lorenzo to be an abused child. Ms. Kimbrough appealed this decision, which was upheld by the appeals court. On March 6, 2000, the Stark County Family Court granted permanent custody to Robin Blackshear, the child's biological father.

The trial court held that an unborn fetus is a person under Ohio's criminal code. Ms. Kimbrough appealed on this basis, arguing that a fetus is not a child, and that the General Assembly did not intend to include fetuses under the definition of a child in its child abuse statute. Since her use of cocaine which caused the injury to Lorenzo, occurred during pregnancy, while Lorenzo was a fetus, not a born child, Ohio's child abuse statute (R.C. 2151.031 (D)) cannot be used to remove him from her custody.

The Supreme Court of Ohio disagreed, saying, "We do not agree with Kimbrough in either how she has framed the issue or her interpretation of the statute." The issue, the court said, is not whether a fetus is a child, but whether the plain language of the statute applies to Lorenzo and the facts of the case. R.C. 2151.031 (D) defines an abused child as any child who, because of the acts of his or her parents, suffers physical or mental injury that harms, or threatens to harm, the child's health or welfare. It is clear," the court held, "that the action taken by Kimbrough caused Lorenzo injury both before and after his birth. It is clear that after his birth, Lorenzo was 'a child' as defined in R.C. 2151.011 (B) (6) (c)."[63] Whether fetuses have rights is not the question: born children certainly do, and the state has the right and obligation to protect children. "It is clear," the court continued, "that there can be no more sacred or precious right of a newborn infant than the right to life and to begin that life, where medically possible, healthy and uninjured."[64] Because the mother's prenatal drug use harmed Lorenzo, he is per se an abused child and can be removed from his mother's custody on that basis.

Two judges, Cook and Pfeifer, dissented. Their dissent was not based on the way the majority framed the case. The dissenters agreed with the majority that the issue is not whether fetuses are children, because Lorenzo is a born child. Whether he was injured prenatally, when he was a fetus, or postnatally, once born, is irrelevant. Rather, the dissenters took issue with the fact that the majority simply assumed, without any evidence, that the mother's prenatal cocaine use harmed, or threatened to harm, Lorenzo. A positive result on a newborn's drug screen is, they said, probative evidence of in utero exposure. But that is all it is. Whether that exposure actually harmed the child, or threatened to harm him, is a separate question, and one that requires medical evidence—evidence that was not provided in this case. The testimony that Lorenzo was jittery after birth came from a social worker, not a medical professional, who observed him shake briefly twice during a 5–15 minute period on the day he was born. There was no medical testimony connecting this symptom with the prenatal exposure

63. Ibid.

64. Ibid.

to cocaine. Moreover, the next day, Lorenzo's doctor noticed "not much jittering," and the following day he indicated that Lorenzo was "doing fine—no jitteriness." Judge Cook said that he would remand the case for determination of whether Lorenzo's prenatal exposure to cocaine either harmed, or threatened to harm, him, as required by the statute for him to qualify as an abused child.

The dissent was clearly correct in requiring medical evidence as regards actual harm or the threat of harm before removing a newborn from its mother. But while such evidence is necessary, is it sufficient to justify removal from custody? What if Lorenzo had suffered neurological damage as a result of his mother's prenatal cocaine use? Should it follow from that that he should be removed from his mother? I cannot see why it should. Removing him after birth is not going to prevent neurological damage that has already occurred. The justification for removing him from his mother's custody should not be damage already inflicted by prenatal drug use, but rather his mother's ability to take care of him.

Some may assume that because Ms. Kimbrough has a history of drug abuse (she had already given birth to one cocaine-exposed child before Lorenzo), she therefore cannot be a good mother. But this assumption seems unwarranted. Before separating mother and child, and risking harm to the child due to the separation and placement in foster care, it should be demonstrated that she is incapable of caring adequately for Lorenzo. Moreover, even if there is reason to suspect that she is incapable of being a good mother, before taking him away from her permanently, surely a period of observation would be in order. The question that was never addressed, either by the majority or the dissent, is whether the harms to Lorenzo from being taken away from his mother at birth, and placed into foster care, might outweigh any harms that would be caused by allowing him to stay.

It is instructive to contrast Ohio's approach to prenatal drug use with that of New York. In its decision in *Matter of Nassau County Dept. of Social Services v. Denise J.*,[65] the New York Court of Appeals (New York's highest court) held that a positive toxicology screen on a newborn was not sufficient evidence of neglect. In this case, the mother, Denise J., had a history of cocaine abuse and had been admitted to several drug rehabilitation centers. Denise's mother had custody of two of Denise's children because her drug use made her incapable of caring for them. After she gave birth to Dante in November 1990, both mother and son tested positive for cocaine, leading the Nassau County Department of Social Services (DSS) to seek temporarily to remove Dante from Denise's care. Family Court dismissed the petition, apparently because DSS had not provided any medical evidence about Denise's drug use, and directed the hospital to release Dante to his mother's custody.

DSS then brought a consolidated child protective proceeding against Denise on behalf of Dante and her daughter, Dantia (born in 1987). At the fact-finding hearing, DSS introduced into evidence two medical reports showing a positive toxicology for cocaine from Dante and positive toxicology for cocaine and opiates from Denise. In addition, DSS presented evidence of Denise's prior history of drug abuse and her admission that she may have smoked a cigarette containing cocaine at a Halloween party, while she was pregnant with Dante.

Denise's lawyers presented two experts who testified that she provided a clean, well-ordered environment for her children, that she interacted appropriately with

65. 87 N.Y.2d 73, 661 N.E.2d 138, 637 N.Y.S.2d 666.

her children, and that she had passed four random drug tests. They maintained that Denise had not been a regular user of controlled substances since the latter half of the 1980s, and that she was voluntarily receiving counseling at a general education and support program run by the Family Service Association.

Family Court found that a positive toxicology screen for a controlled substance in the newborn was sufficient for a determination of neglect. Denise was placed under the supervision of DSS for a 1-year period, but she was permitted to retain custody of Dante and Dantia. The Appellate Division affirmed, relying on additional evidence in the record for its factual findings of neglect.

The Court of Appeals ruled that the Family Court erred in concluding that Dante's positive toxicology alone was sufficient for the findings of neglect. It noted that New York's Family Court Act sets forth two predicates for a finding of neglect: actual physical, emotional, or mental impairment; or the imminent danger of such impairment. Actual impairment cannot be demonstrated by a positive toxicology test since many children exposed prenatally to cocaine and other controlled substances are not impaired.

What about imminent danger? As we saw, the Ohio Supreme Court held that prenatal cocaine use "threatened harm," even if no actual harm was done. This justified classifying Lorenzo as an abused child, who could be removed from his mother's custody. By contrast, the New York Court of Appeals held that the mother's prenatal drug use by itself could not establish "imminent danger." The danger to which a born child might be exposed after birth, and from which the state ought to protect him, has to do with the likelihood that the parent will abuse or neglect the child, and that question cannot be settled solely by the mother's prenatal drug use (although it is relevant to parental fitness). Thus, a positive toxicology report, in conjunction with other evidence, may support a finding of neglect. In this case, the record contained other evidence of neglect, including the fact that two of Denise's children were already in her mother's custody. However, the DSS did not attempt to permanently or even temporarily remove the children from Denise's custody. All it sought to do was to place her under DSS supervision for 1 year. Given the evidence presented of neglect, this seems a limited and reasonable intervention.

Compulsory Cesarean Sections

When a commonly performed procedure (such as cesarean section) poses little risk to the woman (or even reduces maternal mortality or morbidity), and may be the only way to secure live birth, physicians may feel an obligation to the fetus to act as its advocate and to get the woman to consent to lifesaving surgery. Admittedly, refusal in such circumstances is rare. Most women, faced with the possibility of fetal damage or death, readily consent to the treatment their doctors recommend. Occasionally, however, a woman rejects a physician's recommendation, perhaps on religious grounds, perhaps because she does not think that surgery is necessary, or perhaps because she is afraid of surgery. The courts have long held that competent adults may refuse lifesaving medical treatment. But does the right to refuse treatment for oneself include a right to refuse treatment necessary to save another's life? These cases pose agonizing dilemmas for physicians. Nancy Rhoden writes, "They pit a woman's right to privacy and bodily integrity . . . against the possibility of a lifetime of devastating disability to a being who is within days or even hours of independent existence."[66]

With a few notable exceptions,[72] most commentators have argued that pregnant women should not be forced to undergo medical treatment for the sake of preserving the life or health of their fetuses.[73] Attitudes among practicing physicians seem to be more split. A study published in 1987 found considerable support among heads of fellowship programs in maternal-fetal medicine for legal intervention of various kinds into the management of pregnancy. Almost half of those surveyed supported involuntary detention of pregnant women whose behavior endangers their fetuses. About the same number thought that the precedents set by the courts for emergency cesareans should be expanded to include other procedures, such as intrauterine transfusion, as these become part of standard medical care.[74]

Because women so rarely refuse cesarean deliveries in the face of acute fetal distress, it is difficult to find data on how often doctors in the United States perform them without consent. However, such cases are not unknown. In one case, the placenta of a woman in labor detached prematurely from the inner wall of the uterus (a condition known as abruptio placentae), presenting an imminent threat to fetal survival. The mother repeatedly refused to give consent to a cesarean section, and the attending physicians felt that there was no time to attempt to secure a court order. Despite her refusal of consent, she did not actively resist when given general anesthesia. The physicians then delivered a severely stressed but otherwise healthy infant by cesarean section.[75]

The temptation simply to ignore the mother's refusal is understandable. Doctors are naturally reluctant to stand by and watch a baby who would be fine if delivered surgically die, or perhaps worse, suffer profound neurological damage. If they turn out to be right—the baby's life is saved and it is clear that the baby would have died if they had not operated—it seems harsh to blame them. If the woman herself is later glad that the doctors ignored her refusal, if she is *grateful* to them for having saved her life and that of her child, it does not seem that anyone else can say that they acted wrongly. Nevertheless, I will argue that these conditions cannot be guaranteed in advance, and therefore doctors are not morally justified in ignoring the refusals of competent patients.

In at least one case, a woman was not subjected to a forced cesarean, but was criminally charged after refusing a cesarean section. In December 2003, Melissa Rowland was brought from Florida to Utah by an adoption agency to give up for adoption the twins she was carrying. On December 25, she contacted a hospital by telephone, complaining of no fetal movement, and was told to go to a hospital immediately. She did not. On January 2, she was seen by a doctor at another hospital that she should have an emergency cesarean section, due to oligohydramnios (abnormally small amount of amniotic fluid), fetal growth retardation, and repetitive fetal heart rate decelerations.[67] She refused, saying that she did not want to be "gutted

66. Nancy K. Rhoden. 1987. "Cesareans and Samaritans," *Law, Medicine & Health Care* 15 (3): 118–125, at. 118.

67. Susan Haack. 2008. "The Rights and Responsibilities of Pregnant Women," *Ethics & Medicine: An International Journal of Bioethics* 24 (3), Fall. Published on http://www.cbhd. org/content/rights-and-responsibilities-pregnantwomen-0. Accessed March 16, 2010.

from breast bone to pubic bone." She went to another hospital on January 9 to see whether the fetuses were still alive. No heart beat could be found on one of the twins by external monitor. She left the hospital, against medical advice. Finally, she returned to one of the hospitals on January 13, where she delivered by cesarean section a stillborn male, and a girl, who survived, but tested positive for cocaine and alcohol.[68] An autopsy revealed that the dead twin probably could have been saved if the cesarean had been performed when the doctor recommended it. Rowland was charged with murder, a charge that was later dropped. She pleaded guilty instead to two charges of child endangerment for using drugs during pregnancy.

Susan Haack defends the decision to prosecute Rowland, arguing that, "The maternal decision to carry a child to term creates a beneficence-based fiduciary obligation on the part of the mother (and physician) to act in the best interest of the unborn child, and to sacrificially care for and nurture that child . . . Why should pregnancy, a state of heightened responsibility, exempt women from accountability for irresponsible and illegal behavior? . . . Yes, women should be free to make informed choices in the context of their beneficence-based responsibilities, but such freedom should not exempt them from culpability when their autonomous decisions harm others."[69]

Was Rowland fully competent and thus accountable for her actions? That is doubtful. She suffered from mental illness (which is why the murder charge was dropped), was often homeless, and had tried to kill herself twice. Katha Pollitt describes Rowland as "not exactly a poster child for pregnant women's rights." She was a substance abuser who had four previous children, two of whom were given up for adoption, and one who was taken away by child protective services after Rowland punched her in a supermarket.[70] However, it is not the case that there is no reasonable alternative to the use of legal sanctions in such cases, as Haack maintains. Instead, we can implement policies that attempt to prevent such situations. Pollitt writes:

> Melissa Rowland's case is one that never should have happened. Instead of arranging her auto-da-fé, whether for murder or child endangerment, the State of Utah should be asking itself how it can improve services for poor, pregnant, mentally ill substance abusers—and maybe take a look at adoption agency practices, too. When doctors and nurses take the time to know their patients and treat them with empathy and respect, patients usually follow their advice.[71]

Cases like that of Melissa Rowland are extremely rare. More common are cases in which the woman's refusal of a cesarean section is ignored or overridden. The justification is premised on the assumption that such a delivery is necessary to protect the health of the baby (and perhaps that of the mother as well). However, we may be skeptical of the claim of necessity in light of the skyrocketing rate of

68. Ibid.

69. Ibid.

70. Katha. Pollitt. 2004. "Pregnant and Dangerous." *The Nation*, April 8. http://www.thenation.com/doc/20040426/pollitt. Accessed March 16, 2010.

71. Ibid.

cesarean deliveries: from approximately 5% in the mid-1960s to nearly 32% in 2005.[72] Nearly 40% of hospitals in the United States ban vaginal birth after cesarean section (known as VBAC); the VBAC rate is only 7.8%. Many American women who have had one cesarean delivery (perhaps indicated by breech birth or fetal distress) have no alternative to cesarean delivery in a subsequent pregnancy. This is the case, despite ACOG's recommendation that a trial of labor is appropriate for women who have had a low transverse uterine incision from a previous cesarean delivery and who have no contraindications for a vaginal birth.[73]

Some experts estimate that more than half of the 1 million cesarean operations performed each year in the United States are unnecessary.[74] This means that there is a substantial chance that a woman compelled to accept a cesarean for the sake of the fetus will have been forced to undergo an unnecessary operation. Consider the case of Amber Marlowe, who went into labor on January 14, 2004. After a routine sonogram, doctors at Wilkes-Barre General Hospital in Pennsylvania decided that the baby looked too big for a vaginal delivery and told her she needed a cesarean. Mrs. Marlowe was not convinced; she had delivered her previous six babies, including some large ones, vaginally. Fetal monitoring showed that the fetus was not in distress. The doctors spent hours trying to convince her to change her mind. When they were unsuccessful, they sought, and got, a court order for a medically necessary cesarean section. Against physician advice, Amber and her husband, John, checked out of Wilkes-Barre and went to another hospital, where she delivered a healthy 11-pound girl vaginally.[75]

Physician fallibility is only one reason why we should be reluctant to take the management of a pregnancy out of the woman's hands. Another reason is the increased risk to the woman from surgical delivery. Admittedly, cesarean sections are now relatively safe. Maternal mortality after cesarean section is extremely low, about 6 in 100,000 for planned cesarean sections, and about 18 in 100,000 for emergency cesarean sections, and usually is due to blood clots, infections, or the complications of anesthesia.[76] Nevertheless, cesarean section is major surgery, and, as such, is associated with higher rates of maternal mortality,[77] morbidity, and increased pain

72. CDC. 2007. "Births: Final Data for 2005," *National Vital Statistics Reports*, 56 (6). http://www.cdc.gov/nchs/data/nvsr/nvsr56/nvsr56_06.pdf. Accessed February 23, 2010.

73. ACOG Practice Bulletin: Vaginal Birth After Previous Cesarean Delivery. 2004. http://www.acog.org/acog_districts/dist9/pb054.pdf. Accessed March 16, 2010.

74. Gina Kolata. 1989. "New York Is First State to Try to Curb Caesareans," *New York Times*, January 27. http://www.nytimes.com/1989/01/27/nyregion/new-york-is-first-state-to-try-to-curb-caesareans.html?scp=4&sq=reduce+cesarean+birth+rate&st=nyt. Accessed January 23, 2011.

75. Lisa Collier Cool. 2005. "Could You Be Forced to Have a C-Section?"
Baby Talk magazine, May. http://www.advocatesforpregnantwomen.org/main/publications/articles_and_reports/could_you_be_forced_to_have_a_csection_1.php. Accessed March 16, 2010.

76. Web MD. 2011. "Cesarean Section – Risks and Complications." http://www.webmd.com/baby/tc/cesarean-section-risks-and-complications. Accessed January 23, 2011.

77. It is unclear how much higher the risk of mortality is from a cesarean delivery. According to Wikipedia, "Caesarean Section," the UK National Health Service places the risk of death

than vaginal delivery. The question, then, is not simply whether the interests of the fetus should be considered, but how to weigh its interests against those of the pregnant woman. How much of a risk is she ethically and legally required to take with her own life and health to safeguard the life and health of her fetus?

Courts have sometimes cited *Roe v. Wade* as authority for a court-ordered cesarean.[78] This betrays a misunderstanding of *Roe v. Wade* and subsequent abortion cases.

The Implications of *Roe v. Wade*

In *Roe v. Wade*, the Supreme Court held that the constitutional right of privacy, which protects a woman's decision to terminate a pregnancy, is not absolute. It can be balanced against other state interests, including the interest in protecting potential life. That "important and legitimate" state interest becomes "compelling" at viability, permitting states, if they choose, to prohibit abortions after viability, except when necessary to preserve the life or health of the mother. One commentator, noting that *Roe v. Wade* gives to the state "substantial authority to protect fetal life," concludes that this authority extends to nonabortion cases. John Myers writes:

> The state's interest in viable fetal life permits it to forbid abortion, an act designed to extinguish life. It follows from this that the state is empowered to proscribe other acts calculated or likely to lead to the same result. Furthermore, since the interest in preservation of fetal life authorizes intervention to prevent destructive acts, it should also authorize limited compulsion of action which is necessary to preserve fetal life.[79]

On this basis, Myers argues that the Georgia Supreme Court was correct in ordering a cesarean delivery in *Jefferson*. "The evidence was clear that fetal death would result unless the surgery was ordered. While maternal risk in cesarean delivery is not inconsequential, the certainty of fetal death outweighed that risk . . ."[80] Ironically, in this case, there was no "certainty of fetal death." The surgery was not performed, the placenta previa corrected itself, and Mrs. Jefferson gave birth vaginally to a healthy baby girl. Myers acknowledges the possibility of medical error, but says, "... the reality of medical error must not be allowed to stand in the way of essential fetal treatment. As medical science progresses, errors in prediction will decrease."[81] I am not suggesting that doctors should ignore clinical indications for cesarean

for the mother at 3 times that of a vaginal birth. However, the Wikipedia entry points out that this can be misleading, since women with severe health problems or high-risk pregnancies may require cesarean deliveries which can distort the mortality figures. http://en.wikipedia. org/wiki/Cesarean. Accessed January 25, 2011.

78. *Jefferson v. Griffin Spalding County Hospital Authority*, 247 Fa. 86, 274 S.E.2d 457 (1981).

79. John E. B. Myers. 1984. "Abuse and Neglect of the Unborn: Can the State Intervene?" *Duquesne Law Review* 23(1): 1–76, at 18.

80. Ibid., at 75.

81. Ibid., at 70, footnote 373.

deliveries because they *might* be wrong. Rather, the number of times the doctors who have sought compulsory cesareans *have* been wrong should make us examine more carefully their claims of knowledge. How accurate are their instruments for predicting that a cesarean is necessary for fetal well-being? Generally, diagnoses of placenta previa by ultrasonagraphy are exceptionally uncontroversial and accurate. Yet doctors can mistake a more benign partial placenta previa for a complete one, or the placental position may change between the time the sonogram was taken and delivery. Moreover, as noted previously, the rate of cesarean sections has skyrocketed in recent years. Myers' prediction that progress in medical science will result in fewer errors in prediction is at odds with the increased number of cesarean sections and unnecessary cesarean sections.

The most common fetal indication for surgical delivery is prediction of fetal distress, based upon electronic fetal monitoring (EFM). But fetal monitors have an astonishingly high false-positive rate, due in part to the fact that the problem screened for—fetal hypoxia during labor of sufficient severity to cause fetal damage—occurs only rarely in a population of healthy, normal women. As the incidence of a condition decreases in frequency, it becomes increasingly likely that positive diagnoses are really false positives. The false-positive rate for predicting cerebral palsy is 99%, according to the American College of Gynecologists and Obstetricians (ACOG). Although the use of EFM has become routine (used in about 85% of labors), it has not reduced cerebral palsy or perinatal mortality.[82] Despite this, facing the risk of a brain-damaged child and a multimillion-dollar lawsuit, doctors may opt for cesarean delivery on the basis of EFM.

The upshot of a policy of allowing doctors to take whatever steps they believe to be necessary to protect the fetus is an increase in maternal risk. Myers thinks that this is justified so long as the risk to the fetus from not performing the operation is greater than the risk to the woman from performing it. Several commentators[83] have argued that this sort of "trade-off" between maternal and fetal health is precisely what *Roe v. Wade* and subsequent abortion decisions do not permit. For example, in *Colautti v. Franklin*,[84] the Supreme Court invalidated a Pennsylvania statute requiring that after viability doctors use the method least likely to harm the fetus unless an alternative was necessary to preserve the woman's life or health. The Court held that by using the word *necessary*, Pennsylvania impermissibly implied that a different technique must be *indispensable* for the woman's health. This flaw was compounded by the failure to "clearly specify . . . that the woman's life and health must always prevail over the fetus's life and health when they conflict."[85] Rhoden observes that this means that a woman cannot be compelled to undergo an even slightly greater

82. ACOG Refines Fetal Heart Rate Monitoring Guidelines. 2009. http://www.acog.org/from_home/publications/press_releases/nr06–22–09–2.cfm. Accessed March 16, 2010.

83. For example, Lawrence J. Nelson, Brian P. Buggy, and Carol J. Weil, "Forced Medical Treatment of Pregnant Women: 'Compelling Each to Live as Seems Good to the Rest,'" *Hastings Law Journal* 37 (May 1986); and Nancy K. Rhoden, "The Judge in the Delivery Room: The Emergence of Court-Ordered Cesareans," *Law, Medicine & Health Care* 15 (3): 1951–2030. December 1986.

84. *Colautti v. Franklin*, 439 U.S. 379 (1979).

85. Ibid., at 400, cited in Rhoden, "The Judge in the Delivery Room" (see note 83), p. 1990.

risk for the sake of the viable fetus. The Court again upheld this principle in *Thornburgh*.[86] The Court struck down Pennsylvania's amended statute on the ground that it, like the old statute, "failed to require that maternal health be the paramount consideration."[87] Nelson, Buggy, and Weil summarize the Court's position: "Even though the state's interest in protecting fetal life becomes compelling at viability, this interest is *not* sufficiently compelling under the Constitution to support a statutory requirement that the mother bear *any* increased risk to her health in order to save her viable fetus."[88]

McFall v. Shimp and the Duty to Rescue

The principle that pregnant women should not be compelled to undergo any additional risks for the sake of the unborn, even after viability, can be given an equal protection basis. Outside pregnancy, there are virtually no circumstances in which the body of one person could be required to save the life of another. One famous case is *McFall v. Shimp*,[89] in which Robert McFall, who was dying of aplastic anemia, asked the court to order his cousin, David Shimp, the only family member with potentially compatible bone marrow, to donate bone marrow to him. Bone-marrow extraction is not an especially risky procedure—far less risky than major surgery—but it is painful and invasive. Shimp apparently believed that the medical risk to him was greater than his cousin's doctors assessed it. On a balancing-interests approach, McFall's interest in survival might well outweigh Shimp's interests in avoiding pain and minimal risk. The court rejected this approach. Although the court found Shimp's behavior to be morally reprehensible, it refused to order him to donate. The court emphasized that there was no legal duty to rescue others, and it stated that to require this would change every concept and principle upon which our society is founded. The court said:

> For a society which respects the rights of *one* individual, to sink its teeth into the jugular vein or neck of one of its members and suck from it sustenance for *another* member, is revolting to our hard-wrought concepts of jurisprudence. Forcible extraction of living body tissue causes revulsion to the judicial mind. Such would raise the spectre of the swastika and the Inquisition, reminiscent of the horrors this portends.[90]

McFall and Shimp were only cousins, but there is no doubt that the outcome would have been the same even had they been father and child. Angela Holder states, "In no case is an adult ever ordered to surrender a kidney, bone marrow, or any other

---

86. *Thornburgh v. American College of Obstetricians & Gynecologists*, 737 F.2d 283 (3rd Cir. 1984), *aff'd* 106 S. Ct. 2101 (1986).

87. Ibid., p. 300. Cited in Nelson et al, "Forced Medical Treatment" (see note 83), p. 744.

88. Nelson et al, "Forced Medical Treatment" (see note 84), p. 745.

89. *McFall v. Shimp*, 10 Pa. D. & C.3d 90 (1978).

90. Ibid., p. 92 (emphasis in original).

part of his body for donation to his child, to another relative, or to anyone else."[91] In fact, it is doubtful that a parent could be legally compelled to donate a pint of blood necessary to save his or her child's life.

The case of minor children is slightly different, since they are often not capable of giving consent. This is not necessarily a bar to donation, since some courts have allowed parents to authorize an incompetent sibling to donate a kidney to a sibling suffering from renal failure, using a substituted judgment basis.[92] Other courts have rejected the claim that the test is whether the incompetent would consent to donate if he could do so, and have simply refused to authorize the transplant on the grounds that it is not in the best interest of the incompetent.[93] While courts have disagreed about whether parents may *authorize* donation on behalf of minor children, there is agreement that such authorization cannot be *compelled*. In one case, Tamas Bosze, a Chicago bar owner, was told that only a marrow transplant could save his son, Jean-Pierre, from dying of leukemia. The boy's only potential donors were twin half-siblings born out of wedlock to the father's former girlfriend. Bosze sued the woman in an attempt to compel her to have the children tested for tissue compatibility. She refused, on the ground that this would not be in the twins' best interest. A court upheld her decision. In so doing, the court upheld the principle that no one is legally required to donate a body part to another, not even when this is needed to save a life. (Shortly thereafter Jean-Pierre Bosze died.[94]) As we saw in Chapter 2, individuals may not be legally compelled to be "Good Samaritans." This principle of our legal system must be remembered in assessing compulsory cesareans. To force women to undergo major surgery, even relatively safe major surgery, is to impose an unequal and unjustified burden on pregnant women. Even if we accept—as I do—the premise that women have *moral* obligations to the children they plan to bear, and even if these moral obligations include undergoing risks and making sacrifices to secure the health and well-being of the children they have decided to bear, it is quite another matter to think that these moral obligations should be legally coerced. I think we can agree that it would be appallingly selfish for a woman to expose her nearly born baby to the risk of an irreversible handicap simply to avoid an abdominal scar. But even in such a case, the woman should not be legally compelled to undergo surgery.

The aforementioned argument is based on the injustice of imposing burdens on pregnant women that are not imposed on other people. But what if the burdens were not unequally imposed? Would the state be justified in legally compelling all citizens, men and women, to undergo bodily risk and invasion where necessary to save a life? The answer to this question depends on one's general political outlook. Those who lean toward a more libertarian perspective will be opposed to "Good Samaritan" laws in general and will find the idea of compulsory donation of bodily parts especially repellent. Those who take a more communitarian approach may

91. Angela Holder. 1985. *Legal Issues in Pediatrics and Adolescent Medicine*, 2nd edition (New Haven: Yale University Press), p. 171.

92. See, e.g., *Hart v. Brown*, 29 Conn. Supp. 368, 289 A.2d 386 (1972); *Strunk v. Strunk*, 445 S.W.2d 145 (Ky. 1969).

93. See In re *Richardson*, 284 So.2d 185 (La. Ct. App. 1973); In re *Pescinski*, 67 Wis.2d 4, 226 N.W.2d 180 (1975).

94. Lance Morrow. 1991. "Ethics: Sparing Parts," *Time*, June 17, pp. 54–58.

argue that all members of a community have a duty to make sacrifices for the good of the whole. For example, requiring healthy adults to make occasional blood donations might be considered justifiable. Communitarians might also argue that women should be legally compelled to undergo cesarean sections, where this is necessary to spare the child lifelong disability or death, given the relatively small objective risk to the woman and the enormous benefit to the child.

I cannot undertake a full-scale treatment of the merits of these opposing political theories. Fortunately, this is not necessary. Even communitarians should oppose compulsory cesareans, because, regardless of whether they could be justified in theory, there are overwhelming practical objections to them. For example, most doctors, even those who favor legal intervention in some cases, balk at using physical force to perform the surgery.[95] However, the potential for physical compulsion is implicit in legal coercion. Doctors who seek court orders should think about what they are willing to do to ensure that these are carried out. Francis Kenner, a Colorado woman who was told during labor that she needed a cesarean because of fetal distress, became more cooperative after the judge ordered a cesarean section. This was fortunate because, as her physician noted, "had the patient steadfastly refused it might not have been either safe or possible to administer anesthesia to a struggling, resistant woman who weighed in excess of 157.5 kg."[96] George Annas asks, "Do we really want to restrain, forcibly medicate, and operate on a competent, refusing adult? Such a procedure may be 'legal,' especially when viewed from the judicial perspective that the woman is irrational, hysterical, or evil-minded, but it is certainly brutish and not what one generally associates with medical care."[97]

The Case of A. C.

Perhaps the most brutish example of a forced cesarean was one performed on a dying woman in June 1987. Angela Carder (known as "A. C." in the court papers) was approximately 25 weeks pregnant, when she learned that the cancer she had had as a teenager, and had thought was in remission, had reoccurred. On Thursday, June 11, she was admitted to George Washington University Hospital. At first, the doctors were guardedly optimistic about her condition. Angela had repeatedly done better than expected in her long battle with cancer. She had been told at the age of 13 that she had only a few years to live. So, on Friday, June 12, the possibility of participating in a new NIH chemotherapy protocol was discussed. But by the following Monday, it seemed that Angela's condition was terminal. Her long-term-care physician, Dr. Jeffrey Moscow from the National Institutes of Health, told Angela that this time she should not expect a cure or have hope for "long-term survival." Angela agreed to palliative

95. Rhoden, "The Judge in the Delivery Room" (see note 83), footnote 273, p. 2004, citing a statement by Dr. Norman Fost, Presentation on Fetal Therapy at The Hastings Center, Conference on Abortion and Scientific Change, Hastings-on-Hudson, New York (May 24, 1985).

96. W. A. Bowes and B. Selgestad, "Fetal versus Maternal Right: Medical and Legal Perspectives," 58 *American Journal of Obstetrics & Gynecology* (1981), p. 209. The case is In re *Unborn Baby Kenner*, No. 79 JN 83 (Col Juv. Ct. March 6, 1979).

97. George Annas, "Forced Cesareans: The Most Unkindest Cut of All," *Hastings Center Report* 12(3): 16–17, 45, p. 45.

radiation and/or chemotherapy to relieve her pain and to try to reach 28 weeks in her pregnancy, at which time the fetus's chances of viability would be greatly increased.

Angela's health rapidly deteriorated, and by Monday evening, she was transferred to the intensive care unit and intubated (had a tube placed in her airway to help her breathe). The next morning, her condition worsened. She was in a great deal of pain. A priest was called to give the last rites. Her husband, parents, and doctors all agreed that keeping Angela comfortable while she died was what she wanted, and that her wishes should be honored.

On Tuesday morning, George Washington University, through its general counsel, Vincent Burke, asked a local trial judge to come to the hospital to decide what, if any, interventions should be performed on behalf of the fetus. Judge Emmett Sullivan of the District of Columbia Superior Court summoned volunteer lawyers and convened an emergency hearing in the hospital. According to Nettie Stoner, Angela's mother, they were called from Angela's bedside to a "short meeting." They were not told that it was a court hearing, nor that it would take them away from their daughter all day.

Much of the hearing was an attempt to determine what Angela's wishes with regard to the pregnancy were. Angela was at that point heavily sedated in order to maintain her ventilatory function and was unable to carry on a meaningful conversation. Angela's attending physician, Louis Hamner, testified that the night before, when Angela was alert and awake, she had agreed to have a cesarean section at 28 weeks. Her doctors did not think an earlier cesarean section would be advisable. "Much prior to that, the prognosis was poor enough that we would be extremely uncomfortable intervening."[98]

Angela's doctors did not think that her fetus was viable. This was based partly on its gestational age but also on Angela's condition. Asked what the prognosis would be for the fetus if the court ordered intervention, Dr. Hamner replied that, generally, fetuses at 26 weeks have between 50% and 60% chance of survival. However, because this fetus had been exposed to multiple medications, its chances for survival were lower.[99]

Dr. Maureen Edwards, a neonatologist and director of nurseries at GWU Hospital, was more optimistic. Acknowledging that it was very difficult to give a prognosis for a particular neonate or fetus, Dr. Edwards nevertheless projected a 50%–60% chance of survival for the fetus, and only a 20% chance of serious handicap. However, Dr. Edwards had not examined Angela and apparently had no specific knowledge of the condition of the fetus, nor any knowledge of the medicines to which the fetus had been exposed. Despite this, Judge Sullivan accepted her prognosis for the fetus over that of Angela's doctors.

According to Dr. Hamner, Angela understood that premature delivery has an increased risk of cerebral palsy, neurological defects, hearing loss, and blindness. It was his belief that Angela, having gone through so much illness and pain in her own life, did not want to bring a baby into the world who would have to undergo these problems. The guardian *ad litem* for the fetus, Barbara Mishkin, argued that such quality-of-life considerations were not a determining factor in deciding what medical care should be provided to the so-called Baby Does, and so "the possible

98. In re *Angela Carder*, Testimony and Proceedings, no. 87-609, June 16, 1987, p. 33.

99. Ibid., p. 15.

disability of this particular baby ought not to be a determining factor here."[100] Ms. Mishkin argued that this case did not pose the problem of choosing between the life of the mother and the life of the fetus, because the life of the mother was already lost. At the same time, the state has an obligation as *parens patriae* to protect the life of a viable fetus: "Even in *Roe* v. *Wade* where the mother does have the possibility of making the decisions, the mother's decision-making on that score ceases at the point of viability, and we are beyond that point now, so my sense is that this is not a question of the woman's right to refuse treatment. This is the question of the state's obligation to protect this baby."[101]

Angela's lawyer, Robert Sylvester, protested that the mother's right to her choices and privacy does not cease with viability. He cited *Colautti* and *Thornburgh* as establishing the principle that maternal health must be the physicians' primary consideration. To perform a cesarean on Angela in her very weakened state, he said, would be in effect to terminate her life. The judge acknowledged that the performance of a cesarean might very well hasten Angela's death, but he noted that she was only expected to live another 24–48 hours anyway. The decision was a difficult one, but, given the choices, he concluded that the fetus should be given an opportunity to live.

Dr. Hamner went to Angela's bedside and found her arousable. He told her about the proceedings and the judge's ruling, and he asked her whether she would consent to a cesarean section to save the baby even though it might shorten her life. Her answer was yes. This conversation was reported to the court. Dr. Hamner went back to Angela's room to verify his previous discussion with her. This time he made it clear that *he* would not perform the operation without her consent, but that it would be done in any case. Because of the tube in her windpipe, Angela was unable to speak, but she mouthed very clearly several times, "I don't want it done."[102]

Her lawyer suggested that the judge's decision should be amended to show that there was now an utterance from Angela that she did not want the procedure done. Despite testimony from Dr. Weingold that Angela was responding, understanding, and capable of making decisions, the fact that Angela had given unexplained contradictory responses within a short period of time was taken by Ms. Mishkin to indicate either that Angela was not capable of making a reasoned or competent decision, or that she had been unduly influenced by her husband and mother. It was suggested that she may have been trying to spare her mother, who is in a wheelchair, from raising a baby she did not want. Mrs. Stoner had testified that she would never put the baby up for adoption, that she would do the best she could, "but we don't want it. Angela wanted that baby. It was her baby. Let that baby die with her."[103]

Under the circumstances, Angela's change of mind does not seem evidence of "incompetence to decide." Anyone might veer back and forth, given such a terribly difficult decision. On the one hand, she wanted the baby very much, which would incline her toward taking all steps to ensure its survival. On the other hand, she had

100. Ibid., p. 65.

101. Ibid., p. 70.

102. Ibid., p. 92.

103. Ibid., p. 60.

expected to give birth to a healthy baby whom she and her husband would raise. Now she was being asked whether she was willing to submit to surgery that might shorten her life, and would certainly increase her suffering, in order to give birth to an extremely premature, potentially severely handicapped infant, whom she would not survive, and whom others would have to raise. These factors might understandably have led her to change her mind regarding the cesarean.

Judge Sullivan maintained that he was unsure what Angela really wanted. Yet he never went to Angela's bedside to find out what she wanted. He said that he did not do so out of fear of worsening her condition, which is ironic, in view of his willingness to order a procedure that he recognized had the potential to shorten her life.

Despite professions of not knowing what Angela really wanted, the attorneys for the hospital, fetus, and District of Columbia said that it could be assumed that she did not want the cesarean performed. As Richard Love, assistant corporation counsel for the District of Columbia, conceded, "I don't think we would be here if she had said she wants it."[104] However, this did not matter, since they did not regard Angela's wishes as determinative anyway. The fact that her death was imminent and the fetus was viable was sufficient, they argued, to establish a compelling state interest that could override the patient's wishes.

Angela's lawyer made a last attempt to get the District of Columbia Court of Appeals to block the order as she was being wheeled into surgery. A hearing was held over the telephone, under extremely adverse conditions. All parties were not in the same room to use the phone. There was difficulty hearing because of outside noises from traffic, hospital personnel coming in and out, and so forth. In fact, the scene was precisely what George Annas had predicted would occur under such conditions in an article that appeared in the *New England Journal of Medicine* only a month before.[105] The three judges hearing the matter were unfamiliar with the relevant law, as became evident when Elizabeth Symonds, representing the American Civil Liberties Reproductive Freedom Project, cited *Thornburgh* and *Colautti* in support of the claim that the state has no authority to impose any regulations that would increase the risk to the woman's life and health.

JUDGE NEBEKER: The authority you first rely on, is that decision in the factual context of this case?
MS. SYMONDS: They were in abortion context. I believe the—
JUDGE NEBEKER: It's critical we know that. I thank you for telling us. With the time constraints, we don't have the time to start reading.[106]

The court denied the request for a stay, allowing the hospital to go ahead with the operation. The baby, Lindsay Marie Carder, died approximately 2½ hours later. (Despite this, the guardian *ad litem* for the fetus continued in subsequent briefs to insist that the fetus was "viable." Apparently, she considers a fetus to be viable if it survives birth for any period of time, no matter how brief. This seems a bizarre

104. Ibid., p. 97.

105. George J. Annas. 1987. "Protecting the Liberty of Pregnant Patients," *New England Journal of Medicine* 320: 1213–124.

106. In re *Angela Carder*, no. 87-609, District of Columbia Court of Appeals, June 16, 1987, p. 6.

interpretation of viability.) Two days later, Angela died. The surgery was listed as a "contributing factor."[107]

On November 10, 1987, a three-judge panel of the District of Columbia Court of Appeals upheld the emergency order. The panel said that the general principle that the state ordinarily may not infringe upon the mother's right to bodily integrity did not apply because "she had, at best, two days left of sedated life; the complications arising from the surgery would not significantly alter that prognosis. The child, on the other hand, had a chance of surviving delivery..."[108]

Was it certain that Angela would definitely die within a few days? Her cancer specialist, Dr. Moscow, did not agree with this extremely pessimistic prognosis. He had recommended that Angela receive radiation and chemotherapy, because he thought that she had a chance of partial remission, and possibly a few more months of life. Dr. Moscow was not even informed of the June 16 hearing, and so had no opportunity to testify as to her condition. But even if it were true that Angela had only hours to live, it was her life, and her decision. As George Annas pungently observes:

> [The judges] treated a live woman as though she were already dead, forced her to undergo an abortion, and then justified their brutal and unprincipled opinion on the basis that she was almost dead and her fetus's interests in life outweighed any interest she might have in her own life or health. This is what happens when judges (and hospital lawyers that call them) forget what judging is all about and combine rescue fantasy with dehumanization of the dying.[109]

This egregious judicial error was corrected on March 21, 1988, when in response to a request from 40 organizations, including the American Civil Liberties Union, the American Medical Association, and the American College of Obstetricians and Gynecologists, a three-judge panel of the District of Columbia Court of Appeals vacated the order. Without comment, the judges announced that the full court would hear new arguments at a later hearing.

The full court issued its opinion April 26, 1990. It agreed with the vacating of the order of the trial court on the ground that the judge had improperly used a balancing analysis, weighing the rights of A. C. against the interests of the state. Instead he should have determined whether A. C. was competent to refuse the surgery. If she was, then it should not have been performed. "[T]he right to bodily integrity is not extinguished simply because someone is ill, or even at death's door."[110] If she was incompetent, or the court was unable to determine competency, then her wishes should have been determined through the substituted judgment procedure.

107. In re *Angela Carder*, no. 87-609, Amended Brief on the Merits, p. 22. The Death Certificate of Angela Carder lists as a contributing cause of death the "status post-Cesarean section."

108. In re A.C., 533 A.2d 611, 617 (D.C.App. 1987).

109. George J. Annas. 1988. "She's Going to Die: The Case of Angela C," *Hastings Center Report* 18 (1): 23–25, p. 25.

110. In re: A.C., *Appellant*, No. 87-609, District of Columbia Court of Appeals (en banc) (Decided April 26, 1990), p. 1130.

Citing *McFall v. Shimp*, Judge John A. Terry, who wrote the majority opinion for the court, stated that courts do not compel one person to permit a significant bodily intrusion upon his or her bodily integrity for the benefit of another person's health: "Even though Shimp's refusal would mean death for McFall, the court would not order Shimp to allow his body to be invaded.... a fetus cannot have rights in this respect superior to those of a person who has already been born."[111] The court declined to specify whether, or under what circumstances, the state's interests can ever prevail over the interests of a pregnant patient. "We do not quite foreclose the possibility that a conflicting state interest may be so compelling that the patient's wishes must yield, but we anticipate that such cases will be extremely rare and truly exceptional. This is not such a case."[112]

Less Invasive Cases

Carder makes it clear that the state cannot force a woman against her will to undergo a cesarean section, even to save a viable fetus. What about less invasive procedures, such as blood transfusions? Jehovah's Witnesses refuse transfusions, based on their religious conviction that this is forbidden by the Bible.[113] They believe that anyone who "eats" blood will be deprived of the opportunity for everlasting life and the resurrection of the body.

It is difficult for non-Witnesses to understand the opposition to blood transfusions. No other "People of the Book" interpret the relevant passages of the Bible as do Jehovah's Witnesses. However, the reasonableness of their belief is irrelevant. As Justice Warren Burger said in his dissent in *Georgetown*, the right to refuse treatment is not limited to "*sensible* beliefs, *valid* thoughts, *reasonable* emotions, or *well-founded* sensations."[114]

Does *pregnancy* change the moral and legal situation of Jehovah's Witnesses? The pregnant Witness exposes not merely herself, but also her unborn child, to the risk of death. In numerous cases, courts have held that the right to practice religion freely does not include liberty to expose children to ill health or death. The Supreme Court has said, "Parents may be free to become martyrs themselves. But it does not follow they are free ... to make martyrs of their children."[115] There are numerous cases of

111. Ibid., p. 1123.

112. Ibid., p. 1142.

113. "And whatsoever man there be of the house of Israel, or of the strangers that sojourn among you, that eatest any manner of blood: I will even set my face against that soul that eateth blood, and will cut him off from among his people ..." (Lev. 17: 10–14), cited by Ruth Macklin, "Consent, Coercion, and Conflicts of Rights, " *Perspectives in Biology and Medicine* 20:3 (Spring 1977), pp. 360–371, p. 361.

114. *Application of President and Directors of Georgetown College*, 331 F.2d 1000, 1010 (D.C. Cir. *cert. denied* 377 U.S. 978 (1964).

115. *Prince v. Massachusetts*, 321 U.S. 158 (1944), p. 170.

court-ordered blood transfusions for children of Jehovah's Witnesses.[116] In fact, not only may courts override the decisions of parents who withhold necessary medical treatment from their children out of religious conviction, but the parents may be subject to criminal charges.[117] If courts can override parental refusal of treatment for born children, may they do the same for nearly born fetuses?

A transfusion is far less risky and invasive than a cesarean section. For this reason, some who are opposed to compulsory cesareans are willing to accept court-ordered transfusions. Neonatologist Alan Fleischman holds that " . . . it is acceptable for physicians to bring pressure to bear on the woman to accept the procedure, including the coercive step of seeking court adjudication. However, coercive measures should stop short of physically restraining or forcibly sedating a woman who continues to refuse treatment despite a court order that grants physicians permission to override her refusal."[118] Dr. Fleischman's coauthor, philosopher Ruth Macklin, would allow persuasive efforts, emotional appeals, and other noncoercive means to convince a woman to accept a low-risk medical procedure for the sake of her fetus, but she holds it unacceptable to invoke the force of law to override her refusal.

How should we decide between these two positions? One factor is the value we place on autonomy, understood here as the right of competent adults to make decisions about their own bodies and medical treatment. Macklin seems to be advocating an absolutist position on the value of autonomy, while Fleischman is willing to balance autonomy against other important values, such as the life and health of the nearly born fetus. However, it is not entirely clear that respecting a person's refusal of treatment necessarily upholds his or her autonomy. It depends on the reasons for refusing treatment. In some of the cases involving Jehovah's Witnesses, there is evidence that the patients wanted the transfusions necessary to save their lives but felt that they could not consent to them, on religious grounds. A court order allows them to have the transfusion they fervently desire without consenting to it. Some Witnesses apparently feel that the responsibility is therefore out of their hands, and thus does

116. See, e.g., In re *Green*, 448 Pa. 338, 292 A.2d 387 (1972); *Wallace v. Labranz*, 411 Ill. 618, 104 N.E.2d 769 (1952); *State v. Perricone*, 37 N.J. 483, 181 A.2d 751 (1962).

117. There have been a number of cases of people who rely exclusively on faith healing being convicted of manslaughter or neglect in cases where their children have died. For example, in July 1990, in Boston, Massachusetts, two Christian Scientists, David and Ginger Twitchell, were convicted of involuntary manslaughter in the death of their 2-year-old son, Robyn, who died in 1986 of a bowel obstruction. See David Margolick, "In Child Deaths, A Test For Christian Science," *New York Times*, August 6, 1990. http://www.nytimes.com/1990/08/06/us/in-child-deaths-a-test-for-christian-science.html. Accessed January 25, 2011. See also Jerry Casey, "Faith-healing deaths: Previous stories," The Oregonian, June 18, 2009. http://blog.oregonlive.com/clackamascounty/2009/06/faithhealing_deaths_previous_s.html. Accessed January 25, 2011.

118. Alan R. Fleischman and Ruth Macklin. 1987. "Fetal Therapy: Ethical Considerations, Potential Conflicts," in William B. Weil, Jr., and Martin Benjamin, eds., *Ethical Issues at the Outset of Life* (Boston: Blackwell Scientific Publications), p. 144.

not violate their religion.[119] Since their refusal is not fully autonomous, a court order overriding the refusal does not necessarily violate the patient's autonomy.[120]

A comparable situation may occur when a woman belongs to a religious sect opposed to cesarean delivery. Mary Jo O'Sullivan, professor of obstetrics and gynecology at the University of Miami School of Medicine, relates the following incident: "The baby's head was way too large. Without a c-section the only way to get the baby out would be to wait until it died and take it apart, piece by piece. I just couldn't do that. Nor was anyone else at the hospital willing to do it."[121] Dr. O'Sullivan finally got a court order authorizing a cesarean, but she was still uncomfortable about forcing surgery. "To my surprise, when I showed the patient the court order, she seemed relieved that the decision was out of her hands."

Despite the desirable outcome in this case, Dr. Nancy Milliken disagrees with Dr. O'Sullivan's decision. "Individuals can't have it both ways," she says. "We can't say: we want the right to make our own health care decisions and then turn around and expect the doctor to *make us* do what's good for us."[122] Not only does this expectation put doctors in the untenable position of having to figure out whether the patient means what she says, it also sets a dangerous precedent. Doctors, already convinced that they know what's *best* for the patient, may delude themselves as to what the patient "really wants." Less articulate and assertive patients may be forced to undergo procedures that violate their deepest religious beliefs. A woman in labor and weak from loss of blood may be in no condition physically to resist a blood transfusion. How are we to tell whether her refusal is authentic? What safeguards can we devise to ensure that her autonomy is not being violated? Ultimately, the criterion of interpretation will be "doctor knows best." Thus, I am led, somewhat reluctantly, to conclude that even if, in the particular case, a court order would not be coercive or violative of autonomy, physicians are not in a position to know this in general. For this reason, doctors should not be encouraged to second-guess the refusals of their competent patients.

As the degree of invasiveness decreases, the argument for intervention becomes stronger. What if the fetus can be protected from serious mental and physical handicap by simply compelling its mother to swallow a vitamin pill? Should our respect for maternal autonomy be absolute and unconditional? Can the risk to the unborn ever outweigh the woman's right to refuse treatment? In considering this question, two things should be kept in mind. First, in the vast majority of cases, the pregnant patient wants to give birth to a healthy baby, and she will cooperate with her obstetrician. Where she refuses, she may have good reasons, even if they are not reasons that are acceptable to her doctor. Only rarely is noncooperation due to stubbornness or silliness or indifference to the welfare of the baby. Second, it is important to realize in such cases that legal coercion is not the only method of protecting the not-yet-born child.

119. See, for example, *Application of President and Directors of Georgetown College* (note 115).

120. This is suggested in Bruce L. Miller, "Autonomy and the Refusal of Lifesaving Treatment," *Hastings Center Report* 11 (4): 22–28.

121. Ronni Sandroff, "Invasion of the Body Snatchers: Fetal Rights vs. Mothers' Rights," *Vogue* (October 1988), p. 330.

122. Ibid.

Other professionals may be brought in, to make sure the woman understands the full implications of her decision for her baby. Often a more creative approach on the part of health care providers will enable a resolution acceptable to all.[123]

Respect for autonomy is only one reason against a coercive approach. In addition, court orders can have a destructive effect on the physician–patient relationship.[124] Moreover, as John Robertson and Joseph Schulman point out in their discussion of pregnant women with phenylketonuria (PKU), coercive measures may offer little protection to the not-yet-born child.[125] The measures most likely to benefit the nearly born fetus, such as court-ordered cesareans, are also the most invasive and violative of the woman's right to bodily integrity. Less invasive measures, such as the restrictive PKU diet, are more easily justifiable, but difficult to impose without the consent and cooperation of the pregnant woman. Thus, although coercive measures might be justified where the risk to the woman is very low and the benefit to the baby very great, such cases are virtually nonexistent. The most desirable approach, as Robertson and Schulman correctly conclude, and the one that should be taken in all but the most rare and exceptional cases, is "education, counseling, and assuring access to treatment."[126]

123. For example, see my 1989 article, "Preterm Labor and Prenatal Harm," *Hastings Center Report* 19 (2): 32–33.

124. American College of Obstetricians & Gynecologists Committee Opinion Number 55, "Patient Choice: Maternal-Fetal Conflict" (October 1987). See also ACOG Committee Opinion Number 321, "Maternal Decision Making, Ethics, and the Law," November 2005.

125. John A. Robertson and Joseph D. Schulman. 1986. "Pregnancy and Prenatal Harm to Offspring: The Case of Mothers With PKU," *Hastings Center Report* 17 (4); 23–33.

126. Ibid., p. 32.

5

Assisted Reproductive Technology

Louise Brown was the first human baby born as a result of in vitro fertilization (IVF). Her birth in 1978 in Lancashire, England, opened up a new era in reproductive medicine, in several ways. "Assisted reproductive technology," or ART, which includes IVF, and other related technologies, such as zygote intrafallopian transfer (ZIFT), gamete intrafallopian transfer (GIFT), and introcytoplasmic sperm injection (ICSI), has enabled thousands of couples worldwide to have a biologically related child. But ART is not limited to infertile heterosexual couples. It can also be used by lesbians and gay men to create families, which has had profound social and legal effects. The ability to transfer an egg from one woman to another has separated genetic and gestational parenting, creating legal dilemmas and questions about what it means to be a parent. It has also raised questions about whether there should be financial compensation for genetic material (gamete donation) or reproductive capacity (surrogate motherhood). Assisted reproductive technology has made possible the testing of embryos to prevent the births of children with genetically transmitted diseases, and it has opened the door to the selection, and perhaps one day even the genetic modification, of embryos for nondisease traits. Thus, while ART has become an increasingly accepted treatment for some forms of infertility, controversies over its appropriate use still rage.

The answers to many of these questions depend on how we think about embryos. For example, if embryos are morally equivalent to children, then clearly they cannot be destroyed. Part of the Catholic Church's nearly total rejection of ART stems from the widespread practice of creating surplus embryos and discarding those that are not needed for reproduction. By contrast, on the interest view (see Chapter 1), embryos have even less claim to moral standing than fetuses. As we have seen in Chapter 2, biologists and medical researchers disagree about precisely when the capacity for conscious awareness develops during gestation. However, they agree that the very early embryo cannot be sentient. Prior to the development of the embryonic disc, axis, and primitive streak, which occurs after implantation, approximately 2 weeks after fertilization, there is no possibility of mental activity of any sort. The preimplantation embryo has not yet developed the rudimentary structures of a nervous system, and thus lacks the capacity to experience or suffer. At the same time, the absence of sentience, and thus the lack of moral standing, does not entirely settle the question of what may be done to or with embryos. Even if they lack moral standing, embryos are a potent symbol of human life, deserving of respect. Moreover, embryos used in ART may become children who clearly can suffer and who have a wide range of interests. Thus, the question of acceptable risk is raised here, as it was in Chapters 3 and 4.

The first section provides scientific information for understanding ART, its prevalence, and safety. The second section discusses the need for a moral and legal framework for deciding permissible uses of ART in light of its controversial nature. I present a "procreative responsibility" framework based on John Robertson's procreative liberty account. Such an account emphasizes the importance to people of being able to make their own reproductive decisions, while also recognizing that the core value of the right to reproduce—the creation of families—limits acceptable and responsible choices. The third section explores the question of limits to procreative liberty, that is, whether there are situations in which procreation should be avoided out of concern for the children who would be created. The fourth section discusses some of the dispositional issues that arise when joint reproductive projects end. The fifth section looks at the arguments for and against gamete donation.

THE SCIENCE OF ASSISTED REPRODUCTIVE TECHNOLOGY

About 10% of women in the United States (6.1 million) of reproductive age (15–44 years) have trouble getting and staying pregnant.[1] Couples who want children are generally advised to seek medical help if they are unable to achieve pregnancy after a year of unprotected intercourse or after 6 months if the woman is over 35 years old. Most infertility cases—85% to 90%—are treated with conventional therapies, such as drug treatment or surgical repair of reproductive organs. If these measures do not work, in vitro fertilization and embryo transfer (IVF\ET, or just IVF), and related techniques, such as intracytoplasmic sperm injection (ICSI), and gamete and zygote intrafallopian transfer (GIFT, ZIFT), may be suggested. (The Centers for Disease Control and Prevention [CDC] refers to this group of methods as ART, and I will follow this usage, although sometimes I will simply refer to the most common technique, IVF.) In vitro fertilization may be indicated for women who can produce healthy eggs but who have damaged or diseased fallopian tubes, which prevent the eggs passing from the ovary into the uterus. In vitro fertilization can also help men who have a low sperm count (oligospermia) or low motility, since sperm will not have to travel as far, nor through cervical mucus, if brought together with the egg in a dish.

In Vitro Fertilization

The concept of IVF is simple. The woman is given strong drugs to make her superovulate (produce many eggs). Egg retrievals are performed transvaginally, under anesthesia and ultrasound guidance. A thin needle, which is attached to the side of the ultrasound probe, pierces the top of the vagina, and the eggs are retrieved. They are mixed in a petri dish with sperm, which the man provides by masturbating. (In ICSI, which may be used when there are very few sperm or they are incapable of movement,

1. CDC, Reproductive Health, Infertility, 2009. http://www.cdc.gov/reproductivehealth/ Infertility/index.htm. Accessed July 9, 2010. I have seen higher estimates than the CDC gives, up to 14%.

the sperm is directly injected into an egg.) After about 3 days, when the fertilized eggs get to be clumps of about eight cells each, they may be transferred to a uterus (or the fallopian tubes). Alternatively, the provider may wait until the fifth day after fertilization when the embryos contain over 100 cells each, and are known as blastocysts. Waiting until day five helps to ensure that the embryos are healthy. Over the last few years, fertility doctors have learned that some eight-cell embryos which appear normal on day three are in fact nonviable; that is, they have abnormalities that cause them to stop dividing before the blastocyst stage.

The uterus into which the embryos are transplanted could be the egg provider's uterus, in which case, if she gives birth, she is both the genetic and the gestational mother of the child (or children). Or the embryos could be transferred to another woman's uterus for gestation. In that case, the gestational and genetic mothers will be different, and either (or possibly neither) will be the rearing mother. In vitro ovum nuclear transplantation (IVONT), a still experimental technique, might help women in their 40s, who have not been able to get pregnant with IVF. A woman who is 44 years or older has a 2% chance of getting pregnant using her own eggs. That chance increases to 50% using donated eggs from a younger woman, but this means sacrificing a genetic connection with the child. Scientists have learned that infertility due to aging is often caused by damage to the cytoplasm, the material that surrounds the nucleus of the egg, rather than to damage to the nucleus, which contains the DNA. In IVONT, the nucleus is taken out of the patient's egg and transferred into an egg from a donor which has had the nucleus removed (an enucleated egg). The newly created egg is then fertilized with the sperm of the patient's partner or that of a donor, and the embryo transplanted into her uterus. She is then both the genetic and the gestational mother of the child she bears. Dr. Jamie Grifo, who pioneered the technique, has been able to fertilize eggs created by IVONT and to achieve pregnancy in some patients. However, at this writing there have not been any live births.[2]

In the early days of ART, critics complained both that it was not very successful, and that infertile couples were misled about efficacy. The latter complaint was addressed in 1992, when Congress passed the Fertility Clinic Success Rate and Certification Act (FCSRCA, or the Wyden Act), which requires the CDC to collect data from clinics and submit an annual report to Congress on ART success rates. The first ART Success Rates Report was published in 1997. The Society for Assisted Reproductive Technology (SART), the primary organization of ART professionals, is another source of data about success rates. SART has been collecting data from its member programs since 1985, working closely with the CDC in compliance with the Wyden Act.[3] In 2007, according to the CDC's 2009 Report, there were 483 ART clinics in the United States (over 60% more than there were 10 years ago), and over 52,000 babies born from ART in the United States alone, accounting for slightly

2. Interview with Jamie Grifo on Frontline, aired and published on their Web site June 1, 1999. http://www.pbs.org/wgbh/pages/frontline/shows/fertility/interviews/grifo.html. Accessed July 19, 2010.

3. Society for Assisted Reproductive Technology, http://www.sart.org/WhatIsSART.html. Accessed July 20, 2010.

more than 1% of total U.S. births. There are ART clinics all over the world and more than 3 million babies worldwide have been born using ART.[4]

The success of ART depends on many factors, including the age of the woman and her partner, whether fresh or frozen eggs or embryos are used, and the skill of the practitioners. In 2002, about 28% of IVF cycles in the United States resulted in women giving birth to at least one child. That rate has increased slightly, to 29% in 2007. "To put these figures into perspective, studies have shown that the rate of pregnancy in couples with proven fertility in the past is only about 20% per cycle. Therefore, although a figure of 28% may sound low, it is greater than the chance that a fertile couple will conceive in any given cycle."[5] The largest group using ART (nearly 40%) is women under 35 years old. The percentage of IVF cycles resulting in a pregnancy in this group was 47.6%, and the percentage of cycles resulting in a live birth was 41.3%, according to data from 2008 from SART.[6] If a woman under 35 years of age undergoes multiple rounds of ART, her chances of having a baby are very good, as good as the chances of fertile women in natural conception. There remains a small percentage who cannot get pregnant, despite multiple rounds of ART. Unfortunately, it is not possible to identify those patients in advance.

Health Risks to Women

The drugs used to make women superovulate often cause considerable discomfort, and they may cause more serious health risks, including (very rarely) death. Several small studies conducted in the 1990s suggested that the use of fertility drugs might cause ovarian cancer later in life.[7] However, a number of studies, including a 2009 study of over 54,000 Danish women who visited fertility clinics between 1963 and 1998, have found no increased risk of ovarian cancer.[8] Researchers now believe that use of fertility drugs does not increase a woman's risk of getting ovarian cancer. Rather, women who are infertile because they have endometriosis have an increased risk of ovarian cancer. It is the infertility itself that raises the risk of cancer, not

4. Kirsty Horsey. 2006. "Three Million IVF Babies Born Worldwide," IVF News, June 28, http://www.ivf.net/ivf/three_million_ivf_babies_born_worldwide-o2105.html. Accessed July 15, 2010.

5. Society for Assisted Reproductive Technology (SART). 2010. "Success Rates." http://www.sart.org/detail.aspx?id=1906. Accessed November 1, 2010.

6. SART Clinic Summary Report. 2008. https://www.sartcorsonline.com/rptCSR_Public MultYear.aspx?ClinicPKID=0. Accessed July 19, 2010.

7. Salynn Boyles, "Fertility Drugs, Ovarian Cancer: No Link, Fertility Drugs Appear Safe, Study Says," WebMD Health News," http://www.webmd.com/ovarian-cancer/news/20090205/ fertility-drugs-ovarian-cancer-no-link. Accessed July 15, 2010.

8. Allan Jensen, Heidi Sharif, Kirsten Frederiksen, and Susanne Krüger Kjær. 2009. "Use of Fertility Drugs and Risk of Ovarian Cancer: Danish Population Based Cohort Study," British Medical Journal 338: b249, http://www.bmj.com/cgi/content/abstract/338/feb05_2/b249. Accessed July 15, 2010.

the drugs. Since pregnancy reduces the risk of ovarian cancer, using fertility drugs to get pregnant might reduce their risk.[9]

Health Risks to Offspring

When IVF was first done, it was unknown what the effects would be on the offspring. "Unlike most therapeutic procedures used in medicine, ARTs never underwent rigorous safety testing before clinical use."[10] A number of commentators said that it was immoral to run the risk of producing an abnormal baby.[11] Defenders of IVF replied that animal studies showed that the risk of abnormality with IVF was no greater than with normal conception. Moreover, even if IVF did produce defective embryos, such embryos would be unlikely to implant.

Research into the safety of ART faces significant obstacles. For example, the oldest child conceived by ICSI is not yet out of adolescence, making long-term studies from conception to adulthood impossible.[12] Follow-up studies of patients by clinics is often incomplete because many people seek fertility treatment at clinics far from their homes, and because Americans move around a lot. Another challenge for epidemiological studies of ART safety has to do with the assessment of congenital abnormality:

Importantly, the assessment of offspring conceived by IVF/ICSI is commonly performed by pediatricians as part of a routine neonatal health examination, yet a medical geneticist may have different criteria for disease. Alternatively, the physician may examine these children more closely than naturally conceived children, and inevitably the closer one looks, the greater the likelihood of finding an abnormality.[13]

Early studies indicated that singleton babies conceived through ART did not have a higher rate of birth defects. Some later studies found a correlation between ART and birth defects, although a causal link was not proven. Some fertility doctors have argued that the birth defects were due to the parents' infertility itself, rather than the means taken to overcome infertility. An example is the use of IVF/ICSI for severe male factor infertility caused by congenital absence of the vas deferens (CAVD). Prior to the development of ICSI, men with CAVD had little or no chance of reproducing. But with the advent of ICSI came a serious problem. It was soon discovered that CAVD is caused by defects in the cystic fibrosis transmembrane regulator gene.

9. CancerHelp UK. "Ovarian Cancer Risks and Causes," http://www.cancerhelp.org.uk/type/ovarian-cancer/about/ovarian-cancer-risks-and-causes#fertility. Accessed July 15, 2010.

10. Joseph P. Alukal and Dolores J. Lamb. 2008. "Intracytoplasmic Sperm Injection (ICSI)—What Are the Risks?" *Urology Clinics of North America* 35: 277–288, p. 277.

11. See, for example, Leon Kass. 1979. "Making Babies: The New Biology and the 'Old' Morality," *The Public Interest* 54: 32–60, pp. 29–30.

12. Alukal and Lamb, "ICSI—What Are the Risks?" (see note 10), p. 278.

13. Ibid.

This meant a risk of transmitting to offspring, not merely the father's infertility, but cystic fibrosis, a chronic lung disease in which thick, sticky mucus builds up in the lungs and digestive track, results in life-threatening lung infections and serious digestion problems. "This discovery meant that all patients and their wives undergoing sperm aspiration with ICSI for CAVD required careful genetic screening for cystic fibrosis, and if the wife was a carrier (4% risk of carrier status in the general population), then the embryos should undergo preimplantation genetic diagnosis using polymerase chain reaction, so that only healthy embryos would be replaced."[14] Researchers believe that perhaps 75% or more of all cases of infertility have a contributing genetic basis, although in most cases the defect is not diagnosed. "Put simply, large numbers of couples undergo fertility treatments without a complete understanding of the basis of their infertility or the potential long-term risks for their offspring."[15]

In 2005, a large study published in *Obstetrics and Gynecology* found no difference in the rate of birth defects of babies conceived with the help of fertility treatments and babies conceived without medical assistance. There have been more recent reports of increased risk of congenital abnormalities. A 2008 study that compared data from 281 births conceived with ART with 14,095 births conceived without infertility treatments found that among pregnancies resulting in a single birth, ART was associated with twice the risk of some types of heart defects, more than twice the risk of cleft lip with or without cleft palate and over four times the risk of certain gastrointestinal defects compared with babies conceived without fertility treatments.[16] However, the absolute risk of any individual birth defect remains low. "In the United States, cleft lip with or without palate affects approximately 1 in every 950 births; doubling the risk among infants conceived by ART would result in approximately 1 in every 425 infants being affected by cleft lip with or without palate."[17] The study's authors concluded:

> The underlying biological mechanism by which this intervention might lead to phenotypes affecting diverse developmental pathways is unclear. Our findings could have been because of underlying infertility, small numbers or chance. Until further studies have corroborated our findings or clarified the basis for these findings, the practical application of our results is limited.

Although the underlying mechanism of this effect could not be answered by this study, couples considering infertility treatments should be aware of all

14. Sherman J. Silber. 1998. "ICSI Today," *Human Reproduction* 13, Suppl. 1. http://www.infertile.com/infertility-treatments/icsirev/icsirev.htm. Accessed July 27, 2010.

15. Alukal and Lamb, "ICSI—What Are the Risks?" (see note 10), p. 277.

16. J. Reefhuis, M. A. Honein, L. A. Schieve, A. Correa, C. A. Hobbs, and S. A. Rasmussen, and the National Birth Defects Prevention Study. 2009. "Assisted Reproductive Technology and Major Structural Birth Defects in the United States," *Human Reproduction* 24 (2): 360–366.

17. CDC Press Release. 2008. "National Birth Defects Prevention Study Shows Assisted Reproductive Technology Is Associated With an Increased Risk of Certain Birth Defects," http://www.cdc.gov/media/pressrel/2008/r081117.htm. Accessed July 19, 2010.

the possible benefits and risks posed for children conceived with these treatments.[18]

A team of Swedish researchers looked at information about 27,000 Swedish children born from IVF between 1982 and 2005.[19] They found that 53 IVF children had developed cancer compared to the expected rate of 38 cases of cancer in non-IVF children. This was an increased risk of 42%, which looks large. However, given the rarity of childhood cancer, the absolute risk of an IVF child developing cancer was very low, less than 1%. The researchers said they did not think the increased number of cancers was the result of IVF technology, since if it were, one would expect to see a much higher number of cancers. The increase might be due to a difference in the patient population. Whether children conceived by IVF are prone to develop more diseases as they age is widely regarded as unlikely, though deserving of further study.

However, numerous studies have demonstrated an increased risk of birth defects in multiple births.[20] The main risk for the infants is prematurity. Prematurity is associated with an increased risk of respiratory distress syndrome, intracranial hemorrhage, cerebral palsy, blindness, low birth weight, and neonatal morbidity and mortality. Intrauterine growth restriction, intrauterine death of one or more fetuses, miscarriage, and congenital anomalies are all more common in multiple births. The major factor in multiple births from ART stems from the practice of transferring two or more embryos. This issue is discussed in the section "Limits to Procreative Freedom."

PROCREATIVE LIBERTY AND ITS CRITICS

John Robertson

Perhaps the most influential book on ART is John Robertson's *Children of Choice: Freedom and the New Reproductive Technologies*.[21] That is not to say that his notion of procreative liberty as a framework for assessing ART has been without its critics. Indeed, I have been among them.[22] However, it now seems to me that some of the

18. J. Reefhuis et al., "Assisted Reproductive Technology and Major Structural Birth Defects in the United States" (see note 16), p. 365.

19. Bengt Källén, Orvar Finnström, Anna Lindam, Emma Nilsson, Karl-Gösta Nygren, and Petra Otterblad Olausson. 2010. "Cancer Risk in Children and Young Adults Conceived by In Vitro Fertilization," *Pediatrics* 126 (2): 2009–3225.

20. See, for example, Yiwei Tang, Chang-Xing Ma, Wei Cui, Vivian Chang, Mario Ariet, Steven B. Morse, Michael B. Resnick, and Jeffrey Morse. 2006. "The Risk of Birth Defects in Multiple Births: A Population-Based Study," *Maternal and Child Health Journal* 10 (1): 75–81.

21. John A. Robertson. 1994. *Children of Choice: Freedom and the New Reproductive Technologies* (Princeton, NJ: Princeton University Press).

22. See my review essay, "Procreative Liberty," *Children of Choice: Freedom and the New Reproductive Technologies* by John A. Robertson, *Criminal Justice Ethics* 15 (1) (Winter/Spring 1996): 67–74. Some of the material in this section comes from this essay.

objections are based on misunderstandings of the view, some can be easily handled within the basic framework, and some stem not from the framework itself, but from Robertson's unsatisfactory handling of the nonidentity problem (see Chapter 2 and later discussion in this chapter). Perhaps the biggest misunderstanding of Robertson's views is that the procreative liberty framework ignores or gives short shrift to the interests of offspring, in favor of the interests of would-be parents. In part, this is because the phrase "procreative liberty" suggests that all that matters is the freedom of people to make their own decisions about reproduction. A better term would be "procreative responsibility," which restricts procreative liberty to responsible and defensible choices.[23] Procreative responsibility, which is based on Robertson's concept of procreative liberty, is a powerful framework for resolving the controversies created by reproductive technology and protecting the interests of prospective parents, offspring, and society.

The central idea in procreative liberty is that people should be able to make their own choices about whether to have offspring. Robertson is first and foremost concerned to argue that procreative liberty is a fundamental legal, and indeed, constitutional right, but it is not merely a legal right. Like virtually all fundamental constitutional rights, it has its roots in an important moral value: the value of letting people make their own decisions about intensely personal and important matters, in this case, whether to have offspring, without interference from the state, and without being vulnerable to the religious or non-harm-based moral convictions of others. In that sense, procreative liberty is unashamedly a "quasi-moral, quasi-legal algorithm for considering questions about law and policy in reproductive technologies," as Thomas Murray rather dismissively labels it, as opposed to "a comprehensive moral account of the ethics of initiating parenthood, and implicitly of parenthood in general."[24] Such a comprehensive moral account will need to say more about what helps children and families to flourish, and the obligations that parents have to their existing and future children. In my view, the procreative liberty approach contains the seeds of a more comprehensive account and, with a little fleshing out, can provide the sort of "insightful ethical analysis that illuminates what is morally important about families, parents, and children"[25] that Murray seeks.

"Procreative liberty should enjoy presumptive primacy when conflicts about its exercise arise," Robertson writes, "because control over whether one reproduces or not is central to personal identity, to dignity, and to the meaning of one's life."[26] Here, Robertson deliberately echoes Justice O'Connor's language in the abortion case *Casey*. If being forced to bear a child can strike in a fundamental way at one's dignity and conception of what is important in life, so too can being prevented from becoming a parent. Only the most compelling reasons justify the state interfering in reproductive decisions. Without such reasons, these very personal and intimate choices should belong to the individuals who make them, and who will live with the consequences.

23. I owe the suggestion that I need a better name, as well as the name itself, to Paul Menzel.

24. Thomas H. Murray. 2002. "What Are Families For? Getting to an Ethics of Reproductive Technology," *Hastings Center Report* 32 (3): 41–45, p. 42.

25. Ibid.

26. Robertson, *Children of Choice* (see note 21), p. 24.

Onora O'Neill rejects the idea that reproduction should be protected as a matter of self-expression, or that procreation is an area of life in which we express our most intimate and personal choices. "Reproduction indeed matters to people; it is indeed a part of life in which they express their deepest beliefs. But it does not follow that it is or should be seen primarily as a matter of self-expression, or that it should be protected as we protect self-expression."[27] Her reason is that reproduction aims to bring a third party—a child—into existence. O'Neill is certainly right about the core value in reproduction, namely, the value of having children to care for and raise. That is an essential element in procreative responsibility. But this does not negate the importance for individuals of being able to make their own reproductive choices, that is, to decide whether they will become parents. That choice should be protected because of its centrality in people's lives. Few decisions are as important as the decision whether to become a parent. Exercising this choice and becoming a parent imposes awesome responsibilities, and therefore it is a choice that should not be undertaken "lightly or selfishly but reverently and responsibly."[28] There is no conflict between the basis for protecting procreative liberty and acknowledging the responsibility that comes with this liberty.

Equally, in saying that individuals should be able to make their own reproductive decisions, whether to avoid reproducing or to reproduce, Robertson is not saying that the decision to have a child is merely the "flip side" of the decision to avoid having a child, as Murray charges.[29] Robertson explicitly acknowledges that reproduction brings someone into the world to whom one has serious moral obligations, saying:

> Reproduction always has moral significance because it leads to the birth of another person, whose needs for love, nurturing, and resources have to be met. Clearly, one can act responsibly or irresponsibly in reproducing, because of the impact that one's actions will have on offspring and others, including existing children.[30]

Therefore, the presumptive primacy of procreative liberty does not mean that procreative decisions can never be restricted, still less that all such decisions are morally irreproachable. No right is absolute, including the right to reproduce (or not to reproduce). Even fundamental constitutional rights can be limited. Robertson proposes a two-step procedure for determining when reproductive rights may be legally limited. First, it must be determined whether a "distinctively procreative interest" is involved. If so, the question is whether the harm threatened by reproduction (or nonreproduction) is sufficient to override procreative choice.

What, then, is a distinctively procreative interest? Robertson distinguishes procreative interests from ancillary interests in, for example, the conduct of pregnancy

27. Onora O'Neill. 2002. *Autonomy and Trust in Bioethics*. Cambridge: Cambridge University Press, p. 61.

28. These words come from the marriage ceremony of the Church of England. They describe the decision to marry and seem to me equally appropriate for the decision to have a child.

29. Murray, "What Are Families For?" (see note 24), p. 42.

30. Robertson, *Children of Choice* (see note 21), p.73.

or the mode of childbirth. He goes on to note a certain ambiguity in the concept of reproduction, because reproduction has both genetic and gestational elements. One of the consequences of ART is the ability to separate these elements in a way heretofore impossible. In vitro fertilization allows a woman who has no genetic relation to a fetus to gestate it. Although, strictly speaking, she has not reproduced, Robertson considers her to have had a reproductive experience, since gestation is such an important part of reproduction. However, he distinguishes reproduction in either the genetic or gestational sense from child rearing, which may be the reason for valuing procreation but is not essential to having a procreative interest.

Having stated the nature and value of procreative liberty, Robertson goes on to determine its scope. He begins with the "core values" or "core meanings" of procreative liberty. The core value of the right to reproduce is a right to marry and found a family, widely recognized as a basic human right.[31] Nor is this right limited to married people. Single people also have the right to make their own reproductive decisions, whether to use contraceptives and abortion to avoid having offspring, or to have children. The development of reproductive medicine raised the question, Is the right to reproduce limited to those who are able to reproduce "naturally" via coitus? Or is there a right of infertile people to access to ART? Robertson convincingly argues that there is no reason to limit the right to reproduce to those who can reproduce coitally. "Because the values and interests that undergird the right of coital reproduction clearly exist with the coitally infertile, their actions to form a family also deserve respect."[32] To those who argue that there is no legal right to reproduce if one lacks the physical ability to do so, Robertson offers the analogy of the First Amendment rights of a blind person. The fact that a blind person cannot read visually would not bar the person from using Braille, recordings, or a sighted reader. "Similarly, if bearing, begetting, or parenting children is protected as part of personal privacy or liberty, those experiences should be protected whether they are achieved coitally or noncoitally."[33] This may sound obvious today, but Robertson pioneered the concept of parity between coital and noncoital reproduction.

Adoption and the Right to Have Biologically Related Children

The core value in the right to reproduce is creating children of one's own, that is, biologically related offspring. Some people object to this notion. The core value, they maintain, is founding a family, but this need not involve the passing on of one's genes. One can found a family by adopting a child. I agree, and indeed would argue that the ability to adopt a child is within the scope of procreative responsibility. However, I disagree with those who would deny people the right to medical assistance in order to reproduce on the ground that (as it is usually expressed) there are plenty of children

---

31. See, for example, the Universal Declaration of Human Rights, Article 16 (1948), http://www.un.org/en/documents/udhr/. Accessed July 11, 2010. See also Charter of Fundamental Rights of the European Union, Article 9, 2000. http://www.europarl.europa.eu/comparl/libe/elsj/charter/art09/default_en.htm. Accessed July 11, 2010.

32. Robertson, *Children of Choice* (see note 21), p. 39.

33. Ibid.

in the world who need parents. On this critique of ART, adoption is morally superior to ART, because adoption both provides people who want a family with a child, while also providing children who need parents with a family. This, it is alleged, is better than creating more children in an already overpopulated world.

There are basically two responses to this argument. The first concerns the ease of adoption, an issue that is quite controversial. On one side are those who maintain that it is not as easy as it once was to adopt. Due to the legalization of abortion, access of reliable birth control, as well as social factors, such as acceptability of unwed motherhood, the number of healthy newborn babies available for adoption in the United States began to decrease in the 1970s and 1980s.[34] Frustrated by waits of 2 or more years, many Americans turned to international adoptions, from South and Central America and Asia. On the other side are agencies, such as Adoption Advocacy, who say that it is a misconception that international adoptions are quicker than domestic ones. They claim that "approximately 90 percent of the families working with American Adoptions wait an average of 1–18 months."[35] They also say that it is a myth that it is difficult to adopt a healthy newborn in the United States.[36] At the same time, their domestic adoption page includes the following statement: "The healthy infant adoption is the most sought after and the most difficult to find."[37]

There does seem to be agreement that adoption is quicker if the couple is willing to accept an older child and/or a child with special needs. However, it should be recognized that such children pose additional challenges to the already daunting challenge of parenthood. Not everyone is equipped to handle these challenges. This was evident in the horrifying story in 2010 of a 7-year-old Russian boy adopted by a woman from Tennessee, who was sent alone on a one-way flight back to Moscow with a note saying he was violent and had severe psychological problems.[38] One explanation for a tragedy of this kind is the tendency to sentimentalize adoption as a perfect solution and to downplay the potential problems in adopting older children, especially ones who have been institutionalized. Such an approach is in no one's interest. Older children, children who have been institutionalized, and children with disabilities are likely to need more than average care, care not all people who would be perfectly adequate parents are capable of or willing to provide.

Similarly, people who adopt children of other races—usually white people who adopt black or mixed-race children—also face challenges that parents who adopt children of their own race do not face. In 1972, the National Association of Black Social Workers (NABSW) vehemently opposed "the placement of black children in white homes for any reason. We affirm the inviolable position of black children in black families where they belong physically, psychologically and culturally in order

34. POV. 2000. "First Person Plural. Adoption History." http://www.pbs.org/pov/firstpersonplural/history_southkorea.php. Accessed November 1, 2010.

35. Adoption Advocacy. "Domestic Adoption v. International Adoption." http://www.adoptsc.com/DomesticvsInternational.htm. Accessed November 1, 2010.

36. Ibid.

37. Adoption Advocacy. "Domestic Infant Adoption." http://www.adoptsc.com/domestic.html. Accessed November 1, 2010.

38. Associated Press. 2010. "Boy Sent Back to Russia; Adoption Ban Urged," http://www.msnbc.msn.com/id/36322282/. Accessed November 2, 2010.

that they receive the total sense of themselves and develop a sound projection of their future."[39] They hold essentially the same position today, although the emphasis today is keeping black families together. However, when it is not possible for children to be raised by their birth parents, the NABSW maintains "the importance of finding culturally grounded options for children of African ancestry before giving consideration to placing our children outside of the community."[40]

Even if one rejects the opposition of the NABSW to transracial adoption, the complexities of such adoption must be realistically faced. One interracial adoption site gives questions that couples and families should consider before adopting across racial lines:

- Do I have family and/or close friends of other racial, cultural, or ethnic groups? If not, how can I develop such relationships?
- Am I willing to move to another community, change schools, or join appropriate organizations to find adult mentors and peers of my child's race and culture, if necessary?
- How do I feel about meeting the specific needs my child will have in developing self-identity and esteem?
- How do I imagine supporting my child when he or she experiences racial prejudice and discrimination?
- Can I accept the reality that adopting a child of color will mean our family becomes a family of color?

It is not racist for prospective parents to come to the conclusion that they would not be good candidates for interracial adoption. Yet one sometimes hears that ART is unnecessary because childless couples "can always adopt," and furthermore, an unwillingness to adopt an older child, a child with special needs, or a child of a different race is viewed with suspicion. This, in my view, is deeply unfair. In any event, if the argument in favor of adoption over reproduction is based on the needs of existing children for parents, this argument applies as much to fertile couples as it does to those who need medical assistance to have a child. Why should the responsibility for adopting children fall solely on those unlucky enough to be infertile?[41]

Adopting an infant may be easier in foreign countries, including India, Korea, China, and countries in Africa and South America. One difficulty with foreign adoption is ensuring that the children have been placed for adoption voluntarily. There are reports of women being offered large sums to give up their children, and even reports of baby-stealing.[42] Even when the sums offered are not so large as to border on coercion, many

39. National Association of Black Social Workers. 1972. "Position Statement on Transracial Adoption." http://darkwing.uoregon.edu/~adoption/archive/NabswTRA.htm Accessed November 2, 2010.

40. National Association of Black Social Workers. 2010. "Preserving Families." http://www.nabsw.org/mserver/PreservingFamilies.aspx Accessed November 2, 2010.

41. Peter Singer makes this point in "The Test-Tube Baby at 30," http://www.guardian.co.uk/commentisfree/2009/jan/14/vitro-fertlization-ivf-ethics. Accessed July 16, 2010.

42. Scott Carney, "Meet the Parents: The Dark Side of Overseas Adoption," http://motherjones.com/politics/2009/03/meet-parents-dark-side-overseas-adoption. Accessed July 14, 2010.

women who give up their babies for adoption are under a great deal of pressure. As the sociologist (and adoptive mother) Barbara Katz Rothman has put it, adoption is also someone's loss.[43] While it creates a family, it also destroys a family, namely, the birth family. When adoption is advocated as the only solution, or the best solution, to childlessness, that may create an incentive to create social policies that encourage women to relinquish their babies instead of finding ways for them to keep them.

The second response to the claim that adoption is preferable to infertility treatment has to do with the desire of many people to have a biologically related child, just as they would if they were fertile. Infertile couples often go through a grieving process as they come to terms with the fact that they cannot create a child together, a child who exemplifies their physical union and love for one another. At the end of this process, they may decide that adoption is the best option. Or they may prefer to undergo infertility treatment, either because the woman wants to have the experience of pregnancy, childbirth, and lactation, or because ART enables them to create a child who will be genetically related to one or both of them. Some feminists criticize this as "biologism."[44] I confess I simply do not understand what is wrong with wanting to have a child to whom one is biologically connected—a blood relative. Kinship has profound significance for people all over the world. To acknowledge this is to in no way denigrate adoption, or to suggest that adopted children are less valued or loved. The fact that adoptees who love their adoptive families often nevertheless want information about their biological families, about their roots, and where they come from, is testimony to the power of biology and its connection with identity and selfhood.

Core Values and Penumbral Interests

Having a child to whom one is biologically related is at the core of procreative liberty/responsibility. Beyond the core, there are procreative interests we might characterize as "penumbral,"[45] and here the analysis of the right to reproduce becomes more complicated. For example, is there a right to engage in collaborative reproduction, such as the use of gametes from third parties or gestational carriers? Does procreative liberty include the right to choose the characteristics of one's offspring, for example, by embryo selection or (someday) genetic engineering? Is procreative liberty limited to reproduction, or does it include the right to use one's reproductive capacity for nonreproductive purposes, such as donating gametes or embryos for research? Whether these penumbral interests are protected as part of procreative liberty depends, for Robertson, on how closely they are related to the core meanings and values.

43. Barbara Katz Rothman, *Recreating Motherhood* (New York: W.W. Norton & Co., 1989), p. 82.

44. Susan Sherwin. 1992. *No Longer Patient: Feminist Ethics and Health Care.* Philadelphia: Temple University Press.

45. H. L. A. Hart distinguishes between "core" and "penumbral" meanings of legal terms and rules in Chapter 7, *The Concept of Law* (Oxford: Clarendon Press, 1961).

The Interests of Children and the Nonidentity Problem

Robertson is often criticized for placing too much emphasis on the procreative interests of would-be parents, and not enough weight on the interests of the children resulting from the use of these technologies.[46] This is at the heart of Murray's critique: "The most egregious defect of procreative liberty is its nearly complete disregard of the interests of children created through reproductive technologies."[47] Robertson's critics think that he disregards or discounts the interests of children because he thinks that there is rarely, if ever, a reproductive technology or arrangement that should be prohibited "for the sake of the child." However, to say that he *disregards* the interests of the children who will be created is false. Rather, Robertson thinks that when their interests are taken into full consideration, the disadvantages they are likely to experience are *outweighed* by the benefits to them from coming into existence. If this is not the case, if the child after birth would prefer never to have been born, then Robertson admits that the child's life is wrongful, and the child has been harmed and wronged by birth. But since this is rarely, if ever, the case, it is almost never the case that children are harmed by existence, even when they experience very serious disadvantages. It is for this reason that Robertson thinks that reproduction is almost never irresponsible due to the effect on the child. As he explains:

> The problem is that in many cases of concern the alleged harm to offspring occurs from birth itself. Either the harm is congenital and unavoidable if birth is to occur, or the harm is avoidable after birth occurs, but the parents will not refrain from the harmful action. Preventing harm would mean preventing the birth of the child whose interest one is trying to protect. Yet a child's interests are hardly protected by preventing the child's existence. If the child has no way to be born or raised free of that harm, a person is not injuring the child by enabling her to be born in the circumstances of concern.[48]

In other words, what is at work here is not the procreative liberty framework itself, but rather Robertson's belief that a child cannot be harmed or wronged by birth unless the child, after birth, would have an existence so miserable that he himself would prefer never to have come into existence.

To see the implausibility of Robertson's analysis, consider the example he gives of individuals who plan to have a child, despite the fact that they know they will be abusive parents.[49] Even in this case, he denies that reproduction would be irresponsible, since the child will probably have a life better than no life at all, even if less good than the life he or she deserves. Therefore, the child has not been harmed; no harm to the child, no irresponsibility on the part of the parents. It is not surprising that

46. See, for example, Ann MacLean Massie. 1995. "Regulating Choice: A Constitutional Law Response to Professor John A. Robertson's *Children of Choice*," *Washington & Lee Law Review* 52: 135–171, p. 146.

47. Thomas H. Murray, "What Are Families for? Getting to an Ethics of Reproductive Technology" (see note 24), p. 75.

48. Robertson, *Children of Choice* (see note 21), p. 75.

49. Ibid., p. 76.

most people reject this conclusion. The question is how to explain and justify the claim of parental irresponsibility.

The first thing to note is that the "no harm done" claim follows only in cases in which the child has, in Robertson's words, "no way to be born or raised free of that harm." In this example, it is simply not the case that the child has no other way of being born except as an abused child. Robertson's mistake, as Melinda Roberts[50] points out, is to ignore what the couple *could have done* to prevent the harm. Their choices are not limited to *(1)* having a child they will abuse or *(2)* not having a child. They have a third option: to have the child and not abuse him. It may not be that they can simply *decide* not to abuse their child. They may have to take steps, such as taking a parenting class or getting psychotherapy before the child is born. By taking such steps, they can make life better for *this* child. Thus, this is not an example of the nonidentity problem.

What if there are no parenting classes available, or the prospective parents cannot afford psychotherapy? In the real world, there may not be a third option available to them. If so, perhaps the child really does have no other way of being born. However, the parents are still responsible for their decision to bring the child into the world. They do not get completely off the hook even if there was nothing they could have done to change their behavior. Bernard Prusak makes this point in relation to people who find they cannot provide their child with the love any child needs. Obviously, they ought to try to cultivate the disposition to love the child, but they may not succeed. Prusak writes, ". . . if a parent cannot bring him or herself to love his or her child, I think we must say, not that this parent is absolved by the graces of the formula that ought implies can, but that this parent suffers from morally bad luck—the 'constitutive' bad luck of having a heart indisposed to love—and perhaps should have known better than to have wagered becoming a parent in the first place."[51]

Second, we can reject the idea that the correct standard for responsible procreation is the nonexistence condition, and instead replace it with the decent minimum standard (see Chapter 2). However one interprets a decent minimum, it must include the willingness and capacity to be a good parent, or at least a good enough parent, to one's child. As I argued in Chapter 2, it is wrong, it is irresponsible, to have a child (when procreation is avoidable) if one knows that one lacks either the ability to love the child or the capacity to care properly for him or her. This makes the child abuse case quite different from cases where the disadvantage is poverty or a disability or having an elderly mother. In these cases, the love the parents have for the child, and the determination to give the child as good a life as possible, can very often compensate for the disadvantage. By contrast, a couple who has a child they know they will neglect or abuse do not evince the right parental attitude, and this is as relevant to the assessment of the decision to procreate as is the standard for harm. Thus, procreation would be irresponsible even if the child's life does not fall below a decent minimum, as might be the case if the child is lucky enough to get the love and care he needs

50. See Melinda Roberts. 1998. *Child Versus Childmaker: Future Persons and Present Duties in Ethics and the Law.* Lanham, MD: Rowman & Littlefield, pp. 92–96.

51. Bernard G. Prusak. 2010. "What Are Parents for? Reproductive Ethics After the Nonidentity Problem," *Hastings Center Report* 40 (2): 37–47, p. 42.

from others. The child is still "deprived of the special goods of a healthy parent-child relationship, goods that would contribute greatly to her welfare or well-being . . ."[52]

Third, procreation may be irresponsible, even when the decent minimum standard is reached, if there is a possibility of having a different child under better conditions. If one can give one's child a much better start in life by postponing reproduction until one is older and better equipped to be a parent, or financially more stable and better able to take care of a child, that is a very good reason to wait to have a baby. Sometimes waiting imposes a significant burden on the would-be parents and justifies having a child under less than ideal circumstances. However, if no significant burden is incurred by waiting, then postponing reproduction is the responsible choice, and having a child under disadvantageous conditions would be wrong. Admittedly, it would not be a wrong *to the child* so long as the child has a life above a decent minimum. But neither would it be a wrong to the child to delay reproduction, and not bring the child into the world. The choice, then, is between bringing one of two possible people into the world, neither of whom has a right to be born and neither of whom is harmed by nonexistence. The wrongness of bringing into the world the disadvantaged child is not rights-based or person-affecting; rather, it needs to be explained in terms of an impersonal, comparative principle, which says if you are faced with the choice between procreating at two different times, or in two different situations, you ought, as a responsible person, to choose the time or the situation that will be better for whichever child gets born.

In some cases, we can appeal neither to a person-affecting principle, since the child has no other way of getting born and his or her life is likely to be above a decent minimum, nor to a substitution principle, because no child could be born in a better condition. I will consider such cases in the next section, "Limits to Procreative Liberty." So far, my intention has been to show that with the right approach to the nonidentity problem, procreative decisions can be shown to be irresponsible even in cases where the child has no other way of getting born. The nonidentity problem does not vitiate the notion of procreative responsibility. Prospective parents always should consider the impact of their choices and decisions on the children they bring into the world. In addition, an adequate conception of procreative responsibility must be based on defensible core values. In places in *Children of Choice*, Robertson seems to suggest that the core values in reproduction are totally subjective, that is, just the reproductive goals that individuals happen to have. But reproductive goals might be selfish or warped, in which case they would not have any moral value and should not be socially protected. Reproductive interests themselves can and should be subjected to moral assessment, by practitioners, ethics committees, and society. If they cannot stand up to such assessment, they are not protected by procreative liberty and may be legitimately discouraged or prohibited—even if the children created will not have lives that fall below the nonexistence condition or the decent minimum standard. Robertson explicitly recognizes this when he says:

> Yet can we not posit a core view of the goals and values of reproduction such that all actions that affect the decision to reproduce are not protected? On such a view, *procreative liberty would protect only actions designed to enable a couple to have normal, healthy offspring whom they intend to rear.* Actions that aim to

52. Ibid.

produce offspring that are more than normal (enhancement), less than normal (*Bladerunner* [sic][53]), or replicas of other human genomes (cloning) would not fall within procreative liberty because they deviate too far from the experiences that make reproduction a valued experience.[54]

In other words, when pushed by extreme examples, Robertson does not advocate letting people pursue whatever reproductive goals they might have. Instead, he appeals to a notion of the core values of reproduction, a notion that is objective or intersubjective, rather than subjective. These core values can be used to restrict procreative liberty. In my view, this notion should be used, not just in response to extreme cases, but whenever we attempt to assess reproductive technology or arrangements. Robertson's "core values" turn out to be quite similar to Murray's notion of "human flourishing," which he advocates as the basis for evaluating ART. Neither concept provides a definitive guide for determining when a technology or arrangement would be irresponsible or immoral. Both can be interpreted in different ways by reasonable people. But both focus on the importance of children, parents, and families, and so offer reasons derived from such considerations as possible justifications for limiting procreative choices. The next section examines specific real-life examples and the arguments for limits to procreative liberty.

LIMITS TO PROCREATIVE LIBERTY

Postmenopausal Mothers

Menopause used to be the end of childbearing. Using egg donation, women can give birth into their 50s and even 60s. About 1,000 women over the age of 50 years have given birth in the last decade.[55] Older women can get pregnant using ART at the same rate as younger women, so long as they use eggs from younger women. In other words, it is not the age of the uterus that matters, but the age of the woman who provides the eggs.

Some women enter menopause prematurely, in their 30s or 40s (the average age of menopause is 51[56]). Very few people object to them using egg donation to have children. It is the attempts of senior citizens to become mothers that have sparked the most outrage. In January 2005, a 66-year-old Romanian, Adriana Iliescu, gave birth to a 3.2-pound baby girl, Maria Eliza, conceived using donor eggs and sperm.[57]

53. *Blade Runner*, a 1982 movie directed by Ridley Scott, was about genetically engineered human "replicants," created to do dirty and dangerous work, and the search for the scientist who could reprogram them to live full, human lives.

54. Robertson, *Children of Choice* (see note 21), p. 167. My emphasis.

55. Carey Goldberg. 2005. "Experts Debate Age Limits for Childbearing. Committee Grapples With Needs of Kids vs. Those of Parents," http://articles.chicagotribune.com/2005–04–08/news/0504080308_1_mother-and-child-fertility-ethics-committee. Accessed July 14, 2010.

56. National Institute on Aging, "Menopause," http://www.nia.nih.gov/healthinformation/publications/menopause.htm. Accessed July 21, 2010.

57. Carey Goldberg, "Experts Debate Age Limits for Childbearing" (see note 55).

The world's oldest mother, María Carmen del Bousada de Lara became the world's oldest new mother in December 2006 when she gave birth by cesarean section to two twins, weighing 3.5 pounds each, in a clinic in Barcelona, 1 week before her 67th birthday. (Ms. Bousada is no longer the oldest woman to have given birth. In 2008, Rajo Devi Lohan, age 70, gave birth by cesarean section to a daughter in India. She was reported to be dying at the age of 72, allegedly from the effects of the birth, although I have not been able to find a report of her death.) Ms. Bousada had lied about her age to her doctor at the Pacific Fertility Center in Los Angeles, where the cutoff for egg donation was 55 years of age. In July 2009, she died, at the age of 69 years, from breast cancer, leaving orphaned 2-year-old twins.[58]

The Iliescu case led Arthur Caplan to call for the medical profession or state legislators to set age limits on ART. In an interview, he said that Iliescu hardened him up: "Come on now, you're starting to risk everybody's lives now."[59] What Caplan is referring to is the fact that the risks of pregnancy, including high blood pressure, diabetes, and preeclampsia, a potentially serious disease of pregnancy that can force premature delivery, increase with age. However, while this is generally true, these conditions can also affect younger women, and they do not always surface in older women. A study in the 2002 *Journal of the American Medical Association* on 77 post-menopausal women who attempted donor-egg pregnancies concluded that "there does not appear to be any definitive medical reason for excluding these women from attempting pregnancy on the basis of age alone."[60]

Another reason often offered for age limits on ART is that women in their 50s and 60s may not be capable of the rigors of childrearing. Before they learn to sleep through the night, infants are exhausting, as any new parents can testify. Will older mothers have the stamina to care for babies and young children? Will they be able to run after toddlers to protect them from harm? Will they have the energy to deal with temper tantrums? Will they be hip enough to understand their rebellious teenagers? While these are legitimate concerns, they do not inevitably make having a child late in life irresponsible. As many have pointed out, men have always had this option (and have not received nearly as much criticism for exercising it). Perhaps a lack of sleep is harder on young parents than on older people who may not be sleeping through the night themselves. Perhaps age endows older parents with greater wisdom and patience, making them better parents during the terrible twos and the storms of adolescence. Many older women have had to take on the job of parenting their grandchildren when their children were unable to fulfill this role and have done a pretty good job at it. If they can be good childrearers, it would seem that postmeno-pausal women could also be good (or good enough) parents as well.

Finally, there is the risk of their dying before the child is grown, or even out of infancy, as happened in the cases of Ms. Bousada and Ms. Lohan. Ms. Bousada at least

58. Graham Keeley. 2009. "Oldest Mother, Maria Carmen del Bousada, Dies at 69, Leaving Baby Orphans," *The Times*, July 16. http://www.timesonline.co.uk/tol/news/world/europe/article6714820.ece Accessed November 2, 2010.

59. Goldberg, "Experts Debate Age Limits for Childbearing" (see note 55).

60. Richard J. Paulson, Robert Boostanfar, Peyman Saadat, Eliran Mor, David E. Tourgeman, Cristin C. Slater, Mary M. Francis, and John K. Jain. 2002. "Pregnancy in the Sixth Decade of Life: Obstetric Outcomes in Women of Advanced Reproductive Age," *Journal of the American Medical Association* 288 (18): 2320–2323.

was in good health and fully expected to live another 30 years, long enough for her sons to become independent adults. After all, her mother had lived to be 101 years old. But while her expectation may have been reasonable, the risk of a 66-year-old woman dying is a lot higher than the risk of a 30- or 40-year-old woman dying. Is it fair to the child to be brought into the world with an increased risk of being an orphan? If the woman does not die, but becomes frail or decrepit, is it fair to saddle the child with her care at a young age? Is it fair for children to have such old mothers?

Children may be embarrassed by having parents who look like grandparents, they may regret that their parents lack the energy to run around with them, and they may experience anxiety at the thought of losing one or both parents. These are serious, not trivial, harms. However, when we are considering the burdens imposed on the child by having an elderly mother, we must remember that having a younger mother was never an option for this child. It is life with an elderly mom or no life at all. As Robertson puts it, "the potential harm to a child from being born to older parents must be weighed against the tremendous good of being born at all . . . Even if a child 'faces some earlier-than-usual parental deaths or disability, you could hardly say the child has had a terrible life because that happens.'"[61] Most children who lose their parents early in life deeply regret the loss, but they do not regret having been born in the first place. Moreover, if the concern is that the woman might die before the child grows up, then this should apply equally to younger women who attempt pregnancy even when they have potentially life-threatening conditions, such as cancer, diabetes, or heart conditions. Since this is rarely met with the opprobrium that elderly would-be mothers face, one has to wonder if the objection is really based on the harm to the child, or whether it is based on a "yuck factor"—revulsion at the very idea of a woman old enough to be a grandmother—or great-grandmother—getting pregnant.

Not so long ago, a 40-year-old woman was considered too old to have a baby. Today, many women are having babies after the age of 40. As women are living (and living in good health) into their 80s, 90s, and even 100s, the "orphan" objection may decline in force. Clearly, any woman attempting motherhood at an advanced age ought to have a plan for the care of the children, in case she dies. In fact, all parents of whatever age should have such a plan, since any of us can die unexpectedly. But if she is healthy, with a reasonable expectation of living for another 30 years, and has a plan in case of her death, it is far from clear that it would be irresponsible of her to have a child.

A related issue is the moral and legal obligations of doctors and clinics to accept or refuse patients. At common law, a physician had no duty to treat a patient if there was no prior doctor–patient relationship.[62] Over the years, this "no-duty" rule has been modified. Antidiscrimination laws have limited the circumstances in which physicians may deny medical care. They cannot reject patients on grounds of race, ethnicity, or religion. Nor can they refuse to treat someone on grounds of disability, unless the individual "poses a direct threat or significant risk to the health and safety of others that cannot be eliminated by adequate precautions or reasonable modification of policies, practices or procedures."[63] In addition, physicians are not required to treat

61. Goldberg, "Experts Debate Age Limits for Childbearing" (see note 55).

62. Laurel L. Katz and Marshall B. Paul. 2002. "When a Physician May Refuse to Treat a Patient," *Physicians' News Digest*, February. http://www.physiciansnews.com/law/202.html. Accessed July 21, 2010.

63. Ibid.

patients if they have a moral or religious objection to the treatment. This is usually used by physicians who are morally opposed to abortion, but it could equally justify an upper age limit for ART patients, as long as this is based on a genuine and reasonable concern for the well-being of the woman and any offspring that may be produced and is not a pretext for discrimination. American Society for Reproductive Medicine has held that, in general, physicians and clinics are not morally obligated to help people have children if they have well-founded concerns about the ability of the individuals to care for the children,[64] which could include the concern that the patient will die before the child reaches adulthood. Since they will be partly responsible for the child's existence, they are entitled to refuse to participate in reproductive projects they regard as irresponsible or immoral, and to set an upper age limit for ART, or egg donation. Many clinics in the United States have adopted an upper age limit of 55 years.[65] However, it is also morally justifiable for a clinic to decline to set a hard-and-fast age limit. A 56-year-old woman may be in better physical shape, better able to have a healthy pregnancy, and more likely to live another 30 years, than younger fertility patients. She may have a younger partner or an extended family ready and willing to help raise her children if she unexpectedly dies. A case-by-case approach has been found acceptable by the Ethics Committee of ASRM. It concluded that while postmenopausal pregnancy should be discouraged, there is no medical or ethical reason compelling enough to judge assisted reproduction unethical in every case, solely on the basis of the age of the prospective mother.[66]

Even if a limit of 55 years of age is not morally required, shouldn't there be some limit? Caplan's proposal—no single person over 65 years old and no couples whose ages total more than 130 years should be considered eligible for help having children—is hardly draconian. At the same time, such cases will be so rare (only a handful of women in their 60s have given birth in the last decade[67]) that the value of mandating an absolute age limit, whether by professional regulations or law, seems mainly symbolic, as opposed to a policy necessary for protecting offspring.

The Risk of Transmitting Disease or Disability

Despite some studies showing an increased risk of congenital abnormalities in offspring (see earlier discussion), the consensus, based on retrospective data, is that IVF and IVF/ICSI are safe. At the same time, some individuals have a significantly greater risk than average of transmitting a genetic disease to offspring. In autosomal recessive diseases, such as cystic fibrosis, sickle cell anemia, and Tay-Sachs disease, both parents have to be carriers of the mutation for the disease to be transmitted

64. See Ethics Committee, ASRM. 2004. "Child-Rearing Ability and the Provision of Fertility Services," *Fertility & Sterility* 82 (3), September.

65. Apparently this limit was arbitrarily chosen by Dr. Mark Sauer, noted fertility expert, because his grandmother was 85 years old. He reasoned that if she had had a child at age 55, she would have been around until the child was at least 30. Goldberg, "Experts Debate Age Limits for Childbearing" (see note 55).

66. Ethics Committee of the ASRM. 2004. "Oocyte Donation to Postmenopausal Women," *Fertility and Sterility* 82, Supp. 1: S254–S255.

67. Goldberg, "Experts Debate Age Limits for Childbearing" (see note 55).

to offspring. With each pregnancy, they have roughly a 25% chance of having a child with the disease. (There is a 25% chance the child will be disease-free, and a 50% chance the child will not have the disease, but will be a carrier, that is, able to transmit the mutation.) In autosomal dominant diseases, such as Huntington's and achondroplasia (dwarfism), only one parent need have the defective gene, and the risk of transmission of disease is roughly 50% with each pregnancy. Does the increased risk of transmission of genetic disease or disability make reproduction irresponsible?

On the view of procreative responsibility I have been advocating, prospective parents are morally required to consider the impact of their reproductive decision on any offspring they have. This includes the nature of the disease or disability, its likely severity (if this is knowable), and the degree of risk. In addition, it is morally significant whether transmission of the disease can be avoided. For example, a way to avoid the risk of cystic fibrosis in ICSI is to test the wife or female partner of the man to see if she is a carrier for CF, and if she is, to use prenatal genetic diagnosis (PGD) to test the embryos in order to implant only unaffected ones. This creates, once again, a nonidentity problem. If the parents refuse to have their embryos tested, and as a result a child with CF is born, the parents cannot be said to have harmed or wronged that child, since he or she could not have come into the world without CF. To say why PGD and embryo selection is morally obligatory, we need to appeal to a substitution principle (see Chapter 2). Substitution is required just in case this would enable the birth of a child without the disadvantageous condition, without imposing significant burdens on the procreators. It would impose significant burdens on people who were not undergoing ART to require them to create extracorporeal embryos and test them for genetic disease, and therefore this would be an unreasonable requirement. By contrast, if the couple is using IVF/ICSI to have a child, they are already creating extracorporeal embryos and, in the United States anyway, they would be creating more embryos than can be safely implanted, and so they would have to choose which embryos to implant. The decision to test the embryos for CF seems a no-brainer, but this has been disputed by some members of the disability community.

THE DISABILITY CRITIQUE

Over the past decade, disability activists have been critiquing the "medical model" of disability. According to this model, disability is always something to be avoided if possible, and treated if not, using medical means. One of the effects of the medical model is the widespread use of prenatal testing for a very wide range of disorders, including Down syndrome (trisomy 21). Prenatal testing has become a routine part of prenatal care. Until relatively recently, such testing was only offered to pregnant women over the age of 35 years (or 40 years in the United Kingdom), but in 2007, the American College of Gynecologists and Obstetricians changed its guidelines to recommend offering fetal chromosomal screening to all pregnant women, regardless of age, because of improvements in low-risk, noninvasive screening methods. If the screening indicates increased risk, the woman should have the option of diagnostic testing, that is, amniocentesis or chorionic villus sampling.

Although ACOG was careful to say that it was not recommending that all pregnant women be screened, only that all pregnant women be offered the option of prenatal screening, many disability advocates argue that even offering prenatal screening and diagnosis is premised on the belief that disability justifies abortion. This sends the message to people living with disabilities that their births were a mistake, that the world would be better off without them in it. Not surprisingly, they find this message hurtful and offensive. They maintain that decisions to undergo prenatal testing and to have an abortion are often the result of inaccurate and prejudiced ideas about what it is like to have a disability or to have a child with a disability. Moreover, the problems occasioned by disability are not primarily medical, on this view, but stem from discriminatory social arrangements that can and should be changed. Adrienne Asch movingly writes:

> My moral opposition to prenatal testing and selective abortion flows from the conviction that life with disability is worthwhile and the belief that a just society must appreciate and nurture the lives of all people, whatever endowments they receive in the natural lottery . . . . [T]here is abundant evidence that people with disabilities can thrive even in this less than welcoming society . . . [P]eople with disabilities . . . contribute . . . to families, to friends, to the economy. They contribute neither in spite of nor because of their disabilities, but because along with their disabilities come other characteristics of personality, talent, and humanity that render people with disabilities full members of the human and moral community. [68]

I agree with Asch that life with disability is worthwhile in the vast majority of cases, although in rare cases, the nonexistence condition is met, and it would be better for the child never to have been born. Examples include the severest cases of dystrophic epidermolysis bullosa, Tay-Sachs disease, and Lesch-Nyhan syndrome (see Chapter 3). Since such cases are rare, we may put them aside, and acknowledge that life with disability is generally worthwhile, and that "a just society must appreciate and nurture the lives of all people." However, I see no inconsistency with demanding social justice for people with disabilities and the use of prenatal testing to reduce the incidence of disability. I also maintain that using prenatal testing and selective abortion has nothing whatsoever to do with one's ability to be a good parent.

My view is based on two important ideas: the moral permissibility of abortion and the undesirability of disability. I realize that there are people who reject this view of disability, who prefer the term "differently-abled" to "disabled." This seems to me a kind of dishonesty, a sanitizing of the facts. Fortunately, Asch does not engage in this sort of dishonesty. In an early paper, she acknowledges:

> Not all problems of disability are socially created and, thus, theoretically remediable. No matter how much broad and deep social change could ameliorate or eradicate many barriers to fulfillment encountered by today's disabled citizens, in no society would it be as easy or acceptable to have a disability as not to have one. The inability to move without mechanical aid, to see, to hear, or to learn is not inherently neutral. Disability itself limits some options. Listening to the radio for someone who is deaf, looking at paintings for someone who is blind, walking upstairs for someone who is quadriplegic, or reading abstract articles for someone who is intellectually disabled are precluded by impairment alone. Physical pain, the inconveniences and disruptions occasioned by medical treatments, or routines of medication, rest, restricted diet, and exercise programs are

68. Adrienne Asch. 1999. "Prenatal Diagnosis and Selective Abortion: A Challenge to Practice and Policy," *American Journal of Public Health* 89 (11): 1649–1657, p. 1652.

not desirable aspects of life. It is not irrational to hope that children and adults will live as long as possible without health problems or diminished human capacities.[69]

One might think that if there is nothing wrong with wanting one's future child to be free of disability, and if there is also nothing wrong with abortion, there would be nothing wrong with having an abortion to avoid having a child who will be disabled. But this is precisely what Asch wishes to deny. She thinks that there is something wrong with terminating a wanted pregnancy because of "fetal indications." Asch's focus, it should be noted, is not primarily with the decisions prospective parents make regarding testing and subsequent abortion, but rather with the policies and practices of health professionals. In particular, Asch opposes the routinization of prenatal testing because it carries with it the suggestion that the lives of children born with disabilities will be so terrible that they—and everyone else—would be better off if they had never been born.

As a defender of procreative liberty, I certainly agree that prospective parents should be able to make their own decisions on whether to have prenatal testing. Moreover, health care professionals should make it clear that such testing is not undertaken to preserve the health of the fetus, an idea that may be conveyed by the expression, "We just want to make sure everything is okay with the baby." This suggests that prenatal testing is akin to taking prenatal vitamins—something one does for the sake of *this* fetus. Prenatal testing can only provide information about whether this fetus has a genetic disease, information the parents might use to prepare themselves for the birth of a child with special needs or, more commonly, to make the decision to terminate the pregnancy. If decisions to terminate a pregnancy are unduly influenced by negative attitudes on the part of society in general or the medical profession in particular toward having a child with a disability, then such decisions are not truly voluntary, and procreative liberty is not served.

Many people who oppose selective abortion oppose abortion in general. For them, aborting a fetus because it has been diagnosed with a serious genetic defect is morally equivalent to killing a child who has the same defect. On this generally pro-life view, abortion itself is wrong, whatever the reason for choosing it (except, perhaps, in cases of rape or a threat to the woman's life). But this is not Asch's view. She regards fetuses as having a different moral status than born children, and she thinks that abortion is generally permissible if the reason for abortion is that the woman does not want to be a mother. However, if the woman wants to be a mother, then she should be willing to accept the child she will have, regardless of whatever particular characteristics that child will have. In other words, Asch distinguishes between abortion to prevent having a child (*any* child) and abortion to prevent having *this* child, that is, a child with these characteristics. If one really understood that disability need not prevent a child from having a wonderful life, then, according to Asch, there would be no reason to abort a wanted pregnancy. She thinks that abortion for fetal indications can only be based on either ignorance about what it will be like to parent a child with a disability or prejudice toward individuals who have disabilities.

69. Adrienne Asch. 1989. "Reproductive Technology and Disability," in Sherrill Cohen and Nadine Taub, *Reproductive Laws for the 1990s*. New York: Humana Press, p. 73.

In a more recent article, Asch and David Wassermann turn their attention away from a critique of public policy to a critique of individual decisions to have prenatal testing, followed by selective abortion, arguing that the attitudes expressed by such decisions are inconsistent with the attitudes prospective parents should have toward their future children.[70] They begin by rejecting the view that having a child with a disability such as Down syndrome (the condition most commonly tested for) would impose great burdens on the parents. "The most that can plausibly be claimed is that being or having a child with a disability is at times different and more difficult than being or having a 'normal' child, and that specific impairments are very unlikely to meet specific parental expectations (e.g., a child with Down syndrome is not likely to become a great mathematician like her mother)."[71]

However, if dire predictions about what a child with Down syndrome will be able to do or accomplish are false, so is this characterization. Even an average child, with an IQ of 100, is unlikely to become a mathematician, let alone a great mathematician. The average IQ of a child with Down syndrome is about 50; most have intellectual disabilities in the mild to moderate range. "Many affected children learn to read and write, and some graduate from high school and go on to post-secondary programs or college."[72] This means that most children with Down syndrome do not graduate from high school, and still fewer go to college. They are also likely to have greater than average health problems. Nearly half have congenital heart defects. More than 60% have vision problems and about 75% have some hearing loss.[73] "Many adults with Down syndrome are capable of working in the community, but some require a more structured environment."[74] Many can live semi-independently, but they will not become fully independent adults. As people with Down syndrome live longer (the average life expectancy is 60 years), they may outlive their parents, who need to plan for their children's care after their death. These are all realistic concerns that are as relevant to the decision whether to terminate a pregnancy as the evidence that many families with a child who has Down syndrome are happy and thriving.

Someone who takes a pro-choice position on abortion sees pregnancy as a time in which the individual still has the choice whether to become a parent. The fact that a woman chooses to have an abortion, in order to avoid the birth of a child with a serious disability, does not entail that she would not love a child who had the disability. She undoubtedly would, just as a woman who aborts because she is not ready to be a mother would undoubtedly love her child, if she carried it to term. In both cases, the women may be choosing between two possible futures: having this child under these conditions, and having a different child under different conditions later on. If it is

70. Adrienne Asch and David Wassermann. 2005. "Where Is the Sin in Synecdoche? Prenatal Testing and the Parent-Child Relationship," in David T. Wasserman, Robert Samuel Wachbroit, Jerome Edmund Bickenbach, eds., *Quality of Life, and Human Difference: Genetic Testing, Health Care, and Disability* (New York: Cambridge University Press), Chapter 7.

71. Ibid., p. 175.

72. March of Dimes. 2009. Pregnancy & Newborn Health and Education Center, Down Syndrome. http://www.marchofdimes.com/pnhec/4439_1214.asp. Accessed July 31, 2010.

73. Ibid.

74. National Association for Down Syndrome. 2010. "Facts About Down Syndrome." http://www.nads.org/pages_new/facts.html. Accessed July 31, 2010.

reasonable to want to avoid disability in one's child, why should it be hurtful and discriminatory to prefer to have a child without a disabling condition?

Although I maintain that prenatal testing and selective abortion are morally permissible, they are not morally obligatory, except perhaps in the rarest cases where the nonexistence condition cannot be met. Thus, a couple opposed to abortion, who already has a child with CF, might permissibly "take their chances" with a subsequent pregnancy. Since they would not consider abortion if the fetus were diagnosed as having CF, they decline prenatal testing. It seems to me that they are well within their rights to do so. In general, no one is morally required to terminate a pregnancy, any more than one is morally required not to terminate a pregnancy. So long as the prospective parents intend to love and care for their child, and have a reasonable chance of providing the child with a decent life, they act responsibly in knowingly risking the birth of a child with a serious disability. There is nothing irresponsible in being willing to parent a child with a disability.

While Asch and Wassermann primarily oppose selective abortion, they think their argument also applies to PGD and embryo selection. They do not claim that the two are morally exactly alike. The willingness to terminate a pregnancy that has already begun, and indeed is in the second trimester, appears to express a stronger preference against having a child with a serious disability than simply choosing between embryos, and therefore is morally more objectionable on their view. Nevertheless, they view PGD as still "a form of selection, and we might prefer that parents refrain from embryo diagnosis and simply implant any one (or more) of the viable embryos."[75] However, embryos with genetic defects have a much greater chance of not being viable. They are less likely to implant, and if they do implant, they have a much higher risk of miscarriage. "The chance of healthy pregnancy may double when known genetically normal embryos are utilized. Implantation rates (the chance of each single embryo becoming a gestation) can also be raised greatly with PGD."[76] In light of these facts, the refusal of PGD by a couple undergoing IVF in order to have a child does not make much sense. Even if the couple were willing to lessen their chances of pregnancy (and it is hard to see why they would, given the expense and burdens incurred with IVF), it is unlikely any fertility doctor would go along with such a plan. Indeed, I think it would be irresponsible and unprofessional to do so. Moreover, the issue is not simply increasing the chances of achieving pregnancy and live birth. The more important question is the morality of the decision to have, or risk having, a child with a serious disease, such as CF, when this outcome could easily be avoided. The substitution principle I defended in Chapter 2 requires "individuals facing reproductive decisions not to bring into the world children who will experience serious suffering or limited opportunity or serious loss of happiness, if this outcome can be avoided, without imposing substantial burdens or costs or loss of benefits on themselves or others, by bringing into the world different individuals who will be spared these disadvantages." There is no question that CF imposes serious suffering and limits opportunity. This is so even though the lives of people with CF are often well worth living. People who are undergoing IVF because of infertility

75. Asch and Wassermann, "Where Is the Sin in Synecdoche?" (see note 70), p. 195.

76. The Fertility Institutes, Prenatal Genetic Diagnosis (PGD), http://www.fertility-docs.com/PGD.phtml. Accessed July 29, 2010.

almost always create more embryos than can be implanted, so that a choice between embryos is inevitable. If a couple knows or learns during the infertility workup that they are carriers of CF, I maintain that they have a moral obligation to have their embryos tested and to select unaffected embryos. And even if they prefer to avoid embryo selection, they certainly have no right to insist that their fertility doctor participate in the creation of a child with a serious genetic disease, when this could have been easily avoided.

Multiple Births

In the past two decades, the rate of multiple births in the United States increased dramatically. "The rate of twin births increased by 70% between 1980 and 2004, and the rate of higher-order multiples (triplets or more) increased four-fold between 1980 and 1998."[77] About a third of the increase in multiple pregnancies is due to the fact that more women over 30 years old are having babies. The rest of the increase is due to infertility treatments, including fertility drugs and the transfer of multiple embryos in IVF.[78] Most ART pregnancies in the United States result in a multiple-birth delivery. By comparison, only 1.5% of natural-conception pregnancies result in a multiple birth.[79] While the rate of triplet and higher-order multiple births has declined, the incidence of twin births after IVF remains at a constant rate of 25%–40% in the United States.[80] This is largely due to the fact that IVF specialists continue the practice of transferring more than one embryo. A large part of the explanation for this is that fertility doctors come under considerable pressure from patients to transfer double embryos. Even if the doctors inform patients of the risks, patients are often willing to accept them to avoid the burdens and costs of additional cycles, especially since IVF is often not covered by insurance. In 2008, doctors transferred single embryos in only 5.2% of cycles, even for the women with the best chances of getting pregnant, those under 35 years old.[81]

Despite television reality shows that romanticize "super-multiples," that is, triplets and higher, the higher the number of fetuses in a pregnancy, the greater the risks to both mother and babies. They increase exponentially with super-multiples, but the risks are significantly greater even with twins. For example, although triplets are eight to ten times as likely to die in infancy as singletons, the infant mortality rate for twins is four to five time that of singletons.[82] The risk of cerebral palsy is 47 times greater in

77. March of Dimes. 2009. "Multiples: Twins, Triplets and Beyond," http://www.marchofdimes.com/professionals/14332_4545.asp. Accessed July 22, 2010.

78. Ibid.

79. Alukal and Lamb, "ICSI—What Are the Risks?" (see note 10), p. 279.

80. Aaron K. Styer, Diane L. Wright, Anne M. Wolkovich, Christine Veiga, and Thomas L. Toth. 2008. "Single-Blastocyst Transfer Decreases Twin Gestation Without Affecting Pregnancy Outcome," *Fertility and Sterility* 89 (6): 1702–1708, p. 1702.

81. SART. 2008. Clinic Summary Report (see note 6).

82. David Orentlicher. 2010. "Multiple Embryo Transfers: Time for Policy," *Hastings Center Report* 40 (3): 12–13.

triplet pregnancies than in singleton pregnancies, but still eight times greater in twin pregnancies than in singleton pregnancies.[83] In addition to the increased maternal and fetal risks from twin pregnancies, there are also the considerable economic costs, resulting from longer hospital stays and long-term care of disabled premature twin infants. For all of these reasons, experts in maternal-fetal health agree that the goal in pregnancy should be one healthy baby. This is consistent with the procreative responsibility approach I advocate. If the only way to have a child were to have a child with an increased risk of serious health problems, that could be justified if a decent minimum could be achieved, and the parents were committed to loving the child and giving him or her as good a life as possible. However, where the choice is between having one healthy baby or two or more children with an increased risk of serious disabilities, responsible procreators should choose to have one healthy child. It does not matter that the twins or triplets would have lives above the nonexistence condition or even the decent minimum standard. If the choice is between having one child who is likely to be healthy or having two (or more) children with an increased risk of serious health problems, responsible procreators should choose to have one child.

Does double-embryo transfer increase a woman's chances of getting pregnant and having a live birth? This used to be the rationale for transferring multiple embryos. However, recent studies have demonstrated that elective single embryo transfer (eSET) in women under 37 years of age is just as effective as transferring two or more embryos, while significantly reducing the number of twin births.[84] In response to this data, some European countries have legally restricted the number of embryos that can be transferred in a single cycle. Sweden allows only eSET, although double-embryo transfers are permitted for women at low risk of multiple births. After the law was adopted, the birth rate did not change, but the multiple-birth rate dropped from 35% to 5%.[85] In the United Kingdom, the Human Fertilization and Embryology Authority (HFEA) has restricted the maximum number of embryos that can be transferred to women under 40 years old to two, with no exceptions. For women over 40 years old, a maximum of three embryos may be transferred.[86] In 2008, the HFEA introduced a policy which allows clinics the flexibility to devise their own multiple births minimization strategy, consistent with the national aim of reducing the IVF multiple birth rate to 10% over a period of years.[87]

In the United States, there is no regulatory body comparable to the HFEA. This does not mean, as is sometimes claimed, that ART is unregulated. On the state level, physicians are licensed by medical boards, which can revoke their licenses. On the federal level, the CDC collects data, and the Food and Drug Administration (FDA) controls approval and use of drugs, biological products, and medical devices.

83. IVF-Infertility.com, "The Risks and Complications of IVF Treatment," http://www.ivf-infertility.com/ivf/standard/complications/multiple_pregnancy2.php. Accessed July 19, 2010.

84. Ann Thurin, Jon Hausken, Torbjörn Hillensjö, Barbara Jablonowska, Anja Pinborg, Annika Strandell, and Christina Bergh. 2004. "Elective Single-Embryo Transfer Versus Double-Embryo Transfer in In Vitro Fertilization," New England Journal of Medicine 351: 2392–2402.

85. Orentlicher, "Multiple Embryo Transfers" (see note 82), p. 13.

86. Human Fertilization and Embryology Authority. 2009. "Embryo Transfer and Multiple Births," April 13. http://www.hfea.gov.uk/2587.html. Accessed July 24, 2010.

87. Ibid.

The Clinical Laboratory Improvement Act (CLIA) ensures the quality of laboratory testing. As with all medical specialties, specialists in reproductive medicine are board certified. They are also subject to lawsuits if they commit malpractice, which may be determined by a failure to follow practice guidelines. The ASRM practice committee has issued guidelines on the number of embryos for transfer. Here is its rationale for opposing absolute restrictions on embryo transfer:

> Strict limitations on the number of embryos transferred, as required by law in some countries, do not allow treatment plans to be individualized after careful consideration of each patient's own unique circumstances. Accordingly, these guidelines may be modified according to individual clinical conditions, including patient age, individual quality, the opportunity for cryopreservation, and as clinical experience with newer techniques accumulates.[88]

In 1999, ASRM released guidelines recommending the transfer of only two embryos for women younger than 35 years old with a favorable prognosis and three embryos for women with a poorer prognosis for successful implantation. In 2004, the guidelines were updated to recommend eSET for women under 35 years old with a good prognosis. In 2006, the guidelines were again updated to say that women under 35 years old should be given no more than two embryos during a single implantation procedure "in the absence of extraordinary circumstances."[89] The guidelines were updated again after the story of Nadya Suleman, or "Octomom," as she was referred to in the media.

OCTOMOM

Ms. Suleman, a single mother who previously had six children through ART, underwent another round of IVF and gave birth to eight more babies on January 26, 2009. Her Beverly Hills fertility doctor, Michael Kamrava, claimed that he transferred only six embryos, two of which then divided. (At the Medical Board of California's hearing in October 2010 to consider revoking or suspending Dr. Kamrava's license, Deputy Attorney General Judith Alvarado charged that he actually transferred 12 embryos.[90]) In any event, the transfer of even six embryos would have been contrary to ASRM guidelines, which specify that no more than two embryos should be transferred in a healthy woman under 35 years of age; Ms. Suleman was only 33 years old when she was treated. Even if she was considered to have an unfavorable prognosis, because of earlier difficulties getting pregnant, only three embryos, not six, should have been transferred. It has been suggested that Dr. Kamrava, who is not board certified in

88. The Practice Committee of ASRM and the Practice Committee of SART. 2009. "Guidelines of Number of Embryos Transferred," *Fertility and Sterility* 92 (5): 1518–1519. http://www.asrm.org/uploadedFiles/ASRM_Content/News_and_Publications/Practice_Guidelines/Guidelines_and_Minimum_Standards/Guidelines_on_number_of_embryos%281%29.pdf. Accessed July 20, 2010.

89. The Practice Committee of the Society for Assisted Reproductive Technology and the American Society for Reproductive Medicine. 2004. "Guidelines on the Number of Embryos Transferred," *Fertility and Sterility* 82 (3): 773–774, p. 773.

90. Associated Press. 2010. "Lawyer: Octuplets' Mom Implanted With 12 Embryos," http://today.msnbc.msn.com/id/39738767/ns/today-today_people/#slice-2. Accessed November 3, 2010.

reproductive medicine, transferred such a high number of embryos because his previous experience with getting embryos to implant was quite poor. According to data he filed with SART in 2006, his success rate was under 10%, significantly below the average success rate for women under 35 years old of around 45%.[91]

ASRM expelled Dr. Kamrava in September 2009. On December 22, 2009, the California Medical Board filed a disciplinary complaint against him for "gross negligence" in implanting more embryos in Ms. Suleman than should be transferred any woman, regardless of age. It was "not only in violation of the standard of care, but is beyond the reasonable judgment of any treating physician."[92] The Board later added additional charges, including transferring seven embryos to a 48-year-old woman. "The revised complaint also accuses Dr. Kamrava of failing to refer another patient for cancer screening, despite her history of cancer and finding cysts on her ovaries. The 42-year-old woman was later diagnosed with Stage III ovarian cancer and had to have her uterus, cervix, ovaries, and fallopian tubes removed."[93]

In November 2009, ASRM issued new guidelines with the intention of reducing the number of multiple births.[94] The guidelines were revised in two ways. Regardless of prognosis, no more than one embryo beyond those called for in the guidelines should be transferred, and patients must be counseled on the risks of multiple fetal pregnancies. "Both the counseling and the justification for exceeding the recommended limits must be documented in the patient's permanent medical record."[95] The guidelines are nonbinding, and while ASRM notes that SART "strictly monitors member clinics for adherence to ASRM guidelines,"[96] it does not routinely expel noncomplying members. Moreover, it has been estimated on the basis of CDC reports that 80% of clinics in the United States do not follow ASRM guidelines on embryo transfer.[97] In California, Dr. Kamrava's location, the noncompliance rate is 92%.[98]

91. Matthew Herper. 2009. "Octuplet Doc Kamrava: Running the Worst FertilityClinic in the U.S.?" *The Science Business*, February 13. http://blogs.forbes.com/sciencebiz/2009/02/octuplet-doc-kamrava-running-the-worst-fertility-clinic-in-the-us/. Accessed July 20, 2010.

92. Medical Board of California, *In the Matter of the Accusation Against Michael Kamrava, M.D.*, Case No. 06–2009-197098. http://www.latimes.com/includes/misc/kamravaaccusation.pdf. Accessed July 21, 2010. See also Jenny Booth, "Nadya Suleman Octuplets Doctor Michael Kamrava Accused of Negligence," *The Times*, January 5, 2010. http://www.timesonline.co.uk/tol/news/world/us_and_americas/article6976514.ece. Accessed July 19, 2010.

93. Louise Mallon. 2010. "'Octomom' Doctor Faces Fresh Allegations," *BioNews*. http://www.bionews.org.uk/page_66788.asp. Accessed July 19, 2010.

94. The Practice Committee of ASRM and the Practice Committee of SART, "Guidelines on Number of Embryos Transferred" (see note 88).

95. Ibid.

96. ASRM. 2010. "Oversight of Assisted Reproductive Technology," pamphlet published by the American Society for Reproductive Medicine.

97. Marcy Darnovsky. 2009. "The Baby Business and Public Policy," *Science Progress*, May 5. http://www.scienceprogress.org/2009/05/baby-business-and-public-policy/. Accessed July 20, 2010.

98. Ibid.

This, combined with the Octomom scandal, has led for calls for stricter oversight by some bioethicists. For example, Arthur Caplan wrote in the *Philadelphia Inquirer*:

> If the medical profession is unwilling or unable to police its own, then government needs to get involved. We already have rules governing who can get involved with adoption and foster care. Shouldn't these minimal requirements be extended to fertility treatment? And shouldn't some limit be set on how many embryos can be implanted at one time, along with some rules about what to do with embryos that no one wants to use?
>
> Other nations, such as Britain, keep a regulatory eye on reproductive technologies and those who wish to use them, knowing their use can put kids at risk in ways that nature never envisioned. We owe the same to children born here.[99]

David Orentlicher also favors legal limits on the number of embryos to be transferred. He supports educating prospective parents about the risks imposed by twins, and requiring insurers to cover the cost of IVF, to remove the financial pressure to complete one's family with one cycle, but he thinks that these measures are probably not enough. Following the Swedish example, he recommends having physicians transfer only one embryo, "unless a transfer of two was justified by the mother's age, poorer-quality embryos, or no prior success with IVF."[100] To ensure compliance, prior approval for transferring two embryos would probably be necessary, he says, although he does not say who would give such approval.

I argued above that prospective parents are morally obligated to accept eSET if that gives them as good a chance, or nearly as good a chance, to have a baby as transferring double embryos. The medical profession also has an ethical obligation to promote eSET in its guidelines. The ASRM guidelines say, "High-order multiple pregnancy (three or more implanted embryos) is an undesirable consequence (outcome) of assisted reproductive technologies (ART)."[101] But it is not simply high-order multiple births that are the problem. The ASRM should also address the risks and costs imposed by twin birth. Moreover, when the guidelines address eSET, they are not forceful enough, saying only, "For patients with the most favorable prognosis, *consideration should be given* to transferring only a single embryo."[102] A more robust approach would be to say: "Unless the chances of conception for a particular patient would be significantly reduced, only one embryo should be transferred."

Requiring that patients be counseled on the risks of multifetal pregnancy is very important. However, counseling should not be limited to merely informing patients of the risks, and letting them make their own decisions. Doctors should try to persuade patients to accept eSET. Here I am relying on what Ezekiel Emanuel and Linda

---

99. Arthur Caplan. 2009. "Ethics and Octuplets: Society Is Responsible," *Philadelphia Inquirer*, February 6.

100. Orentlicher, "Multiple Embryo Transfers" (see note 82), p. 13.

101. The Practice Committee of ASRM and the Practice Committee of SART, "Guidelines on Number of Embryos Transferred" (see note 88).

102. Ibid. My emphasis.

Emanuel have called "the deliberative model" of the doctor–patient relationship.[103] In this model, doctors are not paternalistic. They do not conceal facts or shade the truth to protect their patients. But neither are doctors simply "hired hands" who just give their patients whatever they want. Instead, doctors on the deliberative model are supposed to engage in dialogue with their patients about their health-related goals, and express their own views when they think their patients are taking undue risks or being personally or socially irresponsible. If patients with a favorable prognosis ask to have more than one embryo transferred because they want twins, doctors should refuse to go along with this request. This will be difficult to do, since the reason for wanting twins is a legitimate one: to avoid the financial and physical burdens of additional cycles of IVF. Nevertheless, individuals do not have the right to subject offspring to increased risk of disability to achieve their goal of having more than one child, and physicians should not accede to such demands. A better solution to the problem of cost is for professional organizations to call for better insurance coverage of ART, and to consider reducing their own fees.

The next question is whether the ASRM guidelines should be made into law.[104] On the pro side, it must be acknowledged that compliance with voluntary guidelines is dismal. However, it is not clear that legal mandates are the solution. A mandate without any flexibility regarding double-embryo transfer would be unacceptable to both patients and doctors. The Swedish approach is more stringent than the ASRM guidelines, but both allow doctors to depart from eSET where this is deemed necessary to achieve a pregnancy. The difficulty of making either approach into law is that there is no existing body that could determine whether transferring multiple embryos was medically justified. Adopting the Swedish approach requires more than a law; essentially it means creating the American version of the HFEA. On the other hand, if the limit for the number of embryos transferred is set high enough—say, six—this would do little except prevent another "Octomom." However, given the rarity of such cases, such a law will have little practical effect. Its significance would be primarily symbolic. Given these problems with finding a legal solution to the problem of multiple births, a better approach would be better education of patients and the public about the risks of multifetal pregnancy, better insurance coverage for ART, and the strengthening of professional guidelines with the aim of reducing twin births as well as high-order multiple births. Professional organizations should also censure, and even expel in some cases, clinics and individuals who fail to comply with practice standards.

In any event, twins can also be caused by the use of fertility drugs, which cause more eggs to develop. Since there are no embryos to transfer, restrictions on embryo transfer do not address the twin problem. The only ways to prevent multiple births due to hyperstimulation are either not to hyperstimulate (which reduces the chances of pregnancy), or to monitor the number of eggs through ultrasound, and then to call off the cycle (i.e., not fertilize the eggs) if there are more than two or three that are mature. Selective reduction is another option, although this involves aborting some of the fetuses and, aside from any ethical objections, risks losing the entire pregnancy

103. Ezekiel Emanuel and Linda Emanuel. 1992."Four Models of the Physician-Patient Relationship," *Journal of the American Medicine Association* 267 (16): 2221–2226.

104. For an excellent discussion of this topic, see John Robertson. 2009. "The Octuplet Case—Why More Regulation Is Not Likely," *Hastings Center Report* 39 (3): 26–28.

through a miscarriage. These are difficult, indeed, heart-wrenching choices for patients and doctors, and they are unlikely to be solved by legislation.

DISPOSITIONAL PROBLEMS

Some of the thorniest problems posed by the new reproductive technologies concern who has jurisdiction over extracorporeal embryos in the event of the parents' death or divorce. The technological advance that has created the problem is the ability to freeze embryos for later implantation. This is a great advantage, since it means that patients can have a second or third chance at pregnancy without having to undergo another round of superovulatory drugs and egg retrieval. However, this leaves the problem of what should be done with surplus frozen embryos. Most IVF centers require couples to specify what will be done with their embryos, should they no longer need them for reproductive purposes. They may choose to have them thawed and discarded, donated to another couple, or used in research. However, such advance agreements are not always created, and even if they are, they can be challenged, just like wills and prenuptial agreements. When such cases come before the courts, judges have to decide how to consider extracorporeal embryos. Is the embryo the property of the couple concerned? Or should the embryos be considered to be "preborn children" and a custody model employed? This was the issue in the case of *Davis* v. *Davis*.[105]

Davis v. Davis

Mary Sue Davis and Junior Lewis Davis married in 1980. They very much wanted to have a family, but after Mrs. Davis suffered five tubal pregnancies, she had her fallopian tubes severed to prevent further risk to her. She and her husband thereafter decided to resort to IVF. After six unsuccessful attempts at IVF, the Davises tried to adopt a child, but the birth mother ultimately decided not to put her child up for adoption. They made other attempts at adoption, but these proved prohibitively expensive, and the Davises returned to the IVF program.

In the fall of 1988, Mrs. Davis learned about a new technique, cryopreservation. On December 8, 1988, nine eggs were aspirated from Mrs. Davis by laparoscopy, fertilized with Mr. Davis's sperm, and allowed to mature in vitro to the eight-cell cleavage stage. Two of the embryos were implanted in Mrs. Davis on December 10, 1988, neither of which resulted in a pregnancy. The remaining seven were placed in cryogenic storage for future implantation purposes.

The Davises discussed the fact that the storage life of the embryos probably would not exceed 2 years. (In 1988, no one knew how long frozen embryos would be viable, and the assumption was that they would not last very long in storage. This assumption has turned out to be incorrect. A 2010 restrospective study of nearly 12,000 cryopreserved embryos showed no difference in the chance for pregnancy, even when embryos

105. Junior L. Davis vs. Mary Sue Davis vs. Ray King, M.D., d/b/a Fertility Center of East Tennessee, Third Party Defendant, No. E-14496, September 21, 1989.

were frozen for more than 9 years.[106]) They also considered the possibility of donating to another couple the remaining seven embryos, should Mrs. Davis become pregnant as a result of her implant on December 10, but the couple made no decision about that matter. There was no discussion about disposition of the embryos in the event of future contingencies, such as their deaths or divorce, because they were regarded by the clinic staff as "old customers" and a very stable couple.[107] Nor were they asked to sign any consent forms. "Apparently the clinic was in the process of moving its location when the Davises underwent this last round and, because timing of each step of IVF is crucial, it was impossible to postpone the procedure until the appropriate forms were located."[108]

Junior Davis filed for divorce in February 1989. He testified that he had known that their marriage "was not very stable" for a year or more, but he had hoped that the birth of a child would improve their relationship. Mary Sue Davis testified that she had no idea that there was a problem with their marriage. Mr. Davis's filing papers requested an order enjoining the fertility clinic from releasing the embryos to Mrs. Davis or others for the purposes of thawing and implantation. With divorce impending, Mr. Davis did not want to become a parent. Mrs. Davis contended that she was the mother of the embryos, and that she had the right to try to establish a pregnancy with them. Moreover, she contended that the embryos were "preborn children" with rights of their own.

A circuit court judge, W. Dale Young, ruled in favor of Mrs. Davis. The judge framed the issue not as who should get the embryos, but rather whether the embryos were people or products. Judge Young concluded that the embryos in vitro were people, and therefore that a "best-interest" analysis was the appropriate one. He held that it was in the manifest best interest of these "children" that they be available for implantation and that their mother be permitted to bring them to term.

The judge's decision that the embryos are people was based exclusively on the testimony of one witness, French right-to-life physician Jerome Lejeune. The testimony of the other witnesses was rejected primarily because they all termed the embryos "pre-embryos." The judge held that he could not find the term in any encyclopedia or dictionary, and hence concluded that there is no such term, and that the seven cryopreserved entities were human embryos. Since, in his view, human life begins at conception, the embryos were human beings, with all the rights of other human beings.

A number of commentators have objected to the term "pre-embryo" as a recent verbal invention, created for self-serving reasons. John Marshall, a professor of clinical neurology and member of the Warnock Committee, writes:

> The term "pre-embryo" was not heard of prior to all this debate [on embryo experimentation]. From the time of fertilization up to about the eighth week the entity was called "embryo." Suddenly this term "preembryo" is now in every

106. Ryan Riggs et al. 2010. "Does Storage Time Influence Postthaw Survival and Pregnancy Outcome? An Analysis of 11,768 Human Cryopreserved Embryos," *Fertility and Sterility* 93 (1): 109–115.

107. Oral information from Charles Clifford, attorney for Junior Davis.

108. *Davis v. Davis*, 842 S.W.2d 588, fn9.

paper and every symposium. Some scientists are saying that they had been thinking along these lines already in 1975. It is surprising that if they had been thinking about it as far back as 1975, they never actually used the term until now. It seems like a public relations manoeuvre to make people think that the experts are against *embryo* experimentation, but that it is alright to experiment on the "pre-embryo," as if the latter was somehow different.[109]

Certainly, what term is used does not determine the entity's moral standing. However, it can be argued that the term "pre-embryo" is more accurate than "embryo" in characterizing the initial phase of mammalian and human development. The earliest stages of development after fertilization do not establish the embryo proper, but a feeding layer or trophoblast, which begins to function before the embryonic disc forms. For this reason, the zygote, morula, and early blastocyst stages can be regarded as pre-embryonic stages, with the term "embryo" reserved for the entity that appears at the end of the second week after fertilization, when the primitive streak, the precursor of the nervous system, appears.[110] Moreover, many commentators would argue that the term "pre-embryo" is not only scientifically more accurate, but that certain features of the pre-embryo—its lack of a nervous system, its ability to turn into more than one individual, and its inability to develop into a person without further intervention (transfer to a uterus) justify ascribing to the pre-embryo a different moral status from that of the implanted embryo. The interest view does not regard these features as morally decisive, but nevertheless it is unfair and inaccurate to view the term "pre-embryo" as a mere verbal maneuver, and worse to claim, as did Judge Young, that the term does not exist.

Like so many other right-to-life advocates, Judge Young assumed that the issue was the genetic humanity of the embryos. But no one has ever disputed that the embryos are genetically human. The issue, totally missed by Judge Young, is whether these human embryos have the moral or legal standing of born human beings. John Robertson expresses the point this way: "While the preimplantation embryo is clearly human and living, it does not follow that it is also a 'human life' or 'human being' in the crucial sense of a person with rights or interests."[111] Robertson calls the judge's conclusion that four-celled preimplantation human embryos are children "unprecedented and unwarranted."[112]

George Annas notes that if the judge really believed that he had to decide this case based on the "best interests of the children," he would have had at least to determine whether Mrs. Davis was a fit mother to gestate them. "Given her past history of inability to carry a fetus to term, there is little probability of her successfully gestating any of the seven embryos. Requiring her to hire a surrogate mother to gestate them

109. John Marshall. 1990. "The Case Against Experimentation," in Anthony Dyson and John Harris, eds., *Experiments on Embryos*. London: Routledge, p. 63.

110. John A. Robertson. 1986. "Embryos, Families, and Procreative Liberty: The Legal Structure of the New Reproduction," *Southern California 59 Law Review* 942: 969–970.

111. John A. Robertson. 1989. "Resolving Disputes Over Frozen Embryos," *Hastings Center Report* 19 (6): 7–12, p. 11.

112. Ibid.

would almost certainly enhance their chances to be born."[113] Annas also points out that despite the fact that Judge Young spent all his time deciding that the embryos are people, not property, he ended up treating them like property. "Instead of deciding custody, visitation, and support issues (which he would have to do if the embryos *were* children), he awards them to Mrs. Davis in exactly the way he would award a dresser or a painting.[114]

Judge Young's decision was bad law and bad bioethics. This was recognized by the Tennessee Court of Appeals, an intermediate-level appeals court that overturned Judge Young's decision, and remanded the case to trial court "for entry of an order vesting them with 'joint control and with equal voice over their disposition.'"[115] The case then went to the Tennessee Supreme Court, which granted review "not because we disagree with the basic legal analysis utilized by the intermediate court, but because of the obvious importance of the case in terms of the development of law regarding the new reproductive technologies, and because the decision of the Court of Appeals does not give adequate guidance to the trial court in the event the parties cannot agree."[116]

The Tennessee Supreme Court tackled the question of whether the preembryos should be considered persons or property. At the time, some commentators maintained that these were the only two possibilities currently in the law.[117] The property model is extremely repugnant to many people, not just right-to-lifers, for it suggests that embryos can be bought and sold, as sperm can be sold, or perhaps marketed for use in cosmetics. However, there is an alternative to viewing extracorporeal embryos either as children or as property. George Annas expresses it this way:

> . . . embryos could just as easily be considered *neither* products nor people, but put in some other category altogether. There are many things, such as dogs, dolphins, and redwoods that are neither products nor people. We nonetheless legally protect these entities by limiting what their owners or custodians can do with them. Every national commission worldwide that has examined the status of the human embryo to date has placed it in this third category: neither people nor products, but nonetheless entities of unique symbolic value that deserve society's respect and protection.[118]

This is the view that the Tennessee Supreme Court adopted, saying, "We conclude that preembryos are not, strictly speaking, either 'persons' or 'property,' but occupy

113. George Annas. 1989. "A French Homunculus in a Tennessee Court," *Hastings Center Report,* 29 (6): 20–22, p. 22.

114. Ibid., p. 21.

115. *Davis v. Davis*, 1990 WL 130807.

116. *Davis* (see note 108), p. 590.

117. See, for example, Douglas Cusine, "Experimentation: Some Legal Aspects," in Dyson and Harris (see note 109), p. 123.

118. Annas, "A French Homunculus" (see note 113), p. 20.

an interim category that entitles them to special respect because of their potential for human life."[119]

What are the implications of this view for deciding *Davis v. Davis?* The court began by saying that any agreement between the couple regarding disposition should be presumed valid and enforced. However, in this case, there was no agreement. It might be argued that there was an implied contract to reproduce using IVF, and that therefore the court should uphold such a contract against Junior Davis, "allowing Mary Sue to dispose of the preembryos in a manner calculated to result in reproduction."[120] The court rejected this argument, saying that there was no indication the parties ever considered the embryos to be used for reproduction outside of the marriage. It turned instead to the question of the right of procreational autonomy, which "is composed of two rights of equal significance—the right to procreate and the right to avoid procreation."[121]

John Robertson argues that, in the absence of advance instructions, the party wishing to avoid reproduction—in this case, Mr. Davis—should prevail.

> A way out of the dilemma exists if we consider the irreversibility of the respective losses at issue and the essential fungibility of the embryos. The party who wishes to avoid offspring is irreversibly harmed if embryo transfer and birth occur, for the burdens of unwanted parenthood cannot then be avoided. On the other hand, frustrating the ability of the willing partner to reproduce with these embryos will—in most instances—not prevent that partner from reproducing at a later time with other embryos. As long as the party wishing to reproduce could without undue burden create other embryos, the desire to avoid biologic offspring should take priority over the desire to reproduce with the embryos in question.[122]

The burdens of unwanted parenthood include risks of financial liability, although Mr. Davis's primary objection to becoming a father was not fear of financial liability. Rather, he objected to being deprived of his reproductive rights and also to having a child produced to live in a single-parent home. His own life was shattered when, at 6 years old, his parents were divorced and he and his three brothers were sent to a boys' home. Robertson refers to such considerations as the "psychosocial impact of unwanted biologic offspring" and argues that these should be given appropriate weight in deciding individual disputes. He maintains that Mr. Davis would be irreversibly harmed if embryo transfer and birth occur, as he would be forced to accept the psychosocial and financial burdens of parenthood. By contrast, Mrs. Davis, now remarried and going by the name Mary Sue Stowe, would not be irreversibly harmed by being denied embryo transfer, as she could reproduce at a later time with other embryos. Admittedly, she has undergone many painful, physically tiring, and emotionally taxing procedures. This is not determinative, according to Robertson, "since the burdens of any one additional

119. *Davis* (see note 108), p. 597.

120. Ibid., p. 598.

121. Ibid., p. 601.

122. Robertson, "Resolving Disputes Over Frozen Embryos" (see note 111), p. 8.

retrieval cycle are moderate and acceptable, at least relative to the irreversible burdens of imposing fatherhood on the husband."[123]

The question of whose interests should prevail is extremely difficult to resolve. The procreative liberty of both parties is at stake. If these frozen embryos in fact represented Mrs. Stowe's last chance to give birth, her desire to become a mother should be given as much weight as Mr. Davis's desire to avoid fatherhood. The case would have to be settled by attempting to determine which party would be more badly harmed by frustration of his or her reproductive interests. Robertson suggests that the desire to avoid reproduction should take priority, so long as the party wishing to reproduce could, without undue burden, create other embryos. It seems to me that it would impose an "undue burden" to require Mrs. Stowe to undergo another round of treatment. She has already undergone serious physical burdens and risks, including being subjected to drugs and hormones to induce superovulation, the long-term effects of which have not been determined; laparoscopy, which carries a significant risk of mortality or morbidity; and the possibility of infection, physical damage, or an ectopic pregnancy through the placement of the zygotes in her uterus. In addition to the physical burdens, Mrs. Stowe has undergone severe emotional trauma from her seven failed attempts at IVF. To ask her to undergo yet another treatment cycle in order to have a chance at pregnancy would be unduly burdensome and unfair.

However, the situation changed when Mrs. Stowe decided not to try to have the pre-embryos implanted in her uterus, but to retain custody of the pre-embryos in order to donate them to another childless couple. This move prompted one of the judges on the state appeals court panel to question Mrs. Stowe's motives for still wanting the embryos. "Is this a case of a party wanting to win at any cost?" Judge Franks asked.[124]

From a right-to-life perspective, Mrs. Stowe's motives are noble. Her concern is solely for the welfare of her "preborn children." She is willing to renounce her claim to the frozen embryos, and her chance to become a mother, in order to enhance their chance of live birth. On the interest principle, however, the welfare of the embryos is not the issue, because fertilized eggs do not have a welfare or interests of their own. Nor does the case any longer involve a conflict of interests in reproductive liberty, since Mrs. Stowe no longer has any intention of becoming pregnant with the embryos. Mrs. Stowe's desire to have her genetic offspring brought to birth by someone else, who will then become the rearing parent, should have no weight at all. As the only reproductive interest is Mr. Davis's interest in avoiding paternity, his interest should prevail. The court held that:

> Ordinarily, the party wishing to avoid procreation should prevail, assuming that the other party has a reasonable possibility of achieving parenthood by means other than use of the preembryos in question. If no other reasonable alternatives exist, then the argument in favor of using the preembryos to achieve pregnancy should be considered. However, if the party seeking control of the preembryos intends merely to donate them to another couple, the objecting party obviously has the greater interest and should prevail.

123. Ibid., p. 9.

124. "Chill in Custody Fight." 1990. *The National Law Journal*, June 18, p. 6.

This language created what became known as the "reasonable alternatives exception."[125]

Obviously, it would be better for everyone concerned if such matters never, or rarely ever, reached the courts. The British solution has been to allow storage of embryos only with the effective consent (i.e., written consent that has not been withdrawn) of both parties providing gametes. As Derek Morgan and Robert G. Lee interpret the Act, "Withdrawal of the consent of either donor to the embryo's creation appears to mean that it must be allowed to perish, although this does not appear explicitly stated."[126] Some American commentators have made similar recommendations.[127] The trouble with this solution is that it is unduly biased in favor of the party wishing to avoid reproduction. What if Mrs. Stowe wanted to attempt another pregnancy but was unable to produce more eggs, so that the frozen embryos represented her last chance at having a genetic child? Should her ex-husband be able to thwart her procreative interest for no good reason, perhaps out of spite? The reasonable alternatives exception at least gives the party who wants to reproduce a chance to make his or her case. However, that raises the question, How should the competing procreative interests be weighed? Specifically, what would count as enough of a burden on the part of the party wishing to reproduce with the frozen embryos to outweigh the other party's right not to reproduce? This issue was raised in the New York case, *Kass v. Kass*.[128]

Kass v. Kass

Unlike the Davises, Maureen and Steven Kass had executed informed consent documents regarding the disposition of their frozen embryos, stating that the embryos would be donated for research in the event that the couple no longer wished to use them to instantiate a pregnancy.[129] This should have foreclosed any debate on what would be done with the embryos, but some of the justices at the appellate level questioned whether the documents were precise enough to indicate the true wishes of the parties. Ultimately, the resolution of the case turned on the finding that the contracts were valid and binding. However, the case is interesting because it raises the question of how to interpret the reasonable alternatives exception in cases where there is no contract or there is reason to doubt the contract's validity.

The facts of the case are as follows. Maureen and Steven Kass were married in 1988. Mrs. Kass had been exposed to diethylstilbistrol (DES) while in utero, which caused her to have difficulty conceiving. They underwent 10 unsuccessful attempts to have a child through IVF between March 1990 and June 1993, at a total cost in

125. Jennifer L. Medenwald. 2001. Note, "A 'Frozen Exception' for the Frozen Embryo: The *Davis* 'Reasonable Alternatives Exception,'" *Indiana Law Journal* 76 (2): 507–524, p. 509.

126. Derek Morgan and Robert G. Lee. 1991. *Blackstone's Guide to the Human Fertilisation and Embryology Act 1990*. London: Blackstone Press Limited, pp. 26–27.

127. See Developments in the Law, "Medical Technology and the Law." 1990. *Harvard Law Review* 103, p. 1545.

128. *Kass v. Kass*. 1998. 235 A.D.2d 150, 663 N.Y.S.2d 581.

129. Ibid., p. 584.

excess of $75,000.[130] On May 20, 1993, numerous ova were removed from Maureen Kass. Four embryos were implanted in her sister, who had agreed to be a surrogate for them, and five of the embryos were frozen. On June 4, they were advised that a pregnancy had not resulted, and Mrs. Kass's sister had changed her mind and no longer would agree to be a surrogate. Immediately, the couple decided to divorce and executed an uncontested divorce document in which they reiterated their desires to donate the embryos for biological study and research. Less than a month after executing the uncontested divorce document, Maureen Kass changed her mind. On June 28, 1993, she wrote letters to the hospital and her IVF physician, informing them of marital difficulties and stating her adamant opposition to the destruction of the embryos. She said that she now wanted possession of the "pre-zygotes" so that she could have them implanted in herself in another round of IVF.

At trial, Judge Roncallo ruled that "a husband's procreative rights in a situation involving in vitro fertilization were no greater than in the case of an in vivo fertilization, such that those rights essentially terminated at the moment of fertilization, making the disposition of the pre-zygotes a matter exclusively within the wife's unfettered discretion."[131] He dismissed the informed consent documents, because these said that the disposition of the embryos in the event of divorce would be left to a court. In addition, the uncontested divorce document did not constitute a waiver of Mrs. Kass's right to determine the future of the frozen embryos. The court gave Mrs. Kass "'the exclusive right to determine the fate of the subject pre-embryos,' including their utilization in another attempt to achieve pregnancy."[132] That judgment was stayed while the case went to the appeals court.

The appellate court found that the lower court had erred in its analogy between abortion and the disposition of frozen embryos. The reason a woman cannot be forced to have an abortion, should the father wish to avoid procreation, is her right of bodily self-determination. Where there is no pregnancy, as in the case of in vitro fertilization and the creation of extracorporeal embryos, no right of bodily integrity is implicated, and therefore it does not follow that the woman has the exclusive right to decide the fate of the embryos. The court referred to the framework provided in *Davis v. Davis*, for weighing the right to procreate against the right not to procreate, but said that there was no need to decide whether such an analysis should be adopted in the present case, since the parties had signed an informed consent document and an uncontested divorce document "in which they unequivocally stated their intent as to the manner of disposition of the subject pre-zygotes."[133] Mrs. Kass's "subsequent change of heart cannot be permitted to unilaterally alter their mutual decision."[134]

In a concurring opinion, Justice Friedmann agreed with the result but disagreed with the analysis that yielded it. He said that the IVF document was subject to multiple and conflicting interpretations, and so it could not be used to resolve the dispute. Therefore, the court was faced with precisely the issue in *Davis*, namely, how to

130. Ibid., at 583.

131. Ibid., at 585.

132. Ibid.

133. Ibid., at 586.

134. Ibid., at 590.

dispose of frozen embryos when the parties cannot agree and there is no intelligible written contract declaring their intentions.[135] In such cases, "the objecting party, except in the most exceptional circumstances, should be able to veto a former spouse's proposed implantation."[136] The concurring justices favored the veto approach over the balancing approach because it was clear to them that when the balancing approach is used, ". . . there can be few situations, if any, where the burden upon the party forced to forfeit using particular pre-zygotes to acquire offspring will outweigh the burden upon the party who wishes to avoid reproduction but is compelled by court order to become a parent."[137] The reason for this is that, once lost, the right to avoid reproduction can never be regained. The "irrevocability of parenthood," and the resulting biological and emotional ties it brings, constitutes the primary reason why courts should not undertake to foist parenthood upon an unwilling individual.[138]

In his dissent, Justice Miller argued that the veto approach unjustifiably favors the right to avoid procreation over the right to procreate. "These rights are just as fundamental, and, depending upon the circumstances of a given case, the right to procreate may be just as irrevocably lost as a result of the other party's veto. Simply stated, the competing fundamental, personal rights of both parties must be taken into consideration and balanced utilizing a fact-sensitive analysis."[139]

While a balancing approach gives weight to both aspects of procreative liberty, the reasonable alternatives exception, as presented in both *Davis* and *Kass*, focuses exclusively on whether the party wanting to implant the embryos has other alternatives available to her for parenthood, including more rounds of IVF and adoption. For example, in *Davis*, while the court acknowledged the trauma Mary Sue had already experienced, and the burdens a subsequent round or rounds of IVF would impose, it ultimately discounted all of this "because she would have a reasonable opportunity, through IVF, to try once again to achieve parenthood in all its aspects—genetic, gestational, bearing, and rearing."[140] However, as one commentator points out, ". . . what a 'reasonable alternative' is cannot be determined without taking into consideration all of the pain, trauma, and expense suffered by a party prior to a frozen embryo custody dispute. Factors such as these must be incorporated into the reasonable alternatives exception in order to achieve a true balance of the right to procreate and the right to avoid procreation."[141] At the same time, embryos should not be awarded to one party as a kind of reward for all the pain, trauma, and expense she has suffered in the attempt to procreate. Unless there is a reasonable possibility that the party wishing to implant will be able to get pregnant, and carry a pregnancy to term—something that was dubious in both the *Davis* and *Kass* cases—no procreative interest is served by awarding the frozen embryos to her, assuming she intends to have the embryos

135. Ibid., at 592.

136. Ibid.

137. Ibid.

138. Ibid.

139. Ibid., at 599.

140. *Davis*, 842 S.W.2d at 604.

141. Medenwald, "A 'Frozen Exception' for the Frozen Embryo" (see note 125), at 522.

implanted in herself. Presumably, the use of a surrogate would enable her to achieve genetic, although not gestational, parenthood. If undergoing another round of IVF would impose such physical and financial burdens on her as to make this an unreasonable request, then her right to procreate with the existing frozen embryos, whether she gestated them or used a surrogate, might outweigh the father's right to avoid procreation. It is conceivable, though less likely, that the party wishing to procreate with the frozen embryos would be the man, who could hire a surrogate to gestate them. Once again, the question would be whether he had reasonable alternatives to becoming a father. Since he could contract with a gestational carrier (one who would be inseminated with his sperm), there does not seem to be any reason why he would have to use the embryos he created with his ex-wife in order to have children genetically related to him.

The courts in *Davis* and *Kass* both suggested adoption as an alternative route to parenthood. Earlier I mentioned some of the difficulties couples face in trying to adopt.[142] Certainly, these difficulties should not be downplayed in suggesting that the party wishing to procreate has other alternatives. More important, people who undergo IVF seek a genetic connection with their offspring. Some people disparage this desire, suggesting that parents ought not to care whether the children they raise are related by blood. However, people do value creating offspring who are biologically connected to both parents, and infertile people are simply seeking to replicate as much of the experience they would have had, but for their infertility, as possible. It seems to me that they have as much right to have genetically related offspring as fertile people, and that this should be protected by procreative autonomy. If so, then adoption, while a wonderful way for many people to create a family, should not be deemed an alternative that justifies depriving one of the parties of his or her procreative liberty.

Ideally, disputes over the disposition of frozen embryos will be avoided by well-constructed, unambiguous informed consent documents executed prior to the creation of the embryos. Realistically, there will continue to be such disputes, and sometimes they will come before the courts. When they do, courts should recognize that both aspects of procreative liberty—the right to reproduce as well as the right to avoid reproduction—are fundamental. The crucial point from the perspective of the interest view is that the relevant interests are not those of the frozen embryos, but those of the disputing parties. These cases will rarely be easy to resolve, but without conceptual clarity about the nature and status of extracorporeal embryos, they will be hopeless.

GAMETE DONATION

In vitro fertilization often enables people who cannot reproduce coitally to reproduce using their own gametes, but it also creates the possibility of reproducing using the gametes of other people. Some critics object to involving "third parties," either because this is seen as intruding on what should be an intimate relationship or because of confusion about lineage and psychological problems this could create in offspring. Such objections can be made regardless of whether the gamete donors are paid. Others object only to "commercial gamete donation," sometimes on the ground

142. See also David L. Theyssen. 1999. Note, "Balancing Interests in Frozen Embryo Disputes: Is Adoption Really a Reasonable Alternative?" 74 *Indiana Law Journal* 711.

that this commodifies reproduction. Other objections to payment to gamete donors are that it exploits the donors, especially egg donors, by inducing them to donate their eggs when it is not really in their interest to do so. Still other objections stem from offering larger sums of money to egg donors with particular genetic traits, on the ground that this is a form of eugenics.[143]

A word regarding terminology is in order. Thomas Murray objects to the term "commercial gamete donation." He writes, "Despite the repeated reference to 'donors' of both ovum and sperm, paying individuals for their biological products makes them vendors, not donors."[144] He recommends that the term "AID" (artificial insemination by donor) should really be "AIV" (artificial insemination by vendor). In response, some maintain that paying gamete providers does not make them vendors, because they are not being paid for a product (their gametes); rather, they are being compensated for their time, inconvenience, and risk. I continue to use the term "donation" even when referring to the commercial enterprise, not because I want to prejudge the question of whether payment is for the product or compensation, still less to prejudge the question of moral acceptability, but simply because it is accepted usage.

Sperm Donation

The oldest and most common use of the gametes of a third party is sperm donation, or artificial insemination by donor (AID). The first documented case of using human donor sperm to instantiate a pregnancy occurred in 1884, when a Quaker woman and her merchant husband, 15 years her senior, were unable to conceive. They approached Dr. William Pancoast of Jefferson Medical College in Philadelphia. Extensive examination of the woman revealed no abnormality. Finally, the husband was examined and found to be azoospermic, that is, having no measurable levels of sperm, apparently due to a bout of gonorrhea in his youth. Dr. Pancoast presented the case to his medical students. Semen was collected from the best-looking member of the class and used to inseminate the wife. Without informing either the husband or the wife of the plan, Dr. Pancoast called the wife back to his office under the pretext of doing another examination. She was anesthetized, using chloroform, and artificially inseminated. It was not until it was determined that she had conceived that her husband was told what had been done. At his request, his wife was never informed. She gave birth to a son, the first known child born by donor insemination.[145]

---

143. I discuss these issues in "Payment for Gamete Donation and Surrogacy," *Mount Sinai Journal of Medicine* 71 (4), September 2004: 255–265. Some of the material in this section comes from this article.

144. Thomas Murray. 1996. "New Reproductive Technologies and the Family," in Cynthia Cohen, ed., *New Ways of Making Babies: The Case of Egg Donation*. Bloomington, IN: Indiana University Press, pp. 51–69, p. 64.

145. A. T. Gregoire and Robert C. Mayer. 1965. "The Impregnators," *Fertility and Sterility* 16: 130–134; and Rebecca Taylor. 2005. "Reproductive Technology: From Artificial Insemination to Cloning," lifeissues.net, November 2, 2005. http://www.lifeissues.net/writers/tayl/tayl_02reprotechnology.html. Accessed August 6, 2010.

All of the elements that make this first case of AID shocking—the fact that it was an experimental procedure performed on a woman without her knowledge, much less informed consent, and that it was unquestionably accepted that the husband should have the prerogative to withhold the truth from his wife—are no longer present in sperm donation. Currently, sperm donation is legal in every state in the United States. Both husband and wife must give informed consent to AID, and in most states, the husband of the sperm recipient is the legal father of the resulting child if he consents in advance to the sperm donation. Donor sperm are not allowed by law to be used for IVF in Austria, Germany, Italy, Tunisia, or Turkey.[146] In a few countries (for example, Austria and Norway), sperm donation is permitted in artificial insemination, but not in ART. "No explanation for this prohibition is provided."[147]

Many religious traditions oppose gamete donation even when there is no payment involved. Islam prohibits sperm donation for the same reason it prohibits adoption: confusion about genetic lineage. In addition, it considers AID to be adultery.[148] According to one source, Judaism prohibits sperm donation, especially when the sperm donor is Jewish, although the use of sperm from a non-Jewish donor is sometimes permitted by rabbinical authorities.[149] According to another source, rabbinical authorities disagree, Jewish attitudes toward sperm donation are changing, and it is permissible to use a Jewish sperm donor. In fact, it could be preferable, since using a Jewish donor avoids Halachically forbidden sexual unions.[150] The Roman Catholic Church opposes gamete donation because of its views on the unity of sexual intercourse and procreation. Sexual intercourse without openness to procreation is wrong, the Church claims (hence its opposition to birth control), but equally so is procreation without sexual intercourse (hence its opposition to most forms of assisted reproduction). Even the "simple case" of IVF, where the husband and wife provide the gametes and the resulting embryos are implanted in the wife's uterus, is impermissible, according to Catholic teaching. The wrong is compounded in gamete donation, because the introduction of "a third party" violates the unity of marriage.

A different objection to gamete, specifically sperm, donation comes from Daniel Callahan, who argues that it is intrinsically wrong for someone to become a biological parent, to assist in bringing genetically related offspring into the world, without intending to play a parental role. Callahan likens sperm donation to impregnating and abandoning a woman. In both cases, the impact on the child is the same: an

146. IFFS Surveillance. 2007. *Fertility and Sterility* 87 (4), Suppl. 1, April, p. S28.

147. D. Meirow and J. D. Schenker. 1997. "The Current Status of Sperm Donation in Assisted Reproduction Technology: Ethical and Legal Considerations," *Journal of Assisted Reproduction and Genetics* 14 (2): 133–138, p. 135. See also Claudia Lampic, Agneta Skoog Svanberg, and Gunilla Sydsjö. 2009. "Attitudes Towards Gamete Donation Among IVF Doctors in the Nordic Countries—Are They in Line With National Legislation?" *Journal of Assisted Reproduction and Genetics* 26 (5): 231–238.

148. Meirow and Schenker, "The Current Status of Sperm Donation" (see note 147), p. 134.

149. Ibid.

150. Jewish Sperm Bank, "Biblical Perspective," jewishspermdonor.net: http://www.jewishspermdonor.net/biblical_prospective.html. Accessed August 13, 2010.

unknown, absent father.[151] In response, it is often pointed out that children born from sperm donation usually do have fathers: the infertile men who rear them. To say that they lack fathers seems to denigrate fatherhood from a parental role to mere genetic transmission. There is evidence that children in single-parent households are at a disadvantage (since it is usually more stressful to raise a child on one's own, and often there is less money), but, according to some studies, growing up in a lesbian family does not appear to have a negative impact on quality of parenting or children's psychological development.[152] Many lesbian mothers attempt to mitigate the disadvantages of not having a father by making sure that there are other men in their child's life.

A study coauthored by Elizabeth Marquardt, and published by the conservative Institute for American Values (IAV), of which she is the director, has a different take on the effect of sperm donation on offspring:

> We learned that, on average, young adults conceived through sperm donation are hurting more, are more confused, and feel more isolated from their families. They fare worse than their peers raised by biological parents on important outcomes such as depression, delinquency, and substance abuse. Nearly two-thirds agree, "My sperm donor is half of who I am." Nearly half are disturbed that money was involved in their conception. More than half of them say that when they see someone who resembles them, they wonder if they are related. Almost as many say that they have feared being attracted to or having sexual relations with someone to whom they are unknowingly related. Approximately two-thirds affirm the right of donor offspring to know the truth about their origins. And about half of donor offspring have concerns about or serious objections to donor conception itself, even when parents tell their children the truth.[153]

This study has been criticized by other researchers in the field. One response criticized the methodology, in particular, getting data from an online survey using Survey Sampling International's SurveySpot Web panel. "The authors claim that their sample is 'representative' or 'very nearly representative,' although a more accurate claim would be that it is representative of the 'million plus American households that had signed up to receive web surveys on, well, anything' and who are offered cash

151. Daniel Callahan. 1992. "Bioethics and Fatherhood," *Utah Law Review* 3: 735–746.

152. Susan Golombok, Fiona Tasker, and Clare Murray. 1997. "Children Raised in Fatherless Families From Infancy: Family Relationships and the Socioemotional Development of Children of Lesbian and Single Heterosexual Mothers," *Journal of Child Psychology and Psychiatry* 38 (7): 783–791. A follow-up study of adolescents raised in fatherless families published in 2004 found that there were no serious negative consequences for children with regard to the quality of parenting they experience or their own social and emotional development. See Fiona MacCallum and Susan Golombok. 2004. "Children Raised in Fatherless Families From Infancy: A Follow-up of Children of Lesbian and Single Heterosexual Mothers at Early Adolescence," *Journal of Child Psychology and Psychiatry* 45 (8): 1407–1419.

153. Elizabeth Marquardt, Norval D. Glenn, and Karen Clark. 2010. "My Daddy's Name Is Donor: A New Study of Young Adults Conceived Through Sperm Donation," Institute for American Values. http://familyscholars.org/my-daddys-name-is-donor-2/. Accessed November 4, 2010.

and other rewards for their participation, rather than of the US population as a whole."[154] The authors also criticize the Marquardt study for failing to acknowledge any previous research studies in the field, and they say that "dissemination through the IAV website, rather than through an academically credentialed institution, also suggests a lack of competent peer review at any stage."[155]

However, even if this study has scientific merit (something I am unqualified to judge), it should be noted that the study itself indicates that what most donor offspring—approximately two-thirds—want is information about their biological fathers. This desire can be fulfilled without banning sperm donation, and a growing number of countries, including Germany, the Netherlands, New Zealand, the United Kingdom, and Canada, have prohibited anonymous gamete donation.[156] Some apparently do have serious objections to donor conception itself, but one wonders whether they fully realize the implications of their objections. They may wish that they had not been conceived with donor sperm, just as children born to postmenopausal mothers may wish that their mothers had been younger when they were conceived. But this is not a wish that could have been fulfilled while preserving their identity. Their very existence depends on the practice of sperm donation. Confronted with that stark reality, how many of them could honestly say that they wish that sperm donation had been banned?

In the last 30 years, the freezing and banking of sperm has become a business. There are over a dozen sperm banks in the United States[157] and an estimated 30,000 to 60,000 children are born through AID in the United States alone.[158] In the United States, sperm banks have been regulated by the FDA since 2005, and state agencies often impose licensing requirements as well. These regulations ensure that the sperm is free of transmissible diseases, whether genetic or infectious.

The amount sperm donors get paid varies by location. The Sperm Bank of California's Web site promises $100 "for every ejaculate that meets our minimum sperm count,"[159] although another Web site gives a much lower estimate, typically $35 to $50.[160] This amount is trivial compared with the amount that egg donors receive, partly, no doubt, because the process of retrieving eggs is time consuming, physically burdensome, and not without risk, none of which is true of sperm retrieval, which is done through masturbation. Precisely because egg donors can command much greater sums than sperm donors, the issue of commodification is more salient in egg donation.

154. Eric Blyth and Wendy Kramer. 2010. "'My Daddy's Name Is Donor': Read With Caution," *BioNews*, July 9, 2010. http://www.bionews.org.uk/page_65970.asp. Accessed November 4, 2010.

155. Ibid.

156. Michelle Dennison. 2008. "Revealing Your Sources: The Case for Non-Anonymous Gamete Donation," *Journal of Law and Health* 21: 1–27, p. 9.

157. Sperm Banks, Infertility Resources for Consumers, http://www.ihr.com/infertility/provider/spermbank.html. Accessed August 6, 2010.

158. Marquardt et al., "My Daddy's Name Is Donor" (see note 153).

159. http://www.thespermbankofca.org/pages/page.php?pageid=11. Accessed August 6, 2010.

160. http://www.spermbankdirectory.com/donating-sperm.htm. Accessed August 6, 2010.

Egg Donation

There are several medical conditions that lead women to seek egg donation. They may lack functioning ovaries. Or they may have eggs that are unlikely to fertilize or implant, perhaps because of the age of the women. Some women cannot undergo egg retrieval, usually because scarring due to endometriosis prevents access to their eggs. Finally, egg donation can be used to avoid the transmission of genetic diseases.

The first pregnancy using egg donation was reported in Australia in 1983.[161] When egg donation was first introduced, the eggs came from either close friends or relatives, in a practice known as "known donation," or they came from women who were undergoing IVF themselves. Because the number of eggs retrieved exceeded the number of embryos that could be safely implanted, women undergoing IVF often had extra eggs, which they were often willing to make available for donation. This source greatly diminished when it became possible to freeze embryos (egg freezing is still experimental). Another source of eggs was from patients undergoing tubal ligation. However, the demand for donors soon outstripped these sources and programs began to recruit women from the public at large through advertising. Thus, commercial egg donation came into being.

The main reason for the increasing demand for egg donors is that, for some women, using an egg donor significantly improves their chances of becoming pregnant. As we saw earlier, even postmenopausal women can become pregnant using donor eggs. However, the number of women who want to become pregnant at this stage of life is relatively low. Many more women in their late 30s and early 40s who have delayed childbearing, perhaps in order to pursue careers or perhaps because they have not found partners, want to become mothers. Fertility begins to decline in most women in their late 20s, and it declines at a much more rapid pace at around age 35. As women age, their bodies become less effective at producing mature, healthy eggs, which reduces the chances of becoming pregnant. According to one Web site: "For example, in any given month, your chances of getting pregnant at age 30 are about 20%. At age 40, your chance of getting pregnant in any given month is just 5%."[162] Egg donation is a solution if the infertility results from a problem with egg quality. A 43-year-old woman who uses her own eggs in IVF has a less than 10% chance of giving birth. By contrast, the success rate of women who used an egg donor at age 40 is about 45%. "That's an even better rate than women using their own eggs in their early 30s."[163]

The process of egg donation is very time consuming, often requiring several visits just to be accepted into a program. The prospective donor must undergo physical and gynecological examinations, blood and urine tests, and a psychological examination, and she must participate in discussions of the responsibilities involved in becoming a donor. Because the freezing of eggs is still considered experimental, the

161. New York State Task Force on Life and the Law. 1998. "Assisted Reproductive Technologies: Analysis and Recommendations for Public Policy." New York: The New York State Task Force on Life and the Law, p. 237.

162. Rachel Gurevich, "Getting Pregnant After 35," About.com. http://infertility.about.com/od/causesofinfertility/a/pregnantafter35.htm. Accessed August 13, 2010.

163. Ibid.

"banking" of eggs is not an option. Therefore, the actual donation cycle will not occur until the prospective donor is accepted, is matched with a recipient, and has given her consent.

Most clinics put fairly restrictive limits on acceptable donors. The application provided by one egg donor center specifies that donors must be between 19 and 29 years of age. They must not be adopted (unless the medical records of both birth parents are available). They must not be smokers or recreational drug users. They must be in good health, and not be more than 30 pounds over their ideal weight or have a body mass index of 27 or higher. They must have SAT scores of at least 1100, and if SAT scores are not available, they must provide an official college transcript showing that they had at least a 3.0 (out of 4.0) grade point average. They must have their own transportation to appointments and be available for early morning doctor appointments for about 2 weeks. They must be willing to avoid alcohol and caffeine during the donation process. They must be willing to abstain from sexual intercourse for approximately 2–3 weeks during treatment. They must be willing to abstain from exercise for 2–4 weeks, perhaps up to 8 weeks, depending on their physicians' instructions.[164]

The following is typical of the medical process undergone by donors. First, the physician will prescribe birth control pills for several weeks to temporarily stop the ovaries' normal functioning. This makes it easier to control the donor's response to fertility drugs which will be used later in the cycle. She will be given an injection by the physician or instructed in how to inject the medication daily at home. The medications may cause hot flashes, vaginal dryness, fatigue, sleep problems, body aches, mood swings, breast tenderness, headache, and visual disturbances. Next, medications must be injected over a period of about 10 days to stimulate her ovaries to mature a number of eggs (typically 25–30) for retrieval. Frequent early morning transvaginal ultrasound examinations and blood tests (about every 2–3 days) are needed to monitor the donor's response to the drugs and to adjust the dose as needed. While using injectable fertility drugs, the donor may experience mood swings, breast tenderness, enlarged ovaries, and bloating. Occasionally, these medications result in ovarian hyperstimulation syndrome (OHSS), in which the ovaries swell and fluid builds up in the abdominal cavity. If the hyperstimulation is mild, it will recede after the donor's next menstrual period. If the hyperstimulation is moderate, careful monitoring, bed rest, and pain medication may be necessary. Severe hyperstimulation is infrequent, but it may cause serious medical complications, such as blood clots, kidney failure, fluid accumulation in the lungs, and shock. This condition can be life threatening. It may result in one or both of the donor's ovaries having to be removed. "Despite careful monitoring, up to 33% of IVF treatment have [sic] been reported to be associated with mild forms of OHSS. Severe OHSS has been reported in 3–8% of IVF cycles."[165]

The mature eggs are removed from the ovaries in a minor surgical procedure called "transvaginal ovarian aspiration." It is usually done in the physician's office.

164. The Egg Donation Center of Dallas, Inc. http://www.eggdonorcenter.com/donorapp.pdf. Accessed November 5, 2010.

165. "Risks and Complications of IVF Treatment." 2010. February 14. http://www.ivf-infertility.com/ivf/standard/complications/index.php. Accessed November 4, 2010.

First, the donor will be given painkillers or put under intravenous sedation. Then, the physician inserts a needle through the vagina to aspirate the eggs out of the follicles. According to one description, "The procedure takes 15 to 60 minutes and, except for grogginess and some mild pelvic discomfort, there should be no aftereffects."[166] Some may experience more than mild pelvic discomfort: one egg donor described it (on a Web site for donors) as "feeling like somebody punched you in the stomach." Many donors find the actual retrieval less unpleasant than the side effects from the drugs.

Just as some object to sperm donation, even if the donors are not paid, so too some object to egg donation, even the noncommercial, altruistic variety. In Austria, Germany, Italy, Norway, and Switzerland, the use of donor eggs is illegal.[167] The moral objection to egg donation, according to the Rev. Albert Moraczewski, is based on human dignity, namely, that egg donation is demeaning to women. "A donor woman is not really being treated as a person," he said. "Whether she is paid or acts out of kindness, her egg is being used, so she is not fully treated as a person whose reproductive capacity should be expressed as a result of the love of her husband."[168]

But why is egg donation demeaning? Presumably blood donation is not demeaning; it does not fail to treat the donor as a person. What is the difference? The answer, according to the Vatican, is that egg donation involves a wrongful use of reproductive capacity. However, that simply begs the question. The characterization of egg donation as demeaning does not give a reason why it is wrong (and different from other kinds of bodily donations); rather, egg donation is regarded as demeaning *because* it is considered wrong: a wrongful use of reproductive capacity. Within the context of Catholic teaching, gamete donation is wrong because the only legitimate use of reproductive capacity is a sexual act, open to procreation, between a man and a woman who are married to each other. There is nothing inconsistent or incoherent in this view, but a different view of permissible sexual activity held by many people (including many Catholics) allows for contraception and assisted reproduction. The question is whether there is a "human dignity" argument against egg donation that should be persuasive to people with a more liberal attitude toward sex and reproduction.

While most donors are motivated by altruistic considerations as well as financial ones, very few women would consent to donate eggs to strangers without compensation, because of the arduous nature of the procedure. Many say that egg donation would be impossible if they were not compensated for lost work time, transportation, daycare costs, and the like. However, most donors think that reimbursement for pecuniary expenses alone is not enough. They think that it is only fair that they should receive reasonable compensation for what they go through in order to provide eggs: the inconvenience, burden, and medical risk they have endured.

166. Diane Aronson and Suzanne Levert. 1999. *Resolving Infertility: Understanding the Options and Choosing Solutions When You Want to Have a Baby.* New York: Harper Resource.

167. Joseph G. Schenker. 1977. "Assisted Reproduction Practice in Europe: Legal and Ethical Aspects," *Human Reproduction Update* 3 (2): 173–184, p. 178. See also Liana Müller. "Sperm and Egg Donation." http://www.iet.ntnu.no/~ralf/muller/pubs/eggdonasjon.pdf. Accessed November 5, 2010.

168. Nadine Brozan. 1988. "Babies From Donated Eggs: Growing Use Stirs Questions," *New York Times*, January 18; Sect. A:1.

Opposed to the fairness argument is the commodification objection, which says that to pay donors is to commodify reproduction (or women or eggs or children—these are all variations of the commodification argument). To assess this objection, we need to say what commodification is, and what is wrong with it. Essentially, to commodify something is to give it a market price. That in itself is not a bad thing. We could not buy our groceries or clothes or the morning paper if they did not have a market price. Thus, the commodification argument against egg donation should be interpreted as saying that some things, such as eggs, should not be commodified. However, the question then becomes, why should these things not be given a market price? The rationale is not always forthcoming, and indeed it is sometimes simply assumed. As the guest editors of a special issue on commodification in the *Kennedy Institute of Ethics Journal* put it, "Unfortunately, a great deal of the talk about 'commodification' has been clumsy and sloppy. The term has been used as a magic bullet, as if saying, 'But that's commodification!' is the same as having made an argument."[169]

Debra Satz[170] maintains that the commodification argument rests on the "asymmetry thesis." The asymmetry thesis maintains that markets in women's labor, including egg donation and contract pregnancy, are morally more problematic than other currently accepted labor markets. "Advocates of the asymmetry thesis hold that treating reproductive labor as a commodity, as something subject to the supply-and-demand principles that govern economic markets, is worse than treating other types of human labor as commodities."[171]

The asymmetry thesis is reflected in the law of a number of countries. For example, in Canada it is illegal "to purchase, offer to purchase or advertise for the purchase of sperm, ova, human cells or genes from a donor or a person acting on behalf of a donor."[172] The rationale for the prohibition is ". . . to prevent people from using their gametes as a form of currency."[173] Why should this be prevented? The intuitive idea, at least in part, is that reproductive labor and its products are essentially the sorts of things that should not be bought or sold. Satz calls this "the essentialist thesis" and notes that the thesis itself stands in need of justification. Carole Pateman attempts to justify the essentialist thesis by arguing that reproductive labor is more integrally tied to a woman's identity than her other productive capacities, and therefore to treat it as an alienable commodity is to strike at her own identity.[174] A similar point is made by Suzanne Holland:

For many of us, our sense of the dignity of humanity is fundamentally disturbed by the suggestion that that which bears the marks of personhood can somehow

169. Dena Davis and Suzanne Holland. 2001. "Introduction," *Kennedy Institute of Ethics Journal* 11 (3): 219.

170. Debra Satz. 1992. "Markets in Women's Reproductive Labor," *Philosophy and Public Affairs* 21 (2): 107–131.

171. Ibid., pp. 107–108.

172. Assisted Human Reproduction Act. 2004. http://laws.justice.gc.ca/en/A-13.4/. Accessed August 9, 2010.

173. Health Canada. 2001. http://www.hc-sc.gc.ca/hl-vs/pubs/reprod/overview-apercu/overview-eng.php. Accessed August 29, 2010.

174. Carole Pateman. 1988. *The Sexual Contract*. Stanford, CA: Stanford University Press, p. 207.

be equated with property. We do not wish to have certain aspects of that which we associate with our personhood sold off on the market for whatever the market will bear.[175]

Although Holland formulates the objection in terms of personhood, it seems clear that in this context personhood, identity, and a sense of self are equivalent. Here is Satz's response:

How do we decide which of a woman's attributes or capacities are essential to her identity and which are not? In particular, why should we consider sexuality more integral to self than friendship, family, religion, nationality, and work? Yet we allow commodification in each of these spheres. For example, rabbis or priests may view their religion as central to their identity, but they often accept payment for performing religious services, and hardly anyone objects to their doing so. Does Pateman think that all activities that fall within these spheres and that bear an intimate relationship to a person's identity should be inalienable?[176]

The challenge, then, is to distinguish legitimate activities in which the human body or its abilities are used, from those thought to be illegitimate. As Ruth Macklin has put it, "Every service in our economy is sold: academics sell their minds; athletes sell their bodies . . . If a pretty actress can sell her appearance and skill for television, why should a fecund woman be denied the ability to sell her eggs? Why is one more demeaning than the other?"[177] The Warnock Report stated that it was "inconsistent with human dignity" for a woman to use her uterus for financial profit.[178] John Harris responded by asking, "Why is human dignity seen as attaching to this part of the body, rather than the body as a whole . . . If no general principle about the sale or use of the human body in whole or in part emerges we are entitled to ask why in this special case human dignity is said to be violated."[179]

Holland gives another reason why eggs should not be seen as property. It is that the human body is "inalienable." But what does this mean? To call rights "inalienable" is to say that they cannot be taken away from us. If calling the human body and its parts "inalienable" means that others cannot use my body or body parts without my permission, that is undeniable. But why does this imply that I may not sell my gametes? If "inalienable" just means "may not be treated like property," then Holland has not given a reason why eggs are not property, but rather a tautology.

175. Suzanne Holland. 2001. "Contested Commodities at Both Ends of Life: Buying and Selling Gametes, Embryos, and Body Tissues," *Kennedy Institute of Ethics Journal* 11 (3): 263–284.

176. Satz, "Markets in Women's Reproductive Labor" (see note 170), p. 114.

177. Ruth Macklin. 1996. "What Is Wrong With Commodification?" in Cynthia Cohen, ed., *New Ways of Making Babies* (see note 144), pp. 106–121, pp. 112–113.

178. Mary Warnock. 1985. *A Question of Life: The Warnock Report on Human Fertilization and Embryology.* Oxford: Basil Blackwell, p. 45.

179. John Harris. 1985. *The Value of Life.* London: Routledge & Kegan Paul, p. 144.

The fact that something is a human body part does not make it obviously wrong to sell it. In the novel *Little Women*, Jo sells her hair to raise money to send to her father, who is serving as a chaplain in the Union Army. Surely that was not morally wrong of Jo, nor demeaning to her. Indeed, her willingness to part with "her one beauty" is an unselfish and noble gesture. If selling one's hair is morally permissible, but selling one's gametes is not, what is the moral difference?

It might be thought that I am missing an obvious point. Selling one's hair is not wrong because hair is unrelated to sex and reproduction. Selling one's eggs is akin to selling one's body in prostitution, and "we all know" that prostitution is wrong. Actually, prostitutes do not literally sell their bodies. It is more accurate to say that they rent them out, or rather that they perform sexual acts in exchange for money. Most of us believe that this is wrong, but this belief may be due in part to sexual Puritanism. Perhaps the distaste we feel for prostitution stems (at least in part) from the way prostitutes have typically been regarded in patriarchal societies—as women of no value, undeserving of respect. Imagine a world in which those who provided sexual services were treated with as much respect as psychotherapists, trainers, and masseurs are in our society. Something like this seems to be the case in the Netherlands where prostitution has been legal since 1830, and recognized as a legal profession since 1988. The view in the Netherlands is that prostitution is a profession like any other. "Prostitution is good as long as women (or men) who work as prostitutes do it from their own will, and are not exploited. The sex workers should be respected and their rights protected."[180]

Probably most people are unwilling to adopt the attitude that there is nothing wrong with prostitution, or that it is a profession like any other. (I doubt that even Dutch parents are pleased if their daughters decide to take up this profession.) But even if there is something distasteful about prostitution, there is a vast personal difference between these two kinds of selling, and there is no obvious reason why paying egg donors is incompatible with treating them with respect.

Moreover, as Satz points out, even if women's sexuality and reproduction belongs to a sacred, special realm, a realm worthy of respect, it does not follow that reproductive labor cannot be treated as a commodity.

> We sometimes sell things that we also respect. As Margaret Radin puts it, "we can both know the price of something and know that it is priceless." For example, I think that my teaching talents should be respected, but I don't object to being paid for teaching on such grounds. Giving my teaching a price does not diminish the other ways in which my teaching has value.[181]

Satz argues that there is no distinction between women's reproductive labor and human labor in general, and moreover, that the sale of women's labor is not ipso facto degrading. Her objection to contract pregnancy in particular, and her defense of the asymmetry thesis in general, stems from a concern with gender inequality. Satz writes:

> The asymmetry thesis should be defended on external and not intrinsic or essentialist grounds. The conditions of pervasive gender inequality in our society

180. "Prostitution in Amsterdam," http://www.amsterdam.info/prostitution/. Accessed August 13, 2010.

181. Satz, "Markets in Women's Reproductive Labor" (see note 170), p. 115.

are primary to the explanation of what is wrong with contract pregnancy. I claim that the most compelling objection to contract pregnancy concerns the background conditions of gender inequality that characterize our society.[182]

Since Satz focuses exclusively on contract pregnancy, it is not clear whether she thinks that background conditions of gender inequality provide an argument against commercial egg donation. Indeed, at first glance, the argument seems to go the other way. Justice would seem to require that the women who go through the rigors of egg retrieval be fairly compensated. Why are only egg donors expected to act altruistically, when everyone else involved in egg donation—the doctors, the lawyers, the nurses, the receptionist—receives payment? In light of the sacrifices of time, risk, and burden that egg donors make, it seems only fair that they receive enough money to make the sacrifice worthwhile. To refuse them compensation, or to offer too little, is a form of exploitation.

At the same time, it could be argued that offering women "too much" money may be an attempt to manipulate them into becoming donors. The lure of financial gain may lead them to discount the risks to themselves and to make decisions they will later regret. To take advantage of this is also a form of exploitation. (It is not, I might add, the worst sort of exploitation. Misleading donors about the burdens they might experience, or the financial obligations of the clinic to them, if there are complications, is a much worse exploitation, and unfortunately, all too common.) It might be argued that we should not attempt to protect adults from irrational assessments or choices they will later regret, because this is paternalistic. However, paternalism involves preventing people from doing what they want on the grounds that this is in their best interest. It is not paternalistic to prevent individuals or corporations from taking advantage of other people's susceptibility to temptation.

If there is a risk of exploiting women with offering them either too much money or too little, what is reasonable compensation? When the ASRM Ethics Committee tackled this question, it started from compensation for sperm donation and noted that considerably more time, burden, and risk is imposed by egg donation, justifying considerably more payment. At the same time, the Committee was mindful of the dangers of dangling substantial amounts of money before the eyes of potential donors, leading them to discount the risks to themselves. Balancing these factors, the ASRM guidelines state that amounts above $5,000 need to be justified, and sums above $10,000 go beyond what is appropriate.[183] By and large, most programs seem to fall within these parameters. A survey done by SART found that "the national average for oocyte donor compensation was approximately $4,200 but found notable geographic variations, with the highest average compensation levels occurring in the East/ Northeast ($5,018) and West ($4,820)."[184] However, a study of advertisements for egg

---

182. Ibid., pp. 109–110.

183. Ethics Committee of ASRM. 2007. "Financial Compensation of Oocyte Donors," *Fertility and Sterility* 88 (2): 305–309.

184. Aaron D. Levine. 2010. "Self-Regulation, Compensation, and the Ethical Recruitment of Oocyte Donors," *Hastings Center Report* 40 (2): 25–36, p. 29. Citing S. N. Covington and W. E. Gibbons. 2007. "What Is Happening to the Price of Eggs?" *Fertility and Sterility* 87 (5): 1001–1004.

donors in newspapers found deviation from the ASRM guidelines, with much higher prices being offered to "special donors" with high SAT scores, musical talent or athletic ability, from particular ethnic backgrounds, or with particular physical characteristics. In March 2000, an ad appeared in *The Daily Californian* (the campus newspaper for the University of California, Berkeley), which read, "Special Egg Donor Needed" and listed the following criteria for a "preferred donor": "height approximately 5'6," Caucasian, S.A.T. score around 1250 or high A.C.T., college student or graduate under 30, no genetic medical issues." The compensation was listed as $80,000 "paid to you and/or the charity of your choice." In addition, all related expenses would be paid. Extra compensation was available for someone especially gifted in athletics, science/mathematics, or music. "Although no comprehensive database of these advertisements exists, ads promising as much as $100,000 have appeared in college newspapers."[185]

A problem with a study based on advertisements for egg donors is that the existence of an advertisement does not mean that the money was actually paid. Some fertility doctors suspect that these ads are a "bait and switch": the coed from Princeton who plays the violin and has high SATs calls the clinic, hoping to qualify for a payment of $50,000, only to be told that the offer no longer exists. She is then encouraged to donate eggs for the usual going rate. Aaron Levine, the author of the study, admits that follow-up studies of egg donors do not reveal high levels of compensation.[186] However, payments of up to $50,000 for a few donors have been substantiated. Levine says that even if such amounts "... represent the fringes of the 'market' for oocyte donation and occur only infrequently, they remain ethically problematic."[187]

Part of the reason Canada prohibits the sale or barter of human gametes is to "ensure that a child could not be born as the result of a commercial transaction."[188] To allow such transactions is thought to commodify children. Again, one might ask why it is only the commercial transaction that benefits gamete donors that is prohibited, and not commercial transactions when the money is paid to doctors, lawyers, and clinic personnel. But even if the commodification argument is unsuccessful in general against compensating gamete donors, it has more plausibility when donors with desirable traits are paid considerably more. When donors are paid on the basis of their particular traits, they are not being compensated for their labor. Rather, prospective parents are choosing donors in the hopes of providing their offspring with certain inheritable traits. This is often characterized as an attempt to design one's children, something that many people find worrisome.

A different method for designing children was advertised in 2009 when Dr. Jeff Steinberg, director of The Fertility Institutes in Los Angeles, California, offered

185. Ibid., citing Debora L. Spar. 2006. *The Baby Business: How Money, Science, and Politics Drive the Commerce of Conception.* Boston: Harvard Business School Press.

186. Ibid., p. 34. Citing Andrea L. Kalfoglou and Joel Gittelsohn. 2000. "A Qualitative Follow-Up Study of Women's Experiences With Oocyte Donation," *Human Reproduction* 15 (4): 798–805; Nancy J. Kenney and Michelle L. McGowan. 2010. "Looking Back: Egg Donors' Retrospective Evaluations of Their Motivations, Expectations, and Experiences During Their First Donation Cycle," *Fertility and Sterility* 93 (2): 455–466.

187. Ibid., p. 34.

188. Health Canada, Proposals for Legislation Governing Assisted Human Reproduction (see note 173).

parents the opportunity, starting in 2010, to select their future offspring's hair, eye, and skin color, by genetically testing embryos. After a public outcry, he posted a statement on the clinic's Web site saying that the service would not be offered because the negative societal implications might outweigh the positive aspect of parental choice. Fertility experts were quick to point out that no one can actually do what Dr. Steinberg promised. "The truth is that we cannot (yet) reliably test embryos for eye color, hair color, skin tones and other 'cosmetic' features," warned a statement from the Center for Human Reproduction, a fertility clinic. "It will still take years before all of this will become technically even feasible."[189] Still, this raises the question, when it does become technically feasible, should it be allowed?

Those who oppose both embryo selection for cosmetic traits, and the payment of large sums of money to egg donors, maintain that such practices foster the wrong kinds of parental attitudes, and that this could be harmful to children. Prospective parents should be anticipating having a child to love, not focusing on the traits their child will have. It is one thing to want to have a healthy child, which is the reason for genetic screening of donors, and quite another to be willing to pay huge sums to get a "superior" child. This seems inconsistent with an ideal of unconditional parental love and acceptance. Parents are supposed to love their children just because they are their children, whatever traits they have or lack. They are not supposed to try to "design" their children.

The aforementioned argument assumes that it is possible to design children, and it is concerned about the effect that this might have on them. However, equally, one might be concerned about the impact on children if individuals believe they can "order up" a superior child, and fail in the attempt, after expending a lot of money. Traits are often not inherited in Mendelian fashion, despite what you may have learned in high school biology. In addition, the interaction of genes and the environment (including the uterine environment) makes it very difficult to know in advance what phenotypic traits an individual will have. This is not to deny that traits like appearance, intelligence, or athletic ability have a genetic component, but only to say that they cannot be guaranteed by the choice of an egg donor (who, after all, only provides half the genes). People who pay large sums of money to select donors in order to get specific traits are likely to be disappointed, and this too could have adverse effects on the parent–child relationship.

On the other hand, it is possible that couples who place the ads understand that they cannot determine their children's traits and that they do not have false expectations. Nevertheless, they might say, they want to give their child an advantage, a better chance at traits likely to help the child in life. It is not that they can only love a tall, brilliant, athletic child, they might say, but rather that they are well aware how advantageous such traits can be. Why, they might ask, if they have the money to spend, should they not use it to give their child the best chance in life? When the money is spent on private schools, SAT tutors, music lessons, and expensive summer camps, few seem to object, especially on the ground that the welfare of the child is being threatened.

189. Center for Human Reproduction. "IVF Expert Questions Validity of 'Designer Babies.'" http://www.centerforhumanreprod.com/pdf/designer_baby_030409.pdf. Accessed November 5, 2010.

A different objection is that allowing prospective parents to give their children a "genetic edge" might widen the gap between haves and have-nots. Those who can afford the eggs of "superior" donors will have a better chance at getting superior children, who will in turn pass on their superior genes, creating over time two classes of people, the genetically well endowed and the genetically impoverished. (This argument is usually mounted against genetic enhancement, but it could be used against the selection of egg donors.) However, that objection depends on there being a significant number of advantaged offspring. Only slightly more than 1% of all children born in the United States in a year are conceived through ART. Of these, slightly more than 11% use donor eggs. Even if all of the women using donor eggs were interested in getting specific nondisease traits (which seems unlikely) and even if it were possible to choose traits (which is currently impossible, and remains very unlikely even into the distant future), the numbers of genetically advantaged offspring would be so small as to have a negligible effect on society.

A related objection to paying large sums to certain egg donors is that differential payment is elitist and violates a principle of equality. There is something offensive in the idea that the eggs of Princeton women are worth $50,000, while the eggs of women at SUNY-Albany are worth only $3,000. (John Arras has made the tongue-in-cheek suggestion that perhaps *US News & World Report* should include how much their coeds can get for their eggs in their rankings of colleges.) This provides an additional reason to distinguish between compensation for time, risk, and inconvenience, on the one hand, and payment for eggs, on the other. If payment is justified as fair compensation for the burdens of egg retrieval—"sweat equity"—then larger payments based on the donor's attributes are unjustified. It is as burdensome for a SUNY-Albany student as it is for a Princeton student to go through the egg retrieval process. Basing payment on "sweat equity" has the advantage of not offending against the moral ideal of equality. Moreover, if payment is compensation for the donor's time, risk, and burden, then donors should be compensated regardless of the number or quality of eggs retrieved, which seems fair, whereas this makes no sense if payment is for the product (eggs).

In Canada, where it is illegal to purchase gametes, gamete donors may be reimbursed "for reasonable expenses," which are determined by regulations currently being developed.[190] A similar approach is taken in the United Kingdom. The maximum amount that can be given to egg donors to cover out-of-pocket expenses is 250£. The HFEA also allows "shared egg donation," in which a woman undergoing infertility treatment at a private clinic is superovulated, and then gives half her eggs to a woman who needs egg donation and who pays for both their treatments. This raises the question why only payment in kind should be permitted and not outright payment to women without fertility problems who would be willing to donate, if compensated.

Limiting compensation to out-of-pocket expenses has dramatically decreased the number of gamete donors in both Canada and the United Kingdom, leading to an increase in "reproductive tourism," where women who need eggs go where it is legal

190. Assisted Human Reproduction Canada, Frequently Asked Questions. http://www.ahrc-pac.gc.ca/faq/index.php?qid=63&lang=eng. Accessed August 29, 2010.

to pay egg donors.[191] This increases inequality, since only women who can pay to travel can afford egg donation. Is there room for compromise between those who prefer an altruistic system of egg donation and those who think that egg donors should be paid? Suzanne Holland suggests we take an approach she calls "incomplete commodification":

> With respect to gamete donors, an incompletely commodified approach could recognize that donors are contributing to something that can be seen as a social and personal good (remedying infertility), even as they deserve a degree of compensation that constitutes neither a financial burden ([if they are paid] too little) nor a [temptation to undergo] health risk ([if paid] too much). I see no reason not to follow the suggestion of [the] ASRM [American Society for Reproductive Medicine] and cap egg donor compensation at $5000. . . . Allowing some compensation, but capping it at $5000, would reduce the competition for eggs and perhaps curb the lure of advertising that is targeted to college students in need of "easy money."[192]

If compensation were completely banned, or limited to out-of-pocket expenses, few women would agree to be egg donors. This would be unfortunate for those women who cannot have babies any other way. This is part of the justification for paying egg donors; the other part has to do with treating donors fairly. At the same time, legitimate concerns about equality, the psychological welfare of offspring, and the potential for exploitation of donors justify limiting the amount of payment and tying it to time, risk, and burden, not the genetic traits of donors.

191. Ian Craft, Alan Thornhill, and Andrew Berkley. 2005. "The Truth About Donor Expenses in the UK," *BioNews* 338. http://www.bionews.org.uk/page_37843.asp. Accessed November 5, 2010.

192. Holland, "Contested Commodities at Both Ends of Life" (see note 175), pp. 280–281.

6

Stem Cell Research

Stem cells are found in all multicellular organisms. They are essential for human growth, development, and maintenance. Adult stem cells are specialized in that they can repair only the kind of tissue they are, whether blood stem cells, skin stem cells, and so forth. (Recently, scientists have been able to derive pluripotent stem cells from adult stem cells, but as they exist in the body, adult stem cells are specialized.) Embryonic stem cells are pluripotent; that is, they have the ability to develop into virtually any kind of cell or tissue in the body. This, combined with the fact that they may be capable of living almost indefinitely in culture, without aging or degrading, gives human embryonic stem cells (hESCs) enormous scientific and medical potential. There are four important uses of hESCs:

1. To support basic research on embryonic development and the differentiation of cells. Embryonic stem cells provide a new model for studying the development of the embryo. An embryo starts as a single undifferentiated cell and develops into an organism that has many different types of cells, including blood, nerve, muscle, and skin cells. Research on hESCs will enable scientists to learn more about this process and the ways in which it can go wrong. This will have implications for understanding infertility and its treatment, pregnancy loss and its prevention, and the etiology of birth defects.

2. Drug testing for safety and efficacy. Millions of animals are subjected to painful treatment and death every year in drug testing. This could be avoided if stem cells replaced animal models. Moreover, nonhuman animals, such as guinea pigs, are not always reliable sources of information about what will be safe and effective in humans. For example, thalidomide, which had proved safe in guinea pigs, produced serious birth defects in humans. Even our closest relatives, other primates, are not always reliable predictors of what will be safe and effective drugs in humans. For example, a drug, TGN1412, developed by TeGenero, a German biotech company, and designed for the treatment of arthritis, leukemia, and multiple sclerosis, revealed no safety issues when it was tested on nonhuman primates.[1] In the first clinical trials in humans, however, six subjects

---

1. TGN1412. 2010. http://en.wikipedia.org/wiki/TGN1412.

(healthy young men) had catastrophic systemic organ failure and were hospitalized for several weeks.[2] Parexal International, the Massachusetts company that ran the trial, was criticized for testing it on healthy volunteers instead of ill patients with no other treatment options, and for giving it to all six subjects within a short period of time. In addition, medical ethicists alleged that the Parexal consent form "didn't sufficiently inform the participants of TGN1412's possible dangers or depict the treatment as a new type of drug that can disrupt the body's immune system."[3] The drug has been withdrawn from development.

3. The development of new drugs, by generating better models for diseases, such as Alzheimer's disease.[4]

4. To replace or restore tissues for transplantation or to treat a wide variety of degenerative diseases. For example, hESCs could replace defective insulin-producing cells in the treatment of diabetes. They could be used to create dopaminergic neurons in the treatment of Parkinson's disease. Heart cells could be created for the treatment of heart attacks, and nerve cells for spinal cord injuries. In other words, with the insertion of working cells, the body could in effect heal itself, regenerating damaged tissues and organs.

At present, these possibilities are still theoretical. Although adult stem cells have been used to treat disease for decades, for example, in bone marrow transplants, there are no current cures or therapies using hESCs, and clinical trials are just beginning.

In January 2009, the Food and Drug Administration (FDA) initially approved a Phase I clinical trial (one whose main aim is to test the safety of the therapy, not its efficacy) by Geron, a biotechnology company, of a treatment using hESCs for severe spinal cord injury. The therapy, known as GRNOPC1, was successful in getting rats with induced spinal injuries to walk again. However, the FDA called off the trial in September 2009 when it was discovered that the treatment caused tumors in some of the rats, even though these cysts were microscopic, seemed benign, and were quite ordinary for spinal injuries.[5] For a year, Geron worked at developing new techniques to minimize the formation of cysts, and in August 2010, the FDA gave Geron the go-ahead for a new Phase I clinical trial.[6] Some have questioned whether the first clinical trials of hESCs should be on people with spinal cord injuries, where the

2. Eva von Schaper. 2006. "TeGenero Drug Too Perilous to Test on Healthy People (Update2)," May 2. http://www.bloomberg.com/apps/news?pid=newsarchive&sid=a.kK3_aFltJ4. Accessed September 28, 2010.

3. Ibid.

4. Lawrence Goldstein. 2010. "Why Scientific Details Are Important When Novel Technologies Encounter Law, Politics, and Ethics," *Journal of Law, Medicine & Ethics* 38 (2): 204–211, p. 208.

5. Aaron Saenz. 2009. "Geron Explains Why First Embryonic Stem Cell Clinical Trial Is Stalled," Singularity Hub. http://singularityhub.com/2009/09/02/geron-explains-why-first-embryonic-stem-cell-clinical-trial-is-stalled/. Accessed September 10, 2010.

6. Aaron Saenz. 2010. "Geron Restarts Embryonic Stem Cell Clinical Trials for Spinal Cord Injury." August 2. Singularity Hub. http://singularityhub.com/2010/08/02/gerons-embryonic-stem-cell-clinical-trials-for-spinal-cord-injury-have-returned/. Accessed September 8, 2010.

outcome prediction for any one patient is uncertain. "They sometimes spontaneously get better, and/or physical therapy can work well as do steroids and anti-inflammatory therapy."[7] Professor Lawrence Goldstein, director of the Stem Cell Research Program at the University of San Diego School of Medicine, says that he personally would be more comfortable if the early phase trials of cells derived from hESCs were for disorders where the prognosis is known with a great deal of certainty, allowing for a clearer assessment of the risk/benefit ratio.[8]

Another problem with the Geron trial concerns the meaningfulness of informed consent from subjects who have very recently experienced a catastrophic injury (within the past 1–2 weeks) because of the phenomenon known as "hedonic adaptation," the process that reduces the emotional negative effects of a disruptive event. For example, healthy people tend to think that becoming disabled will have a very negative effect on their happiness or well-being. However, most empirical studies suggest that people tend to adjust fairly well to disability, and much better than they would have predicted prior to becoming disabled.[9] This has implications for the ability to give informed consent in the immediate aftermath of a catastrophic injury. Even assuming a clear prognosis, the ability to weigh the risks and potential benefits of participation in the study may be skewed by the tendency to overestimate the long-term burdens of injury and disability.[10]

In November 2010, the FDA gave approval to Advanced Cell Technologies to inject cells created from human embryonic stem cells into the eyes of 12 patients suffering from advanced cases of Stargardt's macular dystrophy, one of the most common forms of juvenile macular blindness.[11] The disease progressively destroys vision, beginning in childhood, and is presently incurable. Although the study is a Phase 1 trial, intended primarily to test safety, investigators will be looking for signs of improvement in the patients' vision. Presumably this trial does not raise the same concerns about prognosis and informed consent present in the Geron trial.

In some places, researchers have jumped the gun and used stem cells in a clinically inappropriate way. For example, an Israeli boy with a rare, fatal genetic disease, ataxia telangiectasia, or A-T, was given highly experimental injections of fetal stem cells that triggered tumors in the boy's brain and spinal cord.[12] The boy's family had taken him to Russia, where he received injections of neural stem cells into his brain and

7. Lawrence Goldstein. 2010. "Why Scientific Details Are Important" (see note 4), p. 210.

8. Ibid.

9. For a good review of the empirical literature on hedonic adaptation, see Peter A. Ubel and George Loewenstein. 2008. "Pain and Suffering Awards: They Shouldn't Be (Just) About Pain and Suffering," *Journal of Legal Studies* 37 (2): S195–S216.

10. I thank Michelle N. Meyer for pointing out this additional difficulty with the Geron study to me.

11. Rob Stein. 2010. "New Embryonic Stem Cell Experiment," *The Washington Post.* http://voices.washingtonpost.com/checkup/2010/11/new_embryonic_stem_cell_experi.html. Accessed December 7, 2010.

12. Ninette Amariglio, Abraham Hirshberg, Bernd W. Scheithauer, Yoram Cohen, Ron Loewenthal, Luba Trakhtenbrot, Nurit Paz, Maya Koren-Michowitz, Dalia Waldman, Leonor Leider-Trejo, Amos Toren, Shlomi Constantini, and Gideon Rechavi. 2009. "Donor-Derived Brain Tumor Following Neural Stem Cell Transplantation in an Ataxia Telangiectasia Patient,"

spinal cord over several years. When he returned to Israel, he began to have head-aches. A magnetic resonance image (MRI) revealed benign tumors pushing on his brain stem and spinal cord. The tumors were removed in 2006, and his condition has remained stable ever since.[13] The material removed from his spine contained both neurons and glial cells, and both male and female cells. Human leukocyte antigen (HLA) typing revealed that the tumor contained cells from at least two donors. These findings enabled his doctors to determine that the growth in the boy's spinal cord was donor cell derived; that is, it was the result of the stem cell injections.[14] A stem cell specialist, Dr. Marius Wernig of Stanford University, commented that the boy's disease was not conducive to stem cell treatment. "Stem cell transplantations have a humongous potential," Wernig said. But "if people rush out there without really knowing what they're doing . . . that really backfires and can bring this whole field to a halt."[15] Goldstein says, "This tale is clearly cautionary about the dangers of seeking 'cures or treatment' of unknown and unproven safety and value at clinics and hospitals located in countries with lax or absent regulation."[16]

Embryonic stem cell research raises a host of ethical, legal, and policy questions. While some believe that "it has the potential to revolutionize the practice of medicine and improve the quality and length of life,"[17] others question whether research often aimed at understanding and treating chronic diseases of aging should be given a high priority in research funding decisions, as opposed to public health and prevention measures.[18] Another objection is that the research's promise has been exaggerated or hyped, similar to the hyping of gene therapy, which was also touted as having the potential to revolutionize medicine but failed to deliver. Other questions focus on safety and the protection of human subjects. When there are successes with animal models, when is it safe to begin human clinical trials, and on which patients? All of these questions, while important, are not unique to hESC research. What makes this research especially morally controversial is the fact that the derivation of embryonic stem cells destroys the embryo. Whether the research is morally permissible, then, turns on the question of the moral standing of the human embryo. This is not the only ethical issue that needs to be addressed. Other ethical issues include the morality of somatic cell nuclear transfer (cloning), the question of payment to egg donors, the discarded/created distinction, and the creation of human/animal chimeras. But it is the moral status of the human embryo that is most fundamental

Public Library of Science (PLoS) MEDICINE. February 17. http://www.plosmedicine.org/article/info:doi/10.1371/journal.pmed.1000029. Accessed September 17, 2010.

13. Associated Press. 2009. "Fetal Stem Cells Trigger Tumors in Ill Boy," February 17. http://www.msnbc.msn.com/id/29243132/. Accessed September 10, 2010.

14. Ameriglio et al., "Donor-Derived Brain Tumor" (see note 12).

15. Associated Press, "Fetal Stem Cells Trigger Tumors in Ill Boy" (see note 13).

16. Goldstein, "Why Scientific Details Are Important" (see note 4), p. 210.

17. Harold Varmus. 1998. NIH Director's Statement on Research Using Stem Cells, Stem Cell Information. http://stemcells.nih.gov/policy/statements/120298.asp. Accessed September 11, 2010.

18. Rebecca Dresser. 2010. "Stem Cell Research as Innovation: Expanding the Ethical and Policy Conversation," Journal of Law, Medicine & Ethics 38 (2): 332–341, p. 335.

to the embryonic stem cell controversy. Before we can explore the ethical issues, however, it is important to have a handle on the science of deriving hESCs.

THE SCIENCE

Embryonic stem cells are derived from the inner cell mass of very early extracorporeal embryos, technically called blastocysts. They are typically 4–5 days old and at the stage when they are hollow microscopic balls of cells.[19] There are different sources for blastocysts. They could be created specifically for research purposes, either by vitro fertilization (IVF) or by somatic cell nuclear transfer (cloning), discussed later in this chapter. A more likely source of blastocysts is donation from couples who have created IVF embryos to have a child and no longer need or want the embryos for reproductive purposes. These are often referred to as "leftover," "discarded," "spare," or "surplus" embryos, as opposed to "created" embryos, a term used to describe embryos specifically created for research purposes. The embryos can be frozen, so that if the woman does not become pregnant the first time around, there are embryos available for another cycle of treatment. Having spare embryos available means that the woman will not have to go through the discomfort, risk, and cost of repeated rounds of superovulatory drugs. However, many more embryos are created than will actually be used for reproductive purposes, resulting in hundreds of thousands of embryos in storage around the world which, with the couple's consent, could be used for research purposes. Even clinically useless (based on poor morphology) IVF embryos that have reached the blastocyst stage, and would ordinarily be discarded, can yield normal and robust hESCs.[20]

Another possible source of stem cells is parthenogenesis, in which an egg is stimulated to become an embryo without being fertilized or being injected with genetic material from a donor somatic cell. Parthenogenetic stem cells (pESCs) or parthenotes, as they are sometimes called, share with conventional hESCs the ability to differentiate into virtually all tissue types. The advantage of parthenogenesis over IVF is that stem cells can be derived without destroying an embryo. There is no embryo to destroy, because the stem cells come from an unfertilized egg. However, just like the creation of IVF embryos, parthenogenesis requires a supply of human oocytes, which is troubling to some feminists, who worry about the exploitation of women who are asked to donate their oocytes, as well as to those who are concerned about the commodification of reproductive material (see Chapter 5).

In October 2001, scientists at Advanced Cell Technology in Massachusetts attempted parthenogenesis, after attempts to clone human embryos were unsuccessful because growth stopped at six cells. They managed to get six blastocysts by parthenogenesis,

19. National Institutes of Health. 2008. "Stem Cell Information." http://stemcells.nih.gov/info/basics/basics4.asp. Accessed September 8, 2010.

20. Bio-Medicine Online. (2008). "Embryos Discarded During IVF Create Stem Cell Line." http://www.bio-medicine.org/medicine-news-1/Embryos-Discarded-During-IVF-Create-Stem-Cell-Lines-10220-1. Accessed September 8, 2010. See also Paul H. Lerou, Akiko Yabuuchi, Hongguang Huo, Ayumu Takeuchi, Jessica Shea, Tina Cimini, Tan A. Ince, Elizabeth Ginsburg, Catherine Racowsky, and George Q. Daly. 2008. "Human Embryonic Stem Cell Derivation From Poor Quality Embryos." *Nature Biotechnology* 26: 212–214.

but none clearly contained the inner cell mass that yields stem cells.[21] In 2006, a team in Boston demonstrated that selected pESCs can serve as a source of histocompatible tissues for transplantation in mice.[22] Most stem cell laboratories at the time of this writing are either working on adult stem cells or embryonic stem cells. However, some work on pESCs continues. For example, in February 2008, the International Stem Cell Corporation announced that its human parthenogenetic stem cell lines will be used in Germany in studies aimed at the treatment of neural disorders such as Parkinson's disease.[23]

Adult Stem Cells

While embryonic stem cells are generally believed to have the greatest therapeutic potential, because of their ability to become virtually any kind of cell or tissue in the body, most stem cells are not derived from embryos. These are known as adult stem cells. The name "adult stem cells" is misleading, because these cells are not limited to adults, but are found in children, infants, fetuses, and umbilical cord blood. ("Nonembryonic stem cells" is the more accurate term, but I use "adult stem cells" because that is the more common term.) The function of adult stem cells, which have been found in the brain, bone marrow, peripheral blood, blood vessels, skeletal muscle, skin, and the liver, is to replace cells in the body that deteriorate due to injury or disease.[24] Residing in the body's tissues, they may remain quiescent, or nondividing, until there is a need for repair.[25]

In the 1960s, scientists discovered two kinds of adult stem cells in bone marrow: hematopoietic stem cells, which form all the types of blood cells in the body, and stromal cells, which generate bone, cartilage, fat, and fibrous connective tissue. Hematopoietic stem cells are the source of red blood cells, which carry oxygen to the tissues; platelets, which clot the blood; granulytes and macrophages, which fight infections from bacteria, fungi, and nematodes; B-cells, which produce antibodies; and T-cells, which kill inflammation foreign to the body. "The average human needs one hundred million new hematopoietic cells every day."[26] This is made possible by hematopoietic stem cells, which are essential to the body's functioning.

21. Advanced Cell Technology. 2001. [Press release]. http://www.advancedcell.com/press-release/advanced-cell-technology-inc-act-today-announced-publication-of-its-research-on-human-somatic-cell-nuclear-transfer-and-parthenogenesis. Accessed May 2, 2006.

22. Kitai Kim, Paul Lerou, Akiko Yabuuchi, Claudia Lengerke, Kitwa Ng, Jason West, Andrew Kirby, Mark J. Daly, and George Q. Daley. 2007. "Histocompatible Embryonic Stem Cells by Parthenogenesis," Science 315 (5811): 482–486.

23. "International Stem Cell Corporation's Human Parthenogenetic Stem Cells to Be Used in Germany in the Development of Treatments for Neural Disease." March 3, 2008. http://www.medicalnewstoday.com/articles/99234.php. Accessed September 8, 2010.

24. Cynthia B. Cohen. 2007. Renewing the Stuff of Life: Stem Cells, Ethics, and Public Policy. New York: Oxford University Press, p. 14.

25. National Institutes of Health. 2008. "Stem Cell Information" (see note 19).

26. Ibid.

Also in the 1960s, scientists working with rats found two regions of the brain containing dividing cells that become nerve cells. However, scientists thought that new nerve cells are never created in adults. "It was not until the 1990s that scientists agreed that the adult brain does contain stem cells that are able to generate the brain's three major cell types—astrocytes and oligodendrocytes, which are non-neuronal cells, and neurons, or nerve cells."[27]

In June 2008, physicians at four European universities (Barcelona, Bristol, Padua, and Milan) were able to perform a tracheal transplant on a 30-year-old Spanish woman with severe shortness of breath from end-stage airway disease caused by tuberculosis. Her left bronchus—the tube connecting the windpipe to the left lung—was so damaged that she was unable to walk for more than a few steps. Conventional treatment would have required the removal of a lung, but this was rejected by her doctors because it was a very risky procedure that was likely to result in very poor quality of life. Instead, her doctors took a segment of trachea from a cadaveric donor and used it as scaffolding to build a new windpipe. They then injected stem cells from the patient's bone marrow into the new windpipe, in the hope that these cells would turn themselves into windpipe cells with the ability to perform the functions of those cells, such as clearing mucus out of the airway. All of the tracheal cells from the cadaveric donor were removed over a 6-week period until no donor cells remained. Because the new trachea had only the patient's own cells, the problem of rejection was avoided. The operation was successful. Just 4 days after the surgery, the transplanted segment was virtually indistinguishable from adjacent normal bronchi. Lung function tests done within 2 months after the surgery were all normal, and the patient was able to climb two flights of stairs, walk for 500 meters, and care for her children.[28] Professor Martin Birchall of Bristol University, one of the four university centers involved in the surgery, characterized the transplant as demonstrating "the very real potential for adult stem cells and tissue engineering to . . . treat patients with serious diseases."[29] However, a surgeon not associated with the case, Dr. Eric Genden of Mount Sinai Hospital in New York, cautioned against viewing the operation as a panacea for people with diseased or damaged tracheas, pointing to the mixed success he and other teams have had with partial tracheal transplants. So far it has not been possible to replace an entire trachea. Although the results look promising, Dr. Genden comments, "I would take the results cautiously. Time will tell."[30]

Opponents of hESC research often argue that such research is scientifically unjustified and unnecessary, because adult stem cells could be used instead. This claim is based on the idea that adult stem cells have as much potential therapeutic promise as

27. Ibid.

28. Paolo Macchiarini, Philipp Jungebluth, Tetsuhiko Go, M. Adelaide Asnaghi, Louisa E. Rees, Tristan A. Cogan, Amanda Dodson, Jaume Martorell, Silvia Bellini, Pier Paolo Parnigotto, Sally C. Dickinson, Anthony P. Hollander, Sara Mantero, Maria Teresa Conconi, and Martin A. Birchall. 2008. "Clinical Transplantation of a Tissue-Engineered Airway," *The Lancet*. November 19. http://press.thelancet.com/airwaypapersfinal.pdf. Accessed October 31, 2010.

29. Alan Cowell and Denise Grady. 2008. "Europeans Announce Pioneering Surgery," *New York Times*, November 19, p. A8. http://www.nytimes.com/2008/11/20/health/research/20stemcell.html?scp=1&sq=&st=nyt. Accessed September 30, 2010.

30. Ibid.

embryonic stem cells. Defenders of this idea point out that, so far, the *only* successful stem cell therapies in humans come from adult stem cells. Moreover, some studies suggest that adult stem cells have the same, or almost the same, plasticity as hESCs. That is, they have just as much ability to turn into all the different kinds of cells in the body.[31] If that is correct, there would be no scientific reason to use embryonic stem cells in research or medicine.

The new thesis of adult stem cell plasticity was greeted with great surprise, because it went against 35 years of research.[32] Many researchers do not agree that adult stem cells are pluripotent, or as pluripotent as hESCs.[33] Some investigators could not reproduce the studies that claimed to demonstrate pluripotency in adult stem cells, and some called into question the experimental design of the studies allegedly demonstrating adult stem cell plasticity.[34] The debate over the plasticity of adult stem cells has not yet, at this writing, been resolved. While adult stem cells clearly have an important role to play in medicine, and may even be better than embryonic stem cells for the treatment of some diseases, it does not follow that there is no need to do embryonic stem cell research, which is important in both basic science and regenerative medicine. From a medical or scientific perspective, the right thing to do is to continue doing both adult and embryonic stem cell research—unless, of course, it is possible to find a substitute for hESCs, one that has all the plasticity of embryonic stem cells and not does involve destroying embryos. Such a substitute has been suggested, one that does not involve the use of human embryos or even human eggs: induced pluripotent stem cells.

Induced Pluripotent Stem Cells

A new development in stem cell research is the derivation of induced pluripotent stem cells (iPSCs) directly from differentiated adult somatic cells, usually skin cells. This began in June 2006, when Shinya Yamanaka of Kyoto University inserted four genes into cells taken from the tails of mice and created iPSCs,[35] which, a year later, he demonstrated to be truly pluripotent.[36] In November 2007, Yamanaka and his colleagues reported that they replicated their previous mouse success with humans. A retrovirus was used to deliver the genes into cells isolated from the face of a 36-year-old woman and the connective tissue of a 69-year-old man. The genes were the same ones Yamanaka had used earlier with mice, and as with the mice, the genes were able to reprogram the adult cells back to the pluripotent stage, at which they could become virtually any cell in the body. At the same time, a team in the

---

31. Cohen, *Renewing the Stuff of Life* (see note 24), pp. 15–17.

32. Ibid., p. 16.

33. Amy J. Wagers and Irving L. Weissman. 2004. "Plasticity of Adult Stem Cells," *Cell* 116 (5): 639–648, March 5.

34. Cohen, *Renewing the Stuff of Life* (see note 24), p. 16.

35. Gretchen Vogel. 2006. "Four Genes Convey Embryonic Potential," *Science* 313: 27.

36. Constance Holden. 2007. "Teams Reprogram Differentiated Cells—Without Eggs," *Science* 316: 1404–1405.

United States, led by James Thomson at the University of Wisconsin in Madison, was making the same effort. Thomson's group used two of the same genes as Yamanaka's as well as two different genes. Their cells came from fetal skin and the foreskin of a newborn. Their technique reprogrammed only about half as many cells as Yamanaka's, but it was effective enough to create several cell lines.[37] Referring to the methods used by Yamanaka and Thomson, stem cell researcher Jose Cibelli of Michigan State University in East Lansing said, "If their method is as good as the oocyte [in reprogramming somatic cells], we will be no longer in need of oocytes, and the whole field is going to completely change. People working on ethics will have to find something new to worry about."[38] Charles Krauthammer, a former member of the President's Council on Bioethics and opponent of hESC research, wrote in a column, "The embryonic stem cell debate is over . . . scientific reasons alone will now incline even the most willful researchers to leave the human embryo alone."[39]

However, Krauthammer's pronouncement turned out to be premature. While human iPSC gene expression is very similar to hESC gene expression, it is not identical. It is not clear that iPSCs can develop into fully functional somatic cells that can be used to treat disease in human beings. The therapeutic potential of hESCs is still unclear, and the potential of iPSCs is even less understood. There have been some successes with animal models: for example, sickle cell disease has been cured in mice using iPSCs.[40] However, as a microbiologist once told me, slightly tongue in cheek, "Everything works in mice." The serious point is that it is a lot easier to get good results with mice, but such success does not guarantee success in humans. Moreover, as Harvard stem cell researcher George Daley, who works with iPSCs points out, at every stage in iPSC research, comparisons with embryonic stem cells have to be made. Only then will it be possible to determine whether iPSCs are the equivalent of embryonic stem cells.[41]

Some scientists are dubious that iPSCs will ever substitute for embryonic stem cells in therapies for diseases. The reason is that so far scientists have used retroviruses to deliver the reprogramming genes into the cells, but these viruses also pose the risk of transforming target cells into cancerous cells. This might be avoided by changing the techniques for reprogramming cells. Already, scientists are experimenting with methods that avoid using as the method of delivery retroviruses that may cause cancer. The "best option would be to forego introducing genes and to use

37. Gretchen Vogel and Constance Holden. 2007. "Field Leaps Forward With New Stem Cell Advances," *Science* 318: 1224–1225.

38. Ibid., p. 1225.

39. Charles Krauthammer. 2007. "Stem Cell Debate Is Over; George Bush Is Vindicated," *Houston Chronicle*. http://www.chron.com/disp/story.mpl/editorial/outlook/5340219.html. Accessed September 11, 2010.

40. Jacob Hanna, Marius Wernig, Styliani Markoulaki, Chiao-Wang Sun, Alexander Meissner, John P. Cassady, Caroline Beard, Tobias Brambrink, Li-Chen Wu, Tim M. Townes, and Rudolf Jaenisch. 2007. "Treatment of Sickle Cell Anemia Mouse Model With iPS Cells Generated From Autologous Skin," *Science* 318 (5858): 1920–1923.

41. Constance Holden and Gretchen Vogel. 2008. "A Seismic Shift for Stem Cell Research," *Science* 319: 560–563, p. 561.

small molecules to slip through a cell's membranes and into the nucleus to turn on the genes that make the cell revert to a pluripotent state."[42]

In 2010, a team headed by Derrick J. Rossi at Children's Hospital Boston was able to create mRNA molecules in a laboratory and insert them into ordinary skin cells. The mRNA molecules provide the skin cells with the instructions for producing the four key proteins needed to reprogram themselves into iPSCs that appear virtually identical to embryonic stem cells. "Moreover, the same strategy can then coax those cells to morph into specific tissues that would be a perfect match for transplantation into patients."[43]

Some scientists think that iPSCs cannot possibly be used in therapies, even if they could be grown without using cancer-causing viruses. Thomas Okarma, president of Geron Corporation, says that starting with a skin cell that might have been altered because of aging or toxins instead of a "pure crystal clear embryo" would add unpredictable risks.[44] The problem of inducing cancer in subjects would have to be resolved before any clinical trials could go forward. The bottom line is that, at this point, we just do not know whether iPSCs are a substitute for hESCs in stem cell research, and therefore any claim that there is no need to do embryonic stem cell research is, at best, premature.

A possible source of embryonic stem cells is from embryos created by somatic cell nuclear transfer. The use of somatic cell nuclear transfer in hESC research is often referred to as "therapeutic cloning." Cloned embryos would be destroyed in the derivation of stem cells, just like IVF embryos, which is one source of moral controversy. In addition, somatic cell nuclear transfer could, in theory, be used to create whole human beings, not just embryos. This possibility leads some to reject any research using cloned embryos. However, in order to assess the morality of using embryos created by cloning, as opposed to embryos created by IVF, it is important to understand the science behind cloning and the different uses to which somatic cell nuclear transfer might be put.

Cloning: Reproductive Versus Therapeutic

Somatic cell nuclear transfer (SCNT), or simply nuclear transfer (NT), as some are referring to it these days, is a method for cloning embryos. If hESC research someday results in treatments for disease, there would be a great advantage to creating embryos by NT, as opposed to IVF. An embryo cloned from the patient's own somatic cells would have the patient's own DNA, as would the stem cells derived from that cloned embryo, thus circumventing the problem of rejection. Once again, it must be stressed that such possibilities are years away, if they are possible at all.

Nuclear transfer is the technique that was used by British scientist Ian Wilmut to clone Dolly, a lamb, in 1997. Nuclear transfer involves removing the nucleus (which

---

42. Ibid.

43. Rob Stein. 2010. "Scientists Overcome Hurdles to Stem Cell Alternatives," *Washington Post*, September 30. http://www.washingtonpost.com/wp-dyn/content/article/2010/09/30/AR2010093003211.html?referrer=emailarticle. Accessed September 30, 2010.

44. Ibid.

contains the DNA) from a somatic cell. (In the case of Dolly, it was a mammary cell; hence, the name "Dolly" after the busty singer, Dolly Parton.) The nucleus is then transferred by a thin glass needle, or pipette, into an enucleated egg cell, that is, an egg cell which has had its nucleus removed. Although the nuclear DNA is removed from the egg, mitochondrial DNA found in the egg lining remains. If the embryo is proved to contain DNA from the somatic cell donor, and mitochondrial DNA from the egg donor, that is proof that the resulting embryo was actually cloned, and not a parthenote.

Fusion of the somatic cell's nucleus and the enucleated egg cell can be performed chemically, or more often by electroporation, a mechanical method using a large electric pulse to enable the DNA from the nucleus to pass into the egg cell. When NT is used to produce a new individual, as in the case of Dolly, it is known as "reproductive cloning." Nuclear transfer has been used to clone mice, rabbits, sheep, goats, pigs, cattle, cats, and a dog, and even two primates: rhesus monkeys named Neti and Detto.[45]

Reproductive cloning is used in the dairy and cattle industries as a means of reproducing elite animals, who display such traits as high milk production or disease resistance. The biggest problem facing breeders who use NT technology is its inefficiency. However, the overall rate of success for cloning mammals remains below 5%, which scientists believe is due to epigenetic errors—that is, errors in gene expression that are not directly associated with changes in the DNA.[46]

In theory, reproductive cloning could also be used to repopulate endangered animals. A wild ox called a gaur was cloned in 2001, but it died from an infection shortly after birth. An endangered wild sheep, a mouflon, was cloned in Italy in 2001 and is living at a wildlife center in Sardinia. "Other endangered species that are potential candidates for cloning include the African bongo antelope, the Sumatran tiger, and the giant panda. Cloning extinct animals presents a much greater challenge to scientists because the egg and the surrogate needed to create the cloned embryo would be of a species different from the clone."[47] However, in November 2008, scientists from Pennsylvania State University reported that they had recovered DNA from the hair of a woolly mammoth, a species which became extinct some 10,000 years ago. They believe that it would be technologically possible, though tedious and expensive (at least $10 million), to modify the genome of a skin cell of the mammoth's closest living relative, the African living elephant, and then through cloning, turn the modified cell into an embryo, which could be brought to term in an elephant mother "and mammoths might once again roam the Siberian steppes."[48]

45. Alison Van Eenennaam, "Animal Cloning." 2008. http://animalscience.ucdavis.edu/animalbiotech/Outreach/Animal_Clones.pdf. Accessed September 10, 2010.

46. Wakayama Teruhiko. 2007. Production of Cloned Mice and ES Cells From Adult Somatic Cells by Nuclear Transfer: How to Improve Cloning Efficiency? *Journal of Reproductive Development* 53 (1): 13–26.

47. Human Genome Project Information. 2009. "Cloning Fact Sheet." http://www.ornl.gov/sci/techresources/Human_Genome/elsi/cloning.shtml#animalsQ. Accessed September 10, 2010.

48. Nicholas Wade. 2008. "With Mammoth Genes, Scientists Ask: What If?" *New York Times*, November 20, p. A1.

Other scientists are skeptical. Rudolph Jaenisch of the Whitehead Institute in Cambridge called the proposal "a wishful-thinking experiment with no realistic chance for success."[49] However, if it turns out to be possible to resurrect extinct species through genome modification, it might also be possible to do the same for ancient and extinct human species, such as the Neanderthal. That would require preserved body parts with Neanderthal DNA. In 2010, three Neanderthal teeth were discovered in a cave in Poland.[50] The age of one of the teeth, as well as its morphology, suggests that it belonged to a Neanderthal man, aged about 20. That tooth has undergone the most analysis, but the researchers are convinced that the other two teeth also belong to Neanderthals who lived 100,000 to 80,000 years ago. Modifying the genome of a modern human being to create a Neanderthal, even if it were technically possible, would raise many ethical objections. Many people are horrified by the idea of any human reproductive cloning, much less the creation of a species that became extinct about 45,000 years ago. Over 50 countries have passed laws to ban reproductive cloning, and no country has legislated to allow it.[51]

Contrasted with reproductive cloning is therapeutic cloning. Therapeutic cloning is the use of NT to create human embryos for the purpose of deriving hESCs. In its report, *Human Cloning and Human Dignity*, the President's Council on Bioethics rejected the term "therapeutic cloning," in favor of "cloning-for-biomedical-research."[52] The Council's objection to the term "therapeutic" was that it suggests, contrary to fact, that NT cloning already has therapeutic uses. Nevertheless, I continue to use the term "therapeutic cloning," because it is used in virtually all publications, whether mass media or guidelines for research. With the strict understanding that we are talking about research that has only the *possibility* of resulting in medical treatments or cures, and that the development of any therapeutic applications remains some years away, the term "therapeutic cloning" is not misleading.

Until the beginning of the 21st century, most scientists were dubious about the possibility of NT as a means of creating embryos. The first group to clone a human embryo via NT was an American team led by Jose Cibelli, in 2001.[53] They were unable to maintain the embryos in solution long enough to derive stem cells. Only one cloned embryo lived long enough to reach the six-cell stage, and a minimum of 64 cells is needed to derive stem cells from the inner mass. A few years later, Dr. Hwang

49. Ibid., p. A24.

50. Mikołaj Urbanowski, Paweł Socha, Paweł Dąbrowski, Wioletta Nowaczewska, Anna Sadakierska-Chudy, Tadeusz Dobosz, Krzysztof Stefaniak, and Adam Nadachowski. 2010. "The First Neanderthal Tooth Found North of the Carpathian Mountains," *Naturwissenschaften* 97 (4): 411–415.

51. Chamundeeswari Kuppuswamy, Darrlyl Macer, Michaela Serbulea, and Brendan Tobin. 2007. "Is Human Reproductive Cloning Inevitable: Future Options for UN Governance," UNI-IAS Report. http://www.ias.unu.edu/resource_centre/Cloning_9.20B.pdf. Accessed September 10, 2010.

52. The Council also rejected the term "reproductive cloning," in favor of "cloning to produce children," since cloning is not a form of reproduction, if that is taken to mean "sexual reproduction."

53. Alex Vass. 2001. "U.S. Scientists Clone First Human Embryo." *British Medical Journal* 323: 1267.

Woo Suk of South Korea claimed to have successfully derived stem cells from cloned human embryos using NT, but it turned out that Hwang fabricated the evidence.[54] This was a great shock to the scientific community, and it probably set back progress in the field. As the vice president of Advanced Cell Technology, stem cell biologist Robert Lanza, put it, "If it wasn't for Hwang's hoax, there's a good chance we would have had the first human [embryonic] stem cells as early as 2004, and they would have been the real thing, not a sham."[55] It should be noted that Hwang's team did create a stem cell line, although not, as he claimed, from a cloned human embryo. It actually was a parthenote, which also has value in stem cell research, something that has perhaps been overlooked due to the scandal of Hwang's fabricating scientific evidence. (Later, Hwang's team was the first to clone a dog, Snuffy, a feat that has been verified.[56])

In 2005, a group at Newcastle University in the United Kingdom—the first team to be granted a license from the Human Fertilization and Embryology Authority (HFEA) to do therapeutic cloning—took eggs from 11 women, removed the genetic material, and replaced it with DNA from embryonic stem cells. They managed to clone three embryos, two of which lived for 3 days, and one of which survived for 5 days.[57] Despite the enthusiasm greeting the British scientists for their feat, a cautionary note was struck by one of the researchers, Professor Alison Murdoch, who said, "We are talking about several years before we are talking about a cell-based therapy that can go back into the patient."[58]

In January 2008, Stemagen, a company based in La Jolla, California, announced that it had used NT to clone human embryos from adult skin cells, using skin cells donated by two men and eggs donated by three young women undergoing fertility treatment.[59] Of the 21 embryos created by nuclear transfer, five survived and grew into blastocysts containing between 40 and 72 cells. Of these five, three turned out to contain DNA from the skin cell of the man, proving it had been reprogrammed to become an embryo. Even more crucial, one of these three embryos was shown to contain mitochondrial DNA from the woman who donated the egg, the only remaining female DNA in the clone. This provides evidence that, for the first time, human blastocysts were cloned by nuclear transfer, using differentiated adult donor nuclei remodeled and reprogrammed by human oocytes. However, the researchers did not

54. Nicholas Wade and Choe Sang-Hun. 2006. "Researcher Faked Evidence of Human Cloning, Koreans Report." *New York Times*, January 10. http://www.nytimes.com/2006/01/10/science/10clone.html?adxnnl=1&ref=hwang_woo_suk&adxnnlx=1284134462-ItRvLvYBGLk5s0nwawMsjg. Accessed September 10, 2010.

55. Joseph Palca. 2006. "Earlier Work by South Korean Scientist Also Fraudulent." *National Public Radio*. http://www.npr.org/templates/story/story.php?storyId=5147015. Accessed October 12, 2008.

56. Ibid.

57. Associated Press. 2005. "British Scientists Said to Clone Embryo," May 20. MSNBC TV. http://www.msnbc.msn.com/id/7921548/. Accessed October 31, 2010.

58. BBC News. 2005. "UK Scientists Clone Human Embryo," http://news.bbc.co.uk/1/hi/health/4563607.stm. Accessed September 10, 2010.

59. Stemagen. 2008. "Stemagen First to Create Cloned Human Embryos From Adult Cells," http://www.stemagen.com/17jan08.htm. Accessed October 10, 2010.

derive any stem cell lines from the embryos. At this writing, no one has managed to create any embryonic stem cell lines from human embryos created by NT.

THE MORAL STANDING OF THE HUMAN EMBRYO[60]

In addition to the scientific challenges described earlier, hESC research is ethically and politically controversial because, at least at present, deriving embryonic stem cells destroys the embryo, preventing it from developing further. This makes it morally unacceptable to those who regard human embryos as human subjects, who may not be harmed or killed in biomedical research. Thus, at the heart of the debate over embryonic stem cell research is a philosophical question about the moral standing of human embryos in general, and specifically in the context of stem cell research.

The question of the moral standing of human embryos is also central to abortion, as discussed in Chapter 2. However, abortion and hESC research differ in two ways that have opposite implications. First, embryonic stem cells are derived from preimplantation, extracorporeal embryos; that is, embryonic stem cells are derived from embryos that exist outside the body. Thus, the derivation of these cells, and the killing of embryos necessary for their derivation, is completely divorced from pregnancy termination. This means that, unlike abortion, hESC research cannot be justified by appeal to a constitutional right of privacy or bodily self-determination. This suggests that the Supreme Court's ruling on abortion simply does not apply to extracorporeal embryos, and therefore a state could justify its restricting or even banning embryo research by appeal to its legitimate interest in protecting potential life (even though this interest would not justify restricting or banning abortion, prior to fetal viability).[61] However, the second difference between abortion and hESC research is that the blastocyst, which is destroyed in the derivation of stem cells, is morphologically and neurologically very different from a fetus. At the blastocyst stage, the embryo consists of a clump of undifferentiated cells, approximately 0.1 to 0.2 millimeters in size, "smaller than Roosevelt's eye on the face of a U.S. dime."[62] The nervous system is not yet in existence, and therefore there is no possibility of sentience or any kind of feeling or awareness. Indeed, the blastocyst lacks even the beginning of a nervous system. The precursor of the nervous system, the primitive streak, does not develop until about 2 weeks after fertilization, a week after stem cells would be removed. Moreover, at this stage of development, the embryo has no heart, no brain, or any organs. While the fetus, at least after midgestation, may be sentient (see Chapter 2), and thus a subject for moral concern, the blastocyst is "too rudimentary in development to have interests or rights," and an

60. Some of the material in this section comes from my article, "Moral Status, Moral Value, and Human Embryos: Implications for Stem Cell Research," in Bonnie Steinbock, ed., *Oxford Handbook of Bioethics* (Oxford: Oxford University Press, 2007), pp. 416–430.

61. For a discussion of this possibility, see John A. Robertson. 2010. "Embryo Stem Cell Research: Ten Years of Controversy," *Journal of Law, Medicine & Ethics* 38 (2): 191–203, p. 193.

62. University of Kansas Medical Center. 2010. "Stem Cell Research Basics: Early Stem Cells." http://www.kumc.edu/stemcell/early.html. Accessed October 6, 2010.

argument can be made that it "thus should not be protected at the cost of legitimate and important scientific research."[63]

As we saw in Chapter 2, the conservative position on abortion regards it as irrelevant that very early embryos are so tiny, or that their cells are undifferentiated, or that they do not have even the precursor of a nervous system. Rather, their moral status derives from their genetic humanity, that is, from the fact that they are biologically human. A human embryo is not a cat embryo or a dolphin embryo: it is a *human* embryo. Using the criterion of genetic humanity, all (and only) human beings have full moral status and rights.

However, even if we were to accept the genetic humanity criterion, that would *not* settle the question of the moral standing of the human embryo. Every cell in the body has a human genome, but obviously not every cell is a human being. Therefore, even accepting genetic humanity as the right criterion of moral standing, it is not the possession of a human genome that makes a cell a human being, but rather its status as a human *organism*, where an organism is defined as an integrated whole with the capacity for self-directed development. Clearly, a skin cell or a blood cell is not an organism, but a human fetus is. What should we say about a human blastocyst? To put it another way, the question is, at what stage of development does the human organism begin to exist?

The Twinning Problem

Some people think that the answer is obvious, a matter of plain biological fact: the human organism begins at fertilization or conception.[64] Let us call this "the conception view." However, the conception view runs up against what is known as "the twinning problem." As noted in Chapter 2, until the formation of the primitive streak at around the fourteenth day postconception, twinning (the division of the embryo into two or more distinct embryos) is still possible. This means that in the very beginning, the embryo is not identified with one and only one human being. If the early embryo is not uniquely identified with one human being, then the claim that the blastocyst is just one stage in the life cycle of a particular human being is not obviously true. Another way to view the preimplantation embryo is as "a community of possibly different individuals held together by a gelatinous membrane."[65] Therefore, even if one accepts the genetic humanity criterion as the correct criterion of moral standing, it does not follow that human blastocysts are human beings, because it is not clear that they are—yet—human organisms.

That issue aside, it is difficult to believe that anyone really believes that blastocysts have the same moral status as born human beings. Consider the following example, which I have adapted slightly from an article by George Annas, who in turn gives

63. Robertson, "Embryo Stem Cell Research" (see note 61), p. 192.

64. See, for example, Richard M. Doerflinger. 2010. "Old and New Ethics in the Stem Cell Debate," *Journal of Law, Medicine & Ethics* 38 (2): 212–219, p. 212.

65. Ronald M. Green. 2001. *The Human Embryo Research Debates: Bioethics in the Vortex of Controversy*. New York: Oxford University Press, p. 29.

credit for the example to Leonard Glantz.[66] You are alone in a fertility clinic, which contains trays of frozen embryos and also (improbably) someone's 3-month-old baby down the hall. The telephone rings and you are informed that a bomb is set to go off in 5 seconds.[67] You can either grab a tray containing 100 frozen embryos or you can grab the baby—you cannot save both. If you really thought that frozen embryos had the same moral status as babies, you would have to save the embryos; after all, there are 100 of them, and only one baby. But of course no sane person would grab the tray of embryos. That is because, rhetoric to the contrary, no one thinks of frozen embryos as morally comparable to babies.

Respect for Embryos

If this is right, then one might think that we ought to adopt the view that human embryos have no moral standing. They are comparable to human gametes, and therefore using them in research is permissible, with the consent of the progenitors. While this view is tempting, I maintain that it does not accord with some important intuitions. While embryos are clearly not persons, nor even sentient beings, neither are they just stuff, or just tissue. Most people do not regard them this way. They tend to regard human embryos as entitled to respect, as a very early form of human life. Indeed, the idea that human embryos are entitled to special or profound respect has been taken by virtually every commission that has considered the matter.[68] If this makes sense, then the interest view (elaborated in Chapter 1) needs to be supplemented. It says that all and only interested beings have moral standing, but it says nothing about the moral significance of beings without interests, including flags, corpses, and embryos. Thus, there seems to be a need for a third category, which comprises beings that do not have interests of their own and yet are regarded as something more than mere stuff, as entitled to respect.

Dan Callahan has suggested that placing embryos into a third category, in which they are entitled to respect, but not given moral standing or rights, is incoherent. He writes, "An odd form of esteem—at once high-minded and altogether lethal. What in the world can that kind of respect mean?"[69] Callahan concludes that offering "respect"

66. George Annas. 1989. "A French Homunculus in a Tennessee Court," *Hastings Center Report* 29 (6): 20–22, p. 22.

67. In the original Annas/Glantz example, the threat is a fire in the lab. I have changed it to a bomb in response to an objection made by Jan Deckers at the 2005 McGill Bioethics Conference, in Montreal, Canada, that the reason one would save the baby is not that a baby has greater moral status than an embryo, but rather that the baby, being sentient, would suffer from being burned, whereas the embryos would not. While this is true, it is not relevant, as can be seen from the fact that morality requires us to save the baby, even if its death would be quick and it would not suffer.

68. See, for example, Mary Warnock. 1985. *A Question of Life: The Warnock Report on Fertilization and Embryology*. Oxford: Basil Blackwell.

69. Daniel Callahan. 1995. "The Puzzle of Profound Respect," *Hastings Center Report* 25 (1): 39–40, p. 39.

to embryos is really just a way for us to feel less uncomfortable while we prepare to kill them.

The challenge, then, is to flesh out the notion of respect for embryos.

Kantian Respect

To develop further the notion of respect for embryos, we must first distinguish respect for embryos from respect for persons. Respect for *persons,* as Kant instructs us, means never treating persons *merely* as means to our ends, but always treating them as ends in themselves. People sometimes misquote Kant as saying that we are never to treat others as means to our ends, but this is a mistake. Of course we treat others as means to our ends; we can scarcely avoid doing so. A customer uses the bank teller as a means to getting cash, while the teller uses the customer as a means to having a job. This sort of mutual using is not morally objectionable. What *is* ruled out by Kantian respect for persons is treating others *merely* as means to our ends, that is, treating them as *nothing more than* tools to be exploited, ignoring their legitimate projects and interests. How do we avoid treating others merely as means to our ends? Onora O'Neill suggests that Kantian respect for persons entails acting on principles that sustain and extend one another's capacities for autonomous action. "To do that is to share and support one another's ends and activities at least to some extent."[70]

In other words, it is when we ignore other people's (legitimate) projects, goals, and interests, treating them as if they were simply vehicles for us to accomplish our own ends, that we violate Kant's injunction. But this means that Kantian respect can be shown only to individuals who *have* ends and interests. Kantian respect is limited to the kinds of beings who have projects and goals that can be shared, supported, and advanced. Without even the possibility of sentience or conscious awareness, preimplantation embryos have no interests of their own at all, and so they cannot have projects or goals. Therefore they are not, to use the Kantian term, "ends in themselves," and *Kantian* respect cannot be intelligibly applied to embryos. Should we conclude that embryos are mere things, and that we can do whatever we want with them? Surely not. As Harvard professor Michael J. Sandel, who was a member of the President's Council on Bioethics, has put it, "It's a mistake to claim respect is all or nothing, on or off."[71] Respect can be a matter of degree, depending on the kind of entity in question.

70. Onora O'Neill. 1986. "The Moral Perplexities of Famine and World Hunger." In Tom Regan, ed., *Matters of Life and Death: New Introductory Essays in Moral Philosophy.* New York: Random House, pp. 323–324.

71. The quotation comes from an exchange Prof. Sandel had with Robert George during one of the early meetings of the President's Council on Bioethics, February 14, 2002. (E-mail correspondence between Michael Sandel and the author.) For a fuller version of this idea, see his 2004 article, "Embryo Ethics: The Moral Logic of Stem Cell Research," *New England Journal of Medicine* 351 (3): 207–209, and the chapter on the stem cell debate in his 2007 book, *The Case Against Perfection: Ethics in the Age of Genetic Engineering* (Cambridge, MA: Harvard University Press).

One possibility is to accord human embryos an intermediate moral status, as we do animals, such as monkeys or dogs. Because they are not human subjects or persons, they can be used and killed in biomedical research aimed at understanding and treating serious human disease. At the same time, many people would oppose using these animals in, for example, cosmetics research, because such research is not sufficiently serious or important to justify the sacrifice of animals with intermediate moral standing. As Dan Brock expresses it:

> It is incompatible with these animals' intermediate moral status and the special respect they are owed to use and destroy them for a relatively trivial human purpose such as developing cosmetics. Limiting their use and destruction only to research aimed at understanding and treating or preventing serious human disease and suffering is a way of showing them special respect and recognizing that their intermediate moral status implies that they are not mere things and so cannot be used for just any human purpose . . . [72]

If animals can have an intermediate moral status, Brock suggests, so can embryos. In fact, Brock does not believe that human embryos do have "significant intermediate moral status." His aim is merely to show that "even if one does believe they have significant intermediate moral status, that is not incompatible with their use and destruction in the creation of stem cell lines."[73]

Do embryos have an intermediate moral status? If so, it cannot be on the same ground that we might ascribe such a status to monkeys and dogs—namely, their capacity to suffer. However, other reasons, such as the fact that they are alive and have the potential to develop into human persons, just like us, might justify an intermediate moral status. Another reason is that many people view embryos as human beings in the earliest stages of life. We show respect for them and their sincerely held moral beliefs by according embryos some moral status, even if not full moral status.[74]

Moral Standing Versus Moral Value

The intermediate moral status view is appealing. However, I think it is conceptually clearer to distinguish between *moral standing*, which is limited to beings with interests, to whom it matters how they are treated, and how their life goes, and *moral value*, which can be possessed by noninterested beings. The same considerations that lead some people to accord human embryos an intermediate moral status lead me to assign them moral value. A being has moral value if there are good moral reasons to treat it in certain ways and not in others.

72. Dan W. Brock. 2010. "Creating Embryos for Use in Stem Cell Research," *Journal of Law, Medicine & Ethics* 38 (2): 229–237, p. 231.

73. Ibid.

74. These reasons are given in the multicriterial approach to moral status developed by Mary Anne Warren in her 1997 book, *Moral Status: Obligations to Persons and Other Living Things* (New York: Oxford University Press). See also Dresser (note 19), for a similar argument about respecting the views of those with whom we disagree.

The reason for making the distinction between moral status and moral value is that different kinds of reasons are invoked in the case of beings with interests (interested beings) than are invoked in the case of beings without interests (noninterested beings). Interested beings provide us with "golden-rule type" reasons for action—reasons that stem from putting ourselves in their place and reflecting on how we would regard being treated as we now propose to treat them. We can and should consider the interests of affected parties (human or nonhuman animal) in making decisions about what to do. By contrast, our reasons for protecting works of art, ancient oak trees, wilderness areas, and entire species of plants or animals cannot stem from their interests or their welfare, as they do not have interests or a welfare of their own. If there are moral reasons for protecting or preserving nonsentient beings, they are different from the reasons we have to care about sentient beings, with interests of their own. The motivation for distinguishing between moral standing and moral value, and explaining the respect due to nonsentient beings in terms of moral value, instead of an intermediate moral status, is to avoid conflating two very different kinds of moral reasons.

What kinds of entities might have moral value? An example is objects of veneration. Consider a nation's flag. In itself, a flag is just a piece of cloth, with no intrinsic moral value. Nevertheless, the flag has deep significance to many people. (This was especially true in the United States after the terrorist attacks of September 11, 2001, when even people who were not usually "flag-wavers" often wore small pins of the American flag.) Taken symbolically, a flag is not just a piece of cloth. It has moral significance, both to those who regard it as a symbol of the United States, and derivatively to those who do not accept its symbolism, but who respect the views of those who do. For this reason, even non-Muslims, who do not regard the Koran as having special moral significance, can regard the desecration of the Koran as morally wrong, because of its symbolic significance to Muslims, combined with a principle of respect for the religious views of others.

If a venerated object has moral significance, there are typically rules about how it must be handled, displayed, or disposed of. For example, it is not acceptable to dispose of the American flag by throwing it in the garbage. As a U.S. veteran put it, "It deserves more respect than that." This, I take it, is not simply a claim about flag etiquette, but a moral claim. But how are we to understand the moral wrongness of throwing the flag in the garbage? Is it because it hurts the flag to be disposed of in this manner, or because we would not want to be tossed in the trash if we were flags? Of course not. These are golden-rule-type reasons, which are absurd when applied to inanimate objects. But from the fact that we cannot apply such reasons to flags, or try to see things from the flag's point of view, it does not follow that respect for the flag is impossible or meaningless.[75]

Another example of something to which respect is owed is a dead body. In itself, a corpse is simply a piece of decaying organic matter, without thoughts, feelings, goals, projects, or interests. And yet it matters what is done to the dead. Consider the following example. In 2002 a crematorium in Georgia failed to cremate the bodies

---

75. I am not suggesting that respect is the only appropriate attitude to display toward venerated objects. People have burned the flag in political protests, to demonstrate their anger at U.S. policies. This might be morally justifiable, in spite of the fact that the action is offensive to many people. Sometimes offending people is the right thing to do.

entrusted to it, but instead scattered them over the crematory property. Bodies were discovered stacked in a small shed. Georgia's chief medical examiner commented, "I have to say the utter lack of respect in which they were piled on top of one another was very disturbing."[76] The story was widely reported and sparked outrage in letters to the editor and editorials. This outrage reflects a *moral* view: that the dead, even more than symbolic objects like flags, are entitled to respect.

It might be claimed that while the outrage expressed is a moral emotion, it does not support a principle of respect for dead bodies. Rather, it stems from the recognition that survivors have interests in how their deceased relatives are treated. People want their loved ones put to rest, not treated like trash. This is clearly right, but it is not the whole story. It is morally wrong to show disrespect for human remains, even if there are no survivors, or even if the survivors are indifferent to how their relatives are treated. While rituals for disposing of the dead differ from culture to culture, the existence of some kind of ritual is not "optional," as rituals about flags, or even having flags, are. Rituals for disposing of dead bodies are so much a part of human history and culture that they are part of what it means to be human. These rituals are intended both to assuage the grief of the living but also to pay respect to the dead. (We see this when, for example, an unknown infant is found dead in a trash can, and strangers contribute to give the baby a decent burial, even when there are no family members to mourn.)

At the same time, respect for the dead does not rule out autopsy nor does it rule out the use of cadavers in medical school, which is essential to the training of doctors. It does mean that medical students should not toss body parts around like Frisbees—unfortunately, a common practice in the past. Today, many medical schools have a burial/cremation ceremony for the cadavers after they are finished with them, to show gratitude and respect to the no-longer-living individuals who donated their bodies to science.

Dead bodies are owed respect both because of what they are—the remains of the once-living human organism—and what they symbolize—a human person who is no more. Human embryos deserve respect for similar reasons: they are a developing form of human life, as well as a symbol of human existence. The claim here is not the strong claim that a human embryo is sacred or inviolable, which suggests something like a right to life, but the weaker claim that human life in all its stages is worthy of respect.

Some authors, such as Maura Ryan, who acknowledge that human embryos do not have full moral standing and a right to life, nevertheless maintain that it is wrong to use embryos in research, especially research that destroys them. To do so ignores their reproductive potential and treats them as dispensable research material to be used for the benefit of others.[77] Cynthia Cohen responds that this construes the moral significance of early human embryos as solely procreative. However, once we recognize the role that early human embryos have to play in medicine, we recognize

76. Andrew Buncombe. 2002. "Crematorium Worker 'Hid Hundreds of Corpses,'" *The Independent*, February 18. http://www.independent.co.uk/news/world/americas/crematorium-worker-hid-hundreds-of-corpses-661106.html. Accessed October 6, 2010.

77. Maura Ryan. 2001. "Creating Embryos for Research: On Weighing Symbolic Costs," in Paul Lauritzen, ed., *Cloning and the Future of Human Embryo Research*. Oxford: Oxford University Press, pp. 50–66.

that they have a moral significance outside of procreation. She writes, "This does not mean that these embryos are devoid of all moral significance in the research setting. In the context of stem cell research, the moral significance of embryos is *not repro-ductive* but *preservative* and *regenerative*; that is, in that context, embryos serve to restore and renew human life rather than to start it on the way into this world. In such instances, human embryos take on moral significance because of their possible contribution to the restoration of human life."[78]

Cohen is right to point out that embryos can have a regenerative, as well as repro-ductive, purpose, and to maintain that the restoration of human life is at least as important as the creation of new life. However, the *moral significance* of the human embryo cannot be based on its potential uses. Many things contribute to the restora-tion or preserving of human life: food, vitamins, antibiotics, and so on. Yet we are not inclined to say that all of these things have a special moral worth or are entitled to special respect. If embryos have a special moral value that other things, including other human cells, do not, it is not because of the ways in which embryos can be used. Respect for human embryos restrains the uses to which we might put them; it is not the basis for treating them with respect.

The Basis for Ascribing Moral Value to Human Embryos

What then is the rationale for regarding human embryos as having a special moral significance? Two related features are salient: its potential to become a person and its symbolic meaning. I have already argued in Chapter 2 that the potential to become a person does not endow a being with full moral status and rights. But as a potential person, it serves as a symbol of human life, and for that reason, has moral value. As expressed by the Ethics Committee of the American Society for Reproductive Medicine:

> The preembryo is due greater respect than other human tissue because of its potential to become a person and because of its symbolic meaning for many people. Yet, it should not be treated as a person, because it has not yet developed the features of personhood, it is not yet established as developmentally indi-vidual, and may never realize its biologic potential.[79]

Lacking even the most minimal essential of personhood—sentience—embryos are not yet "one of us." At the same time, they are not totally alien either. The embryonic stage is a part of our history as biological organisms. Every human being alive today developed from an embryo.[80] Both because it has the potential to develop into a human

---

78. Cohen, *Renewing the Stuff of Life* (see note 24), pp. 85–86.

79. Ethics Committee of the American Society for Reproductive Medicine. 1994. "The Moral and Legal Status of the Preembryo," *Fertility and Sterility* 62: 32S–4S.

80. Jeff McMahan would not agree that adult human beings were once embryos, but even McMahan agrees that my body—that is, my organism—was once an embryo, even though I was not yet present in it (see Chapter 2). If respect is owed to dead bodies, then respect should be owed to embryos as well, even if they are not "us," but only empty organisms.

person, and because the early embryo is a symbol of human life, human embryos deserve more respect than cells that lack this potential and symbolic significance.

Once we acknowledge that embryos are not the kinds of beings for whom Kantian respect is possible or intelligible, but are owed non-Kantian respect for human embryos, how would such respect be demonstrated? My answer is that we can show non-Kantian respect for human embryos by restricting the uses to which we put them.[81] Respect for embryos rules out frivolous or trivial uses, but this does not mean that we cannot use—and destroy—embryos in stem cell research, which has such great potential for medicine. Søren Holm[82] argues that this does not justify hESC research because it is unlikely that every stem cell line generated will have therapeutic usefulness; many will be used, not in medicine, but in basic research. Holm is correct in saying that at this point we have no way of knowing how many of the stem cell lines that are derived will eventually be used for therapeutic purposes, but wrong, I think, to make such a flat distinction between therapeutic uses and basic research. Basic research is not a trivial or frivolous use of embryos, as the creation of an anti-wrinkle cream (to use his own example) would be. Medicine relies on advances in basic research; there can be no cures and therapies without basic research. It is therefore unreasonable to insist that stem cell lines must "produce major therapeutic benefits"[83] to justify the research and the destruction of embryos.

A related objection comes from Rebecca Dresser, who urges both sides on the stem cell debate to aim for "an economy of moral disagreement"[84] by seeking to develop policies that both sides could accept. For example, for a limited time, only research that does not destroy embryos might be funded by the government, to see whether research using alternative sources works. If it does not, then funding of hESC research might again be made available. Such a policy, Dresser says, would show respect for those holding different positions on the ethics of destroying embryos for research. The trouble with this reasonable-sounding proposal is that alternative sources, like iPSCs, have to be compared with embryonic stem cells in order to demonstrate that using these alternative sources works. To fund iPSC research without at the same time funding hESC research would be counterproductive. A better alternative, and one that Dresser also puts forth, would be to fund hESC research but to cease such funding if it turns out that iPSCs, or some other alternative source of pluripotent stem cells, are shown to be just as good.

To display non-Kantian respect for embryos, the uses to which embryos are put, and for which they are destroyed, must be important, as opposed to frivolous or trivial. They ought not to be used (that is, destroyed) in situations where there is no pressing need, or where their use displays contempt rather than respect for human life. However, determining which uses are "frivolous" and which "morally important" turns out to be more complicated than one might think. For example, when I first began writing on respect for embryos, I gave as an example the use of human

81. Dan Brock independently makes the same point in "Creating Embryos for Use in Stem Cell Research" (see note 72).

82. Søren Holm. 2003. "The Ethical Case Against Stem Cell Research," *Cambridge Quarterly of Healthcare Ethics* 12: 372–383.

83. Ibid., p. 377.

84. Dresser, "Stem Cell Research as Innovation" (see note 18), p. 338.

embryos to create jewelry. What I had in mind was souvenir stands hawking earrings or bracelets made from human embryos. In truth, it is hard to imagine anyone being able to create jewelry from something as small as an embryo, but with the rise of nanotechnology and nanosurgery, this no longer seems so farfetched. What if an artist, moved by the beauty of blastocysts, were able to use human blastocysts to create jewelry that was a work of art? Would that necessarily show disrespect for human life? I confess I do not have an answer to this question.

A very different case was the art project of Yale student Aliza Shvarts, who reportedly inseminated herself as often as possible during a 9-month period, and then took herbs to induce abortion, and displayed the results in a student show. After news media across the country picked up the story, there was widespread outrage. However, it is not clear whether Shvarts every actually inseminated herself or induced any abortions. A professor of obstetrics at Yale Medical School doubted she was ever pregnant, as herbal antiabortifacients are incapable of terminating a pregnancy.[85] Some suggested that the blood in her project was menstrual blood, but subsequent testing revealed that there was no human blood in Shvarts's project, menstrual or otherwise.[86] Clearly, the project was "creative fiction."

Shvarts had her defenders. The Yale Women's Center issued a statement, saying, "Whether it is a question of reproductive rights or of artistic expression, Aliza Shvarts' body is an instrument over which she should be free to exercise full discretion."[87] But this seemed to be a minority opinion among Yale students, most of whom found the idea of getting pregnant deliberately for the purpose of aborting the fetus "disgusting."[88] The project was quickly condemned by national groups on both side of the abortion debate. Wanda Franz, president of the National Right to Life Committee, called her "depraved" and "a serial killer," while Ted Miller, a spokesperson for the abortion-rights group NARAL Pro-Choice America, called the project "offensive and insensitive to the women who have suffered the heartbreak of miscarriage."[89]

While questions about whether artists have the right to display disturbing images and ideas likely to offend are never easy, it seems to me that Shvarts's project, assuming it had used deliberately created and aborted embryos, failed to show appropriate respect. No lives were saved; human knowledge was not advanced. The appeal to art has its limits. As far as I can see, the only value of the project was shock value. I conclude that while the issue of respectful treatment of embryos is a matter on which reasonable people can debate, there are clear cases that cross the line. It is disrespectful to throw darts at corpses in booths at a county fair, it is disrespectful to use

85. Ambika Bhushan. 2008. "Experts Shed Doubt on Shvarts' Claims," *Yale Daily News*, April 23. http://www.yaledailynews.com/news/2008/apr/23/experts-shed-doubt-on-shvarts-claims/. Accessed September 14, 2010.

86. Thomas Kaplan. 2008. "Official: No Human Blood in Studio," *Yale Daily News*, April 24. http://www.yaledailynews.com/news/2008/apr/24/official-no-human-blood-in-studio/. Accessed September 14, 2010.

87. Samantha Broussard-Wilson. 2008. "Reaction to Shvarts: Outrage, Shock, Disgust," *Yale Daily News*, April 18. http://www.yaledailynews.com/news/2008/apr/18/reaction-to-shvarts-outrage-shock-disgust/. Accessed September 14, 2010.

88. Ibid.

89. Ibid.

embryos to be hawked as souvenirs, and it is disrespectful to create embryos to be destroyed in a student art project. None of these examples, however, implies that hESC research is inconsistent with respect for human life. Indeed, given the potential of hESC research to yield medical cures and save lives, it is quite the contrary.

The next question is what restrictions should be placed on using embryos within the context of a morally good purpose, such as basic science or medical research? Specifically, is it permissible to create embryos for research purposes, or should such research use only embryos that were originally created for reproductive purposes, which are then discarded?

THE DISCARDED-CREATED DISTINCTION

If embryos are no longer needed for reproductive purposes, they may be discarded or used in research. These embryos are often called "discarded embryos" and are in contrast with "created embryos," that is, embryos created specifically for research purposes. Of course, both embryos used for reproductive purposes and embryos used in research are created. The difference is that so-called discarded embryos were created as part of a reproductive project, while so-called created embryos have been created specifically for research purposes. Many people think that it is morally permissible to derive stem cells from discarded embryos, but not morally permissible to create embryos specifically for the purpose of deriving stem cells. The embryos will be destroyed in either case. What then is the basis of this claimed moral difference? The argument in favor of using only discarded embryos in research is that these embryos are doomed anyway. If they are not used in research, they will be discarded (or kept perpetually frozen). It seems morally better to use them for a potentially useful purpose, such as scientifically valuable research, than just to throw them away.

In its 1999 Report, the National Bioethics Advisory Commission (NBAC) attempted to explain and justify the discarded-created distinction, in terms of respect for embryos:

> An ethical intuition that seems to motivate the "discarded-created" distinction is that the act of creating an embryo for reproduction is respectful in a way that is commensurate with the moral status of embryos, while the act of creating an embryo for research is not. Embryos that are discarded following the completion of IVF treatment were presumably created by individuals who had the primary intention of implanting them for reproductive purposes.... By contrast, research embryos are created for use in research and, in the case of stem cell research, their destruction in the process of research. Hence, one motivation that encourages serious consideration of the "discarded-created" distinction is a concern about instrumentalization—treating the embryo as a mere object—a practice that may increasingly lead us to think of embryos generally as means to our ends rather than as ends in themselves.[90]

90. National Bioethics Advisory Commission. 1999. *Ethical Issues in Human Stem Cell Research* (Vol. 1). Rockville, MD, p. 56.

In my opinion, this confuses the Kantian respect owed to persons with the kind of non-Kantian respect due to embryos.[91] Of course we may not use *persons* in harmful research to which they have not consented, and one way to explain the wrongness of this is to say that this treats them as mere means to our ends. However, as I argued earlier, embryos are not ends in themselves, and so they are not appropriate subjects of Kantian respect. Embryos do not have moral standing, on the interest view, and there is no moral objection to using them as means.

However, I have also argued that human embryos are owed non-Kantian respect, which restricts the uses to which we may put them to important ones. Does non-Kantian respect for the human embryo require us not to create embryos for research, but to restrict ourselves to discarded embryos? The NBAC Report suggests that this is the case, based on the different intent in creating embryos in each case. To create embryos for the primary purpose of reproduction—making a child—is seen as respectful, while creating embryos for research purposes is not.

One question posed by this analysis is the moral significance of intentions and motives in evaluating actions. Hard-core utilitarians discount the moral significance of intentions and motives, maintaining that moral significance rests solely in outcomes. In this case, the relevant outcome is the same. Whether the embryos were created for reproductive purposes, and then discarded, or for research purposes, the embryos are killed in the derivation of stem cells.

On the other hand, nonutilitarians reject the assessment of actions solely in terms of consequences, holding the motives and intentions of actors to be morally significant.[92] In addition, some would appeal to the principle of double effect, essential in Roman Catholic thought, but accepted by many non-Catholics as well. According to this principle, sometime an action has two effects, one licit, one illicit. The classic example is giving high doses of morphine to a terminally ill cancer patient. The high doses are necessary to control pain, but they may also depress respiration, and cause the patient's death. May one do the action for the sake of the permissible outcome, if it also has an impermissible outcome? A consequentialist would analyze the case solely in terms of what produces the best outcome. Does the goodness of keeping the patient pain-free at the end of life outweigh the badness of the risk that this might shorten the patient's life? In most cases, the answer would be a straightforward "yes."

Those who accept the principle of double effect reason quite differently. Of course they want to be able to relieve pain. However, killing patients is absolutely forbidden, even if the patient is terminally ill, suffering great pain, and wants to die. Therefore, the administration of morphine in high enough doses to kill poses a dilemma for them that it does not pose for the consequentialist. The solution lies in the principle of double effect, which says that when an action has two effects, one good and one

91. Dan Brock offers a similar argument. See his "Creating Embryos for Use in Stem Cell Research" (note 72).

92. I agree that intentions matter in moral assessment. See my 1979 article, "The Intentional Termination of Life," *Ethics in Science and Medicine* 6 (1): 59–64. However, while I believe that intentions are morally relevant, I am not a proponent of the principle of double effect, because I reject the absolutist premise that makes it necessary. For example, I think that it may be permissible to cause or hasten the death of someone whose suffering cannot be ameliorated and who wants to die. If this is right, there is no need to appeal to double-effect reasoning.

bad, the action may be done if the intention is to bring about the good effect, and the bad effect is not intended, but merely foreseen.[93] The primary intention in giving the patient morphine is to relieve pain. That this might shorten the patient's life is foreseen, but not intended, either for its own sake or as a means to ending suffering. Under the principle of double effect, giving morphine is morally licit. It is distinguished from euthanasia, which is absolutely forbidden, because in euthanasia the patient's death is intended, as a means to end his or her suffering. This contradicts the fundamental principle, do not evil that good may come.[94]

We can apply double-effect reasoning to the creation of embryos for reproductive purposes (although as discussed in Chapter 5 the Roman Catholic Church does not apply double-effect reasoning to the creation of extracorporeal embryos, because this not only results in the deaths of embryos but also severs the connection between reproduction and sexual intercourse). The good effect is the creation of a child. The bad effect is the discarding and destruction of embryos when they are no longer needed for reproductive purposes. That bad effect, it might be argued, is not desired for its own sake, or even as a means to having a child. It is merely a foreseen and unfortunate consequence. By contrast, if one creates embryos for use in hESC research, one intends them to be destroyed, perhaps not as an end in itself, but certainly as a means to deriving the stem cells to be used in research. Therefore, it is alleged that it is wrong and disrespectful to create embryos for research in a way that it is not wrong or disrespectful to use discarded embryos.

The principle of double effect is philosophically controversial.[95] Those who reject the principle outright obviously would not accept its use as a rationale for distinguishing between discarded and created embryos.[96] Those who think it has moral significance in some contexts can use it to distinguish between discarded and created embryos only if it can be shown that the destruction of embryos created for research purposes is intended as a means of carrying out the research, while the discarding of embryos created for reproductive purposes is not a means to the reproductive project, but merely a foreseen and unwanted side effect. However, I think it is far from clear that this can be demonstrated.

To see why, consider the reason embryos are discarded in assisted reproduction. Embryos are discarded because more are created than can be safely implanted at one time. By creating excess embryos, we enable the couple another chance at a pregnancy if the first round does not work, both saving the couple the expense of another round

93. For a full explanation of the doctrine of double effect, see the entry in the *Stanford Encyclopedia of Philosophy* (2009). http://plato.stanford.edu/entries/double-effect/. Accessed September 15, 2010.

94. This doctrine, essential to Catholic teaching, stems from The Epistle of Paul the Apostle to the Romans 3:8, King James Bible.

95. H. L. A. Hart (1967) rejects the doctrine in "Intention and Punishment," *Oxford Review* 4; reprinted in *Punishment and Responsibility* (Oxford: Oxford University Press, 1968). Philippa Foot (1967) defends the distinction that motivates the doctrine, between what one intends and what one merely foresees, in "The Problem of Abortion and the Doctrine of Double Effect," *Oxford Review* 5: 5–15; reprinted in Bonnie Steinbock and Alastair Norcross, eds. 1994. *Killing and Letting Die*, 2nd ed. New York: Fordham University Press, pp. 266–279.

96. See, for example, Dan Brock, "Creating Embryos for Use in Stem Cell Research" (note 69).

of IVF and protecting the woman from the burdens of an additional cycle of superovulatory drugs. The creating of spare embryos, most of which will be discarded, is a means to reducing the physical, emotional, and economic burdens imposed by multiple rounds of IVF. To classify it as a merely foreseen and unwanted consequence seems disingenuous. It would be more honest and consistent for those who oppose the creation and destruction of embryos in research also to oppose the creation of spare embryos. This is the situation in Italy, where the creation of a surplus of embryos is prohibited by law. No more than three embryos can be created, and all three must be implanted into the uterus of the mother.[97] However, few countries have such restrictive laws, with the result that there is a great deal of embryo wastage.

Another way to avoid the discarding of embryos that does not rely on restricting the number of embryos that can be created is to have excess frozen embryos donated to other infertile couples, so that all created embryos have the chance to be brought to term. In 1997, Nightlight Christian Adoptions began the Snowflake Embryo Adoption Program,[98] with the aim of "helping some of the more than 400,000 frozen embryos worldwide realize their ultimate purpose—life."[99] According to its Web site, over 220 children have been born through the Snowflake Embryo Adoption program.[100] This is a tiny percentage of the approximately half million embryos stored in freezers throughout the world, the vast majority of which will never be brought to birth. Relatively few individuals who go through IVF opt for embryo donation to another couple, most often because they do not want to bring children who are genetically related to them into the world if they are not going to be their parents.

It seems to me that consistency requires opponents of hESC research, whose opposition is based on the destruction of embryos in the research, to be just as opposed to IVF. While IVF need not involve embryo sacrifice, since the number of embryos created could be restricted to the number implanted (although not all will necessarily be brought to term), as a practical matter it does result in embryo destruction.

It is difficult to explain why opposition to IVF has not materialized, unless it is that infertility treatment is associated with adorable babies and happy parents, while embryo research conveys a very different image, that of Nazi scientists performing experiments on innocent and vulnerable human beings. Neither image is accurate. On the one hand, infertility treatment does not always result in live births, and on the other, hESC research cannot be compared to the cruel and scientifically worthless

97. Francesco Frassoni. 2006. "The Laws Covering In Vitro Fertilization and Embryo Research in Italy," *Bone Marrow Transplantation* 38: 5–6.

98. The Ethics Committee of the American Society for Reproductive Medicine rejects the term "embryo adoption," on the ground that it is inaccurate and misleading. "Adoption refers to a specific legal procedure that establishes or transfers parentage of existing children." ASRM. 2009. "Defining Embryo Donation," *Fertility and Sterility* 92: 1818–1819.

99. Nightlight, Snowflake Embryo Adoption and Donation Program. http://www.nightlight. org/snowflakeadoption.htm. Accessed September 10, 2010.

100. Embryo Adoption Awareness Center. http://www.embryoadoption.org/testimonials/index.cfm.

experiments of Nazi scientists.[101] Moreover, embryo research is essential for improving infertility treatment, enabling those adorable babies to get born, even if cures for disease from hESC research are a long way off or fail to pan out entirely. For this reason, infertility treatment and embryo research cannot be divorced. If infertility treatment is morally permissible, so is the research necessary to make it safe and effective. Moreover, if research using embryos is permissible to enable people to have biologically related children, it should also be permissible for other kinds of important, scientifically valid research.

In my view, there is no moral difference between creating embryos for reproductive purposes, and donating the excess embryos to research, and creating embryos specifically for research purposes. The source of the embryos, whether left over from IVF or created specifically for research purposes, is not morally significant. Both reproduction and research have moral value. Both promote serious human interests. It is the value of these projects that justifies the destruction of human embryos. Neither is a trivial or frivolous enterprise that contravenes the principle of respect for embryos as a form of human life. However, the willingness to restrict hESC research to spare embryos may be justified as a *political* compromise, and as Dresser suggests,[102] the willingness to compromise itself can be a way of demonstrating respect for the views of those with whom one disagrees.

PAYMENT FOR OOCYTES

Should women be paid for donating oocytes for research? As we saw in Chapter 5, there is controversy over whether women should be paid to donate eggs for reproductive purposes. In some countries (e.g., Canada, Denmark, and the United Kingdom), payment for gametes is either prohibited or strictly limited. By contrast, in the United States women who donate their oocytes for reproductive purposes are usually financially compensated, although ASRM recommends that financial compensation be limited to $5,000 per cycle.

In the United States, there is greater resistance to paying oocyte donors if the oocytes are to be used in research. For example, the voter-approved state ballot measure that created the $3 billion California Institute for Regenerative Medicine specifically bans compensating women for eggs donated for research. Dr. Sam Wood, chief executive of Stemagen, complains that the prohibition against payment to egg donors is a stumbling block in their ability to derive stem cell lines. "You need to have enough eggs to make this thing work, and when you have enough eggs it does work," he said. "If these guidelines weren't in place, we'd already have many (stem cell) lines

---

101. The overwhelming number of Nazi experiments, such as those done by the infamous Josef Mengele, had no scientific value whatsoever. All were conducted on prisoners without their consent, and they typically inflicted great injury or death. However, some of the research may have yielded valuable results that could save future lives, raising the question of whether the data from these unethical and immoral experiments should be used today. See Kristine Moe. 1984. "Should the Nazi Research Data Be Cited?" *Hastings Center Report* 14 (6): 5–7.

102. Dresser "Stem Cell Research as Innovation" (see note 18).

and be much closer to a treatment for devastating illnesses for which these are so well suited," Wood said.[103]

The U.S. National Academies, composed of the National Academy of Sciences, a private, nonprofit society of distinguished scholars engaged in scientific and engineering research, as well as the National Academy of Engineering, the Institute of Medicine, and the National Research Council, created the Committee on Guidelines for Human Embryonic Stem Cell Research. The Committee's report, "Guidelines for Human Embryonic Stem Cell Research,"[104] came out in 2005, and was updated in 2007, 2008, and 2010 in light of scientific developments, notably the creation of iPSCs. This document contains a lengthy discussion of the arguments for and against paying oocyte donors (see Chapter 5). As in the case of payment to egg donors for reproductive purposes, those opposed to payment worry about undue inducement and the exploitation of women, or about the commodification of life or reproduction. Those in favor consider it only fair to remunerate egg donors for the time, burdens, and risk of egg donation. They point out that research subjects are commonly paid for their participation in research, so why should egg donors be treated differently? Moreover, since the risks and burdens are the same, regardless of how the eggs are used, there seems to be no reason for discriminating between those who donate oocytes for reproduction and those who donate for research purposes. Accepting this logic, New York's Empire State Stem Cell Board announced in June 2009 that stem cell researchers could use New York State funds to pay women up to $10,000 per cycle to donate oocytes.[105] At the time of this writing, New York is the only state that permits women who donate eggs for research to be compensated.

A pragmatic reason against compensation is simply that it is controversial and might cause some people who are not in principle opposed to hESC research to reject it. Seen this way, the prohibition of payment is a political compromise between those who favor whatever is necessary to enable hESC research to succeed and those who support the research but reject payment for oocytes due to concerns about the commodification of reproduction and exploitation of women. Ideally, they would prefer that no gamete donors be compensated but recognize that they cannot do anything about payments in the reproductive context: the practice is too entrenched. These opponents of compensation are willing to tolerate this inconsistency rather than allow the practice of paying egg donors to spread further than it already has. Moreover, some opponents of compensating donors for oocytes to be used in research maintain that the potential for exploitation is greater in the case of research than reproduction. People seeking egg donors for reproductive purposes typically want white, educated, middle-class donors. By contrast, researchers do not care about the

103. Marcus Wohlsen. 2008. "Scientists: Human Egg Shortage Hurts Stem Cell Research," *Associated Press*, July 31. http://www.ledger-dispatch.com/news/newsview.asp?c=247253. Accessed October 31, 2010.

104. National Research Council (NRC) and Institute of Medicine (IOM) of the National Academies. 2005. *Guidelines for Human Embryonic Stem Cell Research*. Washington, D.C.: The National Academies Press.

105. Libby Nelson. 2009. "New York State Allows Payment for Egg Donations for Research," *New York Times*. http://www.nytimes.com/2009/06/26/nyregion/26stemcell.html. Accessed September 15, 2010.

race or socioeconomic class of their donors because these factors do not influence the suitability of eggs for research purposes. Thus, poor women may be recruited for egg donation, which poses a greater risk that these potential donors will be unduly influenced by the prospect of payment, ignoring the risks imposed by egg donation.

Concerns about exploitation appear to have won the day over concerns about equal treatment in the National Academies' Human Embryonic Stem Cell Research Advisory Committee. In its Final Report in 2010, the Advisory Committee acknowledged the fact that New York had decided to compensate egg donors for research and noted that this was an evolving issue, but they decided ultimately not to change the recommendation that women who donate oocytes for research purposes "should be reimbursed only for direct expenses incurred as a result."[106] However, the interpretation of direct expenses was broadened to mean not only such things as travel, housing, child care, and medical expenses but also lost wages.[107]

CHIMERAS, HYBRIDS, AND CYBRIDS

In Greek mythology, the Chimera had the head of a lion, the body of a goat, and the tail of a snake. The Minotaur, which was part-human and part-bull, was also a chimera, as were centaurs, which had the body of a horse and the torso of a man. But chimeras are not just mythological creatures. Chimeras, mixtures of cells from two different kinds of animals, are widely used in research and medicine. Medical researchers have transplanted human skin, tumors, and bone marrow into mice, in order to study, and hopefully find treatments for, a variety of diseases that afflict humans.[108] Xenotransplantation also creates human-nonhuman chimeras and is surprisingly common, for example, the placement of pig heart valves in humans to treat certain types of cardiovascular disease.

While the creation of nonhuman chimeras has not raised much, if any, ethical concern, the creation of human-nonhuman chimeras has been very controversial. As put in the Guidelines from the National Academies, "Although moral intuitions about the creation of chimeras may vary, it is a subject of deep moral concern to many thoughtful people for whom the creation of animals with certain kinds or quantities of human tissues, such as neural or germ line cells, would be offensive. Accordingly, such research requires careful consideration and review."[109] While this is undoubtedly true, it is also true that many of the concerns about chimeras, especially those reflected in legislation introduced into the U.S. Congress, stem more from science fiction than actual stem cell science.

Chimeras are important in stem cell research because they enable scientists to determine whether the tissues and organs derived from human stem cells actually work.

---

106. Ibid., section 3.4.

107. Final Report of the National Academies' Human Embryonic Stem Cell Research Advisory Committee and Amendments to the National Academies' Guidelines for Human Embryonic Stem Cell Research. 2010. http://books.nap.edu/openbook.php?record_id=12923&page=R1. Accessed September 15, 2010.

108. Cohen, *Renewing the Stuff of Life* (see note 24), p. 112.

109. NRC and IOM. 2005. *Guidelines for hESC Research* (see note 104), p. 50.

While scientists can derive human embryonic stem cells in vitro, and even grow tissues from these stem cells in the laboratory, ultimately they need to find out whether the tissues will grow and function properly inside a living animal. They cannot transplant the tissues into human beings while the risks to these subjects are still unknown. "Therefore," as Cynthia Cohen notes, "stem cell scientists have initiated research that involves inserting different kinds of human stem cells into animals that are at various stages of growth to discover how these human cells function in developing organism and to explore the ways in which they repair and replace diseased or injured tissues."[110] This seems no different from any other use of animal models in medical or scientific research.[111]

In the United States, the first bill to attempt to prohibit the creation of human-nonhuman chimeras was the Human Chimera Prohibition Act of 2005 (S.659), introduced by Senator Sam Brownback (R-KS). In 2007, Senator Brownback and Senator Mary Landrieu (D-LA) introduced a virtually identical bill under a slightly different name, the Human-Animal Hybrid Prohibition Act (S.2358). Another version of the same bill (H.R. 5910) was introduced into the House of Representatives in 2008. None of these bills ever got out of committee. Yet it is worth examining the proposed bills and their rationales for the reasons given in the Guidelines created by the National Academies: first, because this is a "subject of deep moral concern to many thoughtful people," and second, because, given the importance of chimeras to stem cell research, it is essential "to distinguish legitimate concerns from discomfort arising from unfamiliarity."[112]

All of the bills introduced into Congress between 2005 and 2008 were basically the same, except that the word *chimera* was replaced (incorrectly from a scientific perspective) by the word *hybrid*. Although the terms are frequently used interchangeably, chimeras differ from hybrids. While both contain the genetic material of two distinct species, in a hybrid, each cell of the animal's body contains the DNA of both species. Perhaps the best-known naturally occurring example of a hybrid animal is the mule, the result of reproduction between a mare and a male donkey. By contrast, there is no commingling of genetic material in individual cells of a chimera. Scientists have been creating chimeras for years. They have fused goat and sheep embryos to create "geeps," which have characteristics of both goat and sheep. They have also transplanted regions of the brain of quails into the brains of chicken embryos, creating chicks that squawk like quails. While the rationale for this type of experiment might seem questionable, Cynthia Cohen explains, "The aim of these experiments was not frivolous; it was to develop interspecies chimeric models to use in the study of cell migration."[113]

No explanation was given for the change in terminology from "chimera" to "hybrid" in the proposed legislation, but it may be due to the possibility of creating cytoplasmic hybrid embryos (described later). However, the acts prohibited by the proposed bills were, for the most part, nothing that stem cell scientists were remotely

110. Cohen, *Renewing the Stuff of Life* (see note 24), p. 110.

111. Some philosophers have objected to the use of sentient animals in research, but that is a separate issue.

112. NRC and IOM. 2005. *Guidelines for hESC Research* (see note 104), p. 50.

113. Cohen, "Renewing the Stuff of Life" (see note 24), p. 112.

interested in doing. Here is the definition of a human-nonhuman hybrid from H.R. 5910:

(A) A human embryo into which a nonhuman cell or cells (or the component parts thereof) have been introduced to render the embryo's membership in the species Homo sapiens uncertain

(B) A hybrid human/animal embryo produced by fertilizing a human egg with nonhuman sperm

(C) A hybrid human/animal embryo produced by fertilizing a nonhuman egg with human sperm

(D) An embryo produced by introducing a nonhuman nucleus into a human egg

(E) An embryo produced by introducing a human nucleus into a nonhuman egg

(F) An embryo containing at least haploid sets of chromosomes from both a human and a nonhuman life form

(G) A nonhuman life form engineered such that human gametes develop within the body of a nonhuman life form

(H) A nonhuman life form engineered such that it contains a human brain or a brain derived wholly or predominantly from human neural tissues

Under this law, the creation of a human-animal hybrid would be punishable by a maximum of 10 years imprisonment and up to $1 million in fines.

With one exception, which I discuss later, the prohibited acts just listed have nothing at all to do with stem cell research. To my knowledge, there are no stem cell scientists contemplating introducing nonhuman cells into human embryos, or attempting to fertilize human eggs with nonhuman sperm, or nonhuman eggs with human sperm. It is unclear what purpose such research would serve. As stated in the National Academies Guidelines, "Interspecies hybrids are rarely viable and no one proposes to generate interspecies hybrids involving human gametes, even if it were possible."[114] Why, then, write legislation aimed at prohibiting something no one is trying to do, and probably could not be done in any event? Two possible explanations present themselves: sheer ignorance about stem cell research, or worse, an attempt to make it seem as if this is what scientists engaged in stem cell research are doing, or would like to do, thus creating or fanning the flames of hostility to such research.

The exception mentioned earlier comes under (E): producing a human embryo by introducing a human nucleus into a nonhuman egg. In both Australia and the United Kingdom, researchers have started using cow eggs, or more precisely, the cytoplasm from cow eggs, to clone embryos from which hESCs can be derived. Why use animal eggs? Dr. Lyle Armstrong of Newcastle University justified the research this way:

We have already done a lot of the work by transferring animal cells into cow eggs so we hope to make rapid progress. Finding better ways to make human embryonic stem cells is the long-term objective of our work and understanding reprogramming is central to this. Cow eggs seem to be every bit as good at

114. NRC and IOM. 2005. *Guidelines for hESC Research* (see note 104), p. 38.

doing this job as human eggs so it makes sense to use them since they are much more readily available but it is important to stress that we will only use them as a scientific tool and we need not worry about cells derived from them ever being used to treat human diseases.[115]

In the United Kingdom, it is the Human Fertilization and Embryology Authority (HFEA) that determines what kinds of research involving human embryos may be done, through the issuing of licenses. Therefore, the first question the HFEA had to address was, What is the nature of the entities that would be generated? "Are they really human embryos and, therefore, entities that fall under the HFEA remit? If they are not human, what are they?"[116] Two scientists writing on the issue maintain that they are certainly not chimeras, because these embryos would have genetically identical cells, whereas chimeras have genetically distinct cells. Chimeras can be formed in two ways. One is when two fertilized eggs or early embryos are fused together. This can happen in nature or in the laboratory. Alternatively, chimeras can be formed in the lab by taking a mass of embryonic stem cells from one developing blastocyst and injecting them into a second blastocyst. In either case, the resulting chimeric embryo is made up of a combination of genetically distinct cells and tissues, that is, cells and tissues from two different organisms. Something very different occurs when scientists take the nuclear DNA from a human embryo and put it inside an enucleated animal egg, and then allow cell division to occur. In this case, all of the cells in the resulting embryo will be genetically identical. That is why the embryo is not a chimera. Nor is it hybrid, in the conventional sense of an animal that is the offspring of members of two different species. Rather, embryos created from human DNA and nonhuman animal cytoplasm are properly known as cytoplasmic hybrids, or "cybrids."

The question then arises: Is it ethically permissible to create cybrids, embryos that contain both human DNA and animal cytoplasm? According to the U.S. Human-Animal Hybrid Prohibition Act of 2008, "human-animal hybrids are grossly unethical because":

- They blur the line between human and animal, male and female, parent and child, and one individual and another individual.
- Human dignity and the integrity of the human species are compromised by human-animal hybrids.
- The uniqueness of individual human beings is manifested in a particular way through their brain and their reproductive organs/cells.
- With an increase in emerging zoonotic infection threatening the global public health, human-animal hybrids present a particularly optimal means of genetic transfers that could increase the efficiency or virulence of diseases threatening both humans and animals.

115. Cell News. 2008. "UK HFEA Approves Human-Animal Hybrid Embryo Research." http://cellnews-blog.blogspot.com/2008/01/uk-hfea-approves-human-animal-hybrid.html. Accessed September 17, 2010.

116. Justin St John and Robin Lovell-Badge. 2007. "Human-Animal Cytoplasmic Hybrid Embryos, Mitochondria, and an Energetic Debate," Nature Cell Biology 9 (9): 988–992.

None of these rationales is compelling. Indeed, the claim that hybrids blur the line between "male and female, parent and child, and one individual and another individual" is incomprehensible. What does the creation of hybrids or chimeras or cybrids have to do with male and female, parent and child, or one individual and another? That seems to be irrelevant rhetoric.

As for the blurring of species, there are two points to make, one scientific, one normative. The scientific point is expressed in the National Academies Guidelines:

> . . . the popular notion that there are clear and distinct lines between species is a notoriously unreliable categorical scheme. Taxonomies developed since Aristotle do not necessarily countenance the idea of natural kinds, and modern scientists differ in their precise definitions of interspecies boundaries. There is general agreement in the scientific community that these boundaries are to some extent arbitrary.[117]

But even if species' lines were clear and distinct, and the creation of cybrids or chimeras would blur those lines, the claim that this is unethical has not been defended. So far, this is merely a description of what a chimera is, not an argument against them. I suspect that the ethical objection to blurring lines is the "unnatural" or "playing God" objection in different dress.[118] But as John Stuart Mill[119] persuasively argued over a century and a half ago, the fact that something is natural does not make it good; that something is unnatural does not make it bad. Plagues, tornados, and hurricanes are all natural; cities, works of art, and vaccinations against disease are all unnatural. All of medicine is "playing God" in the sense that modern medicine saves lives that otherwise would have been lost. Serious moral objections will have to do better than that.

How valid is the public health objection? Do "human-animal hybrids present a particularly optimal means of genetic transfers that could increase the efficiency or virulence of diseases threatening both humans and animals"? To understand this claim, it is necessary to understand what zoonotic diseases are, how they are spread, and what the connection is between chimeras that could be useful in stem cell research and the spread of zoonotic disease. Zoonotic diseases are infections that can be transmitted from animals to human beings. (Some infectious diseases can be transmitted from humans to animals as well, a situation called reverse zoonosis or anthroponosis, but that is not a public health concern.) They include rabies, tuberculosis, anthrax, hantavirus, and other serious diseases. They are on the rise, due to factors such as international travel, trade in exotic and wild animals, population growth of humans and domestic animals, encroachment of humans and domesticated animals into wildlife habitat, climate change, and concentrated animal husbandry operations in close proximity to human populations.

---

117. NRC and IOM. 2005. *Guidelines for hESCR* (see note 104), pp. 49–50.

118. I address this issue in "Legitimate and Illegitimate Appeals to Nature: Lessons from John Stuart Mill," in Gregory Kaebnick, ed., *The Appeal to Nature* (Baltimore, MD: Johns Hopkins University Press, 2011).

119. John Stuart Mill. 1904. "On Nature." In *Nature, The Utility of Religion and Theism* [1874]. London: Watts & Co. for the Rationalist Press.

Zoonotic infections typically occur when humans are exposed to infected animals. This can happen in a variety of ways, as the introduction of HIV, avian flu, and monkey pox in the human population demonstrate. In the case of HIV, for example, some researchers believe that the virus jumped from chimpanzee to humans through the bushmeat trade—the hunting and killing of chimpanzees for human consumption. When the hunters butchered infected animals, they were exposed to their blood, as were people who ate the animals, thus transmitting the infection. People can be infected with avian flu (H5N1) if exposed to infected dead poultry or poultry feces. Because relatively few humans have been infected with bird flu, it is not now a public health menace, but some experts believe it is only a matter of time before this virus mutates into a human to human form, causing a deadly pandemic. An outbreak of monkey pox in the United States in 2003 started with the importation of infected Gambian rats and other African rodents and spread to prairie dogs through the exotic pet trade.

In all of these cases of zoonotic infection, humans were exposed to sick or dead animals. But none of this has anything to do with the creation of chimeras, cytoplasmic hybrid embryos, or hESC research. In the first place, it is not the creation of a hybrid animal that poses a threat to humans, but the mutation of a virus in one species so that it can infect members of another species. But even if the creation of hybrid animals is a public health concern, it has nothing to do with using animals to test tissue derived from human embryonic stem cells. This poses no health threat to human beings, and indeed can promote public health by determining whether the tissue works safely and effectively in a living animal model. The appeal to public health concerns to support a ban on human-animal chimeras either betrays astonishing ignorance about animal to human viral transmission, or it is simply fear-mongering.

There is one last concern that some people have about human-animal chimeras, which has to do with transplanting neural stem cells, or even nonneural cells which might turn into neural cells, into animal brains. The fear is that it might be possible to create an animal with characteristic human capacities of thought: a Stuart Little, the eponymous hero of the children's story by E. B. White. Before even addressing the ethics of creating such a being, it is important to emphasize how unlikely the "mouse with a human brain" scenario is. Transplanting human neurons into the brain of a mouse almost certainly cannot result in a creature with distinctively human cognitive abilities. Not only are mouse brains much tinier than human brains, they are organized differently.[120]

Neuroscientists believe that it is the architecture of the brain that produces consciousness, not the precise nature of the neurons that make it up. As an analogy, architecture determines whether a building is a cathedral or a garage, not whether the bricks used are red or gray. A mouse brain made up entirely of

120. Henry T. Greely, Mildred K. Cho, Linda F. Hogle, and Debra M. Satz. 2007. "Thinking About the Human Neuron Mouse," *American Journal of Bioethics* 7 (5): 27–40. http://www. lexisnexis.com.libproxy.albany.edu/hottopics/lnacademic/?shr=t&sfi=AC00NBGenSrch& csi=258948&srcpdn=academic&product=universe&after=0:ALL&unix=http://web.lexis-n. Accessed September 17, 2010.

human neurons would still be a mouse brain, in size and architecture, and thus could not have human attributes, including consciousness.[121]

Nevertheless, however unlikely the creation of a mouse with a human brain is, it cannot be absolutely ruled out. Would it be unethical to risk creating such a creature, and if so, why?

One worry is that we human beings would not know how to treat such a creature. Would a Stuart Little be a mouse, which could be experimented on and killed? Or a person, with all the rights and protections owed to human subjects? The fact that we would have to figure out what the moral status of such a creature ought to be is not an overriding reason to prohibit creating such an animal, if there are compelling reasons to do it. Nor is this a completely new ethical issue. We already have to confront the moral status of other primates, who have near-human capacities of thought and language. If it were possible to create a creature with the body of a mouse and the thinking capacity (the mind) of a human person—about which I have serious doubts—it is hard to see why that creature would not just be a person, entitled to all the rights and protection of other persons. To say otherwise seems completely unjustified speciesism.

While Cynthia Cohen rejects the "unnatural" and "crosses species boundaries" arguments against the creation of chimeras, as I have, she takes seriously the argument that the creation of chimeras would or might violate human dignity. She begins by rejecting Ruth Macklin's claim that "appeals to dignity are either vague restatements of other, more precise, notions or mere slogans that add nothing to an understanding of the topic."[122] Cohen defends dignity by pointing to its centrality in Kantian moral thought. For Kant, human beings have an unconditioned moral worth or dignity because they are moral agents, responsible for their actions and choices.

In Chapter 1, I said that I accept the Kantian idea that moral agents have a higher moral status than sentient beings that lack the capacity for moral agency. However, even if *moral agents* have unconditioned moral worth or dignity, this does not show that members of the species *Homo sapiens* are possessed of this moral worth or dignity. Any attempt to ascribe dignity to *all* human beings is bound to fail, if the justification for the ascription stems from moral agency, since not all human beings are moral agents.

Therefore, we need to restrict the claim of dignity or unconditioned moral worth to human beings who are moral agents, or perhaps have the capacity to become moral agents. What implications might this have for restricting the creation of chimeras in stem cell research? Cohen starts from the idea that it would be wrong to deprive beings with a capacity for moral agency from exercising that capacity. That is why slavery is intrinsically wrong, even when it is not accompanied (as it usually is) with the infliction of suffering. The slave is a rational agent, who is not permitted to act as a rational agent, but rather is used as an instrument of another's will. Taking the argument a step further, Cohen argues that it would be wrong to create beings whose

121. Ibid.

122. Ruth Macklin. 2003. "Dignity Is a Useless Concept," *British Medical Journal* 327: 1419–1420, p. 1419.

capacity for rational thought and moral agency would be restricted, and she thinks that this might happen if nonhuman animals with human brains were created through the implantation of human neural cells in nonhuman brains. "The human dignity argument maintains that to carry out such a study would violate human dignity because it would render the resulting chimera incapable of exercising its distinctively human capacities, since its brain would be imprisoned in an animal-like body."[123]

But why would a brain with distinctively human capacities be incapable of functioning in a nonhuman body? The assumption seems to be that a brain with distinctively human capacities of thought could function only in a human body, but what is the rationale for this assumption? It is certainly possible to imagine a human mind in a nonhuman body. Perhaps the idea is that a chimera who lacks the voice box characteristic of members of our species would not be able to speak, and that this might render it "incapable of exercising its distinctively human capacities." However, the capacity for speech is not necessary for thought: think of Stephen Hawking, who has a computer to talk for him, or people (and chimpanzees) who use sign language.

I conclude that Cohen's appeal to human dignity as a justification for prohibiting scientists from implanting human cells into animal brains fails. Still, it must be acknowledged that many people are deeply offended by the very idea of a creature with a human brain in an animal body. Although it is extremely unlikely that this would be the result of transferring human neural cells into an animal's brain, it cannot be ruled out as impossible. A better justification for a prohibition on the introduction of hESCs into animal brains is simply that this is offensive to too many people without a compelling justification for doing it. This sort of prohibition would not significantly set back hESC research. Unless and until there is a compelling reason to transplant human neural cells into animal brains, this seems the sort of compromise that advocates of hESC research should be willing to make.

LAW AND POLICY IN THE UNITED STATES

Religious and moral opposition to the destruction of human embryos has limited embryonic stem cell research in the United States, where much of the work is funded privately. Several states have passed legislation that encourages or even funds embryonic stem cell research, including California, Connecticut, Illinois, Iowa, Maryland, Massachusetts, New Jersey, and New York. Such research is currently illegal in Florida, Louisiana, Maine, Michigan, Minnesota, North Dakota, Pennsylvania, and Rhode Island. Some states, such as Nebraska, prohibit the use of state funds for research that destroys embryos. A number of states prohibit reproductive or therapeutic cloning of human embryos.[124]

Federal funding of embryo research began in 1993 when, under the leadership of President Bill Clinton, Congress passed the National Institutes of Health (NIH) Revitalization Act. For the first time, the NIH was given direct authority to fund human embryo research. In 1994, the NIH established the Human Embryo Research

---

123. Cohen, *Renewing the Stuff of Life* (see note 24), p. 126.

124. The Hinxton Group. 2006. *World Stem Cell Polices.* http://www.hinxtongroup.org/wp_am_exc.html. Accessed October 30, 2010.

Panel (HERP), composed of scientists, ethicists, public policy experts, and patients' advocates, and asked it to consider the moral and ethical issues involved and to recommend ethical guidelines for all future federally funded research on human embryos.[125] (It is a peculiarity of the American legal system that research is often restricted by withholding federal funds, rather than by outright bans on certain kinds of research.)

HERP spent 3 months debating the moral significance of the distinction between using (and destroying) spare embryos from fertility clinics that were destined for disposal (or permanent freezing) and creating embryos for research purposes. Those who thought the distinction was important argued that to create embryos for research treated the embryos as mere means to an end, and therefore showed insufficient respect. Others focused on the reaction of the public, arguing that the issue of creating research embryos be put off until the public became more comfortable with research on spare embryos.[126] Patricia King, professor of law at Georgetown University and policy cochair of the Panel, was concerned about a disparate impact on African American women if there were a demand for eggs for research. Although she recognized the need for some research requiring the deliberate fertilization of oocytes, especially research improving fertility medicine, she "dug in her heels when any wider use was proposed. She was especially unhappy with any permission based merely on an inadequate supply of embryos for research."[127] Opposing Professor King was Dr. Brigid Hogan, a research scientist who argued that research validity required having a population of normal embryos, and this meant research embryos. Dr. Hogan also rejected the notion that creating embryos for research failed to demonstrate appropriate respect. She "insisted that the greatest respect that could be shown the embryo was to conduct research on it that is important and valid."[128] Eventually the Panel recommended that federal funding should be available for research on spare embryos from fertility clinics and also on embryos created specifically for research purposes, "when a compelling case can be made that this is necessary for the validity of a study that is potentially of outstanding scientific and therapeutic value."[129] The kinds of studies the Panel had in mind were ones that would improve infertility treatment, such as examining the effects of teratogens on fertilization and embryonic development. According to Ronald Green, this would not in theory rule out the use of research embryos to derive hESCs, if this were the only way to do research that was potentially of outstanding scientific and therapeutic value. However, the Panel did not consider the use of embryos in hESC research, simply because the research was so little advanced at that time.[130] In any event, President Clinton rejected the panel's recommendation regarding embryos specifically created for research and directed NIH to fund only research using spare embryos.

125. Ronald M. Green. 2001. *The Human Embryo Research Debates: Bioethics in the Vortex of Controversy.* New York: Oxford University Press, p. ix.

126. Ibid., p. 82

127. Ibid., p. 83.

128. Ibid.

129. Ibid., 84.

130. Personal communication from Ronald Green.

Even that was too much for Congress. In 1996, under the leadership of Newt Gingrich, Congress passed a law known as the Dickey-Wicker Amendment. Named for its authors, Representative Jay Dickey, Republican of Arkansas, and Representative Roger Wicker, Republican of Mississippi, the law bans federal financing for any "research in which a human embryo or embryos are destroyed, discarded or knowingly subjected to risk of injury or death." "Congress has actively renewed that ban each year since, thus relegating all human embryo research to the private sector."[131]

The Dickey-Wicker Amendment predated embryonic stem cell research, which really got its start in 1998, when a team headed by James Thomson at the University of Wisconsin, using private funds, successfully created the first human embryonic stem cell lines from surplus IVF embryos.[132] However, the amendment appeared to preclude the use of federal funds for embryonic stem cell research, which would greatly hamper research that had the potential to revolutionize medicine. In January 1999, Harriet Rabb, the top lawyer at the Department of Health and Human Services (DHHS), found a way around the Dickey-Wicker Amendment. She argued that federal funds could not be used to derive stem cell lines, because derivation of stem cells involves embryo destruction, but that federal funds could be used to fund subsequent research on the cells. She maintained that embryonic stem cells were not embryos, and therefore the Dickey-Wicker Amendment did not apply to them. This interpretation was used by the Clinton Administration to allow the funding of research with stem cells that other, privately funded scientists had already derived from spare embryos slated for destruction at fertility clinics.

Many people, even including some supporters of hESC research, found the DHHS's interpretation of the Dickey-Wicker Amendment dubious, and an end-run around Congressional intent. It was opposition to the destruction of human embryos in research that led Congress to pass the Dickey-Wicker Amendment in the first place. To interpret the Amendment as applying only to the actual destruction of embryos, and not to research that requires their destruction, seems, as Republican Senator Sam Brownback put it, a bit of "legal sophistry."[133] Law professor Dena Davis, who supports hESC research, and opposes the Dickey-Wicker Amendment, agrees. She writes:

Dickey-Wicker promises that embryos will not be destroyed with taxpayer's money, thus relieving pro-life citizens of the burden of paying for something they find morally abhorrent. DHHS's interpretation, in contrast, says, "Don't worry—we aren't using your money to destroy embryos, we're just using it to do research on stem cells from embryos that were destroyed in a lab across the street." But if it is abhorrent to participate in embryo destruction, it is equally

131. Kyla Dunn, "The Politics of Stem Cells," NOVA scienceNOW. http://www.pbs.org/wgbh/nova/body/stem-cells-politics.html. Accessed September 8, 2010.

132. James A. Thomson, Joseph Itskovitz-Eldor, Sander S. Shapiro, Michelle A. Waknitz, Jennifer J. Swiergiel, Vivienne S. Marshall, and Jeffrey M. Jones. 1998. "Embryonic Stem Cell Lines Derived From Human Blastocysts." *Science* 282 (5391): 1145–1147.

133. Dunn, "The Politics of Stem Cells" (see note 131).

abhorrent to support research on stem cells that can only be obtained by embryo destruction.[134]

Nevertheless, the DHHS interpretation of the amendment was not challenged by President Bush, even as he ordered new restrictions on federal funding for hESC research. In a televised speech to the nation on the evening of August 9, 2001, President Bush offered a compromise that made no one very happy. He allowed federal funding for some embryonic stem cell research, which offended those opposed to all such research, but limited the funding to research on stem cell lines that had been created prior to his speech. This displeased scientists who said that the existing 22 lines were not sufficient for research. They noted that dozens of other stem cell lines had been created using private funds, some of which were easier to access, easier to maintain in the lab, easier to turn into cell types of interest, and more likely to contribute to human therapies, since they had not come into contact with mouse cells, as had all of the existing stem cell lines approved for research under the Bush policy.[135]

Barack Obama promised to lift restrictions on hESC research during his presidential campaign. In March 2009, shortly after he took office, President Obama issued an executive order entitled "Removing Barriers to Responsible Scientific Research Involving Human Stem Cells." This order explicitly revoked the Bush policy and gave authority to the Secretary of State, through the Director of NIH, to "support and conduct responsible, scientifically worthy human stem cell research, including human embryonic stem cell research, to the extent permitted by law."[136]

In July 2009, new guidelines for hESC research created by NIH went into effect.[137] The guidelines restate the Raab interpretation of the Dickey-Wicker Amendment, namely, that the amendment prohibits NIH funding for the derivation of stem cells from human embryos. However, research using hESCs is eligible for federal funding, if the embryonic stem cells were derived from spare embryos created by IVF. Research using stem cell lines derived from embryos created specifically for research purposes may not receive federal funding, nor can federal funding be used to clone human embryos to derive hESCs. The guidelines further require that the donors of the embryos must give informed consent for them to be used in research, and the donors may receive no payment, cash or in kind, for the donated embryos. Moreover, there must be a clear separation between the decision to create embryos for reproductive

134. Dena Davis. 2010. "Restoring Human Embryonic Stem Cell Research," *Bioethics Forum*, August 31. http://www.thehastingscenter.org/Bioethicsforum/Post.aspx?id=4843&blogid=140&utm_source=constantcontact&utm_medium=email&utm_campaign=bioethicsforum20100901/. Accessed September 9, 2010.

135. Dunn, "The Politics of Stem Cells" (see note 131).

136. The White House. 2009. Executive Order 13505, "Removing Barriers to Responsible Scientific Research Involving Human Stem Cells," March 9. http://www.whitehouse.gov/the_press_office/Removing-Barriers-to-Responsible-Scientific-Research-Involving-Human-Stem-Cells/. Accessed September 5, 2010.

137. National Institutes of Health Guidelines on Human Stem Cell Research. 2009. http://stemcells.nih.gov/policy/2009guidelines.htm. Accessed September 8, 2010.

purposes and the decision to donate embryos no longer needed for this purpose to research.

In its 2005 Guidelines, the National Academies called for the establishment of Embryonic Stem Cell Research Oversight (ESCRO) committees at every institution conducting hESC research, to provide local oversight of hESC research. Every institution that has federal funding must have an Institutional Review Board (IRB) to oversee and approve biomedical and behavioral research involving human beings, with the aim of protecting human subjects. ESCROs do not substitute for IRBS but rather "provide an additional level of review and scrutiny warranted by the complex issues raised by hES cell research."[138] The Guidelines also provide limits to such research, specifying as research that "should not be permitted at this time" the keeping of embryos in culture longer than 14 days or until formation of the primitive streak, whichever occurs first;[139] the introduction of hESCs into nonhuman primate blastocysts; and the breeding of any animal into which hESCs have been introduced.[140]

Embryonic stem cell research was thrown into disarray in August 2010, when a federal judge, Royce Lamberth, ordered a temporary halt to federal funding of embryonic stem cell research, saying that President Obama's executive order expanding such funding violated the Dickey-Wicker Amendment. Critics of the decision noted that it goes against a long-standing interpretation of the Amendment, from the Clinton Administration to the present day, and one to which Congress has never objected. As Professor Hank Greely of Stanford Law School points out, the Dickey-Wicker Amendment is part of the annual Appropriations Act, which lays out the budget for government agencies, and thus is reapproved by Congress each year. "'Every year when Congress re-passes the Appropriations Act, it could have changed the language if it thought the interpretations were wrong,' he explains."[141]

The court order is the result of a lawsuit originally filed in August 2009 against the Department of Health and Human Services (HHS) and the NIH, contending that federal funding for research on human embryonic stem cells is illegal because it requires the destruction of embryos. The suit was dismissed in October 2009 on the ground that the plaintiffs—listed in court documents as two Christian organizations, six individuals, and "embryos"—lacked legal standing, that is, had no tangible interest in its outcome. However, two scientists on the plaintiff list, Dr. James L. Sherley and Dr. Theresa Deisher, who work exclusively with adult stem cells, appealed and were granted standing on the basis that they would be irreparably harmed by competition for federal funding under the Obama policy. In response, the government pointed out that Dr. Sherley has received three NIH grants, out of eight applications,

138. NCR and IOM. 2005. *Guidelines on hESC Research* (see note 104), p. 5.

139. The imposition of a 14-day limit for keeping embryos alive in vitro was first articulated by the Ethics Advisory Board in the United States in 1979, and then incorporated into the Warnock Report in 1985.

140. Final Report of The National Academies' Human Embryonic Stem Cell Research Advisory Committee and Amendments to The National Academies' Guidelines for Human Embryonic Stem Cell Research. 2010. Washington, D.C.: The National Academies Press.

141. Alla Katsnelson. 2010. "US Court Suspends Research on Human Embryonic Stem Cells," Naturenews. August 25. http://www.nature.com/news/2010/100824/full/news.2010.428.html. Accessed September 8, 2010.

and Dr. Deisher has never applied for one. It seems clear that the claim of economic harm was merely a pretext for the plaintiffs to gain standing. The real motivation for the case was the researchers' opposition to embryonic stem cell research, which they characterized as "morally objectionable and unlikely to produce promised treatments or cures."[142]

Judge Lamberth's ruling came as a shock to researchers at NIH and universities around the country, who viewed the Obama policy and its interpretation of the Dickey-Wicker Amendment as settled law.[143] Many scientists were confused about what the ruling meant for their work—whether they could continue under the Bush Administration rules, or whether all research on embryonic stem cells could no longer be funded. The Obama Administration asked Judge Lambeth to stay his ruling barring the federal government from funding ongoing hESC research while the case proceeds through the courts. In its brief, the government said that a halt would cause irreparable harm to experiments and could negate years of scientific progress toward new treatments for a range of diseases. The government said a total of $546 million has been awarded for such research to date, and that the investment could be wasted if the research is halted even temporarily; mice being used in lab experiments, for instance, might not survive until funding resumes.[144] Judge Lamberth rejected the appeal, saying that the government's "parade of horribles" that will supposedly result from the preliminary injunction was incorrect. Two days later, however, the U.S. Court of Appeals ruled that federal funding of embryonic stem cell research could continue while the court considers the case.[145]

The simplest, most direct way to ensure federal funding for hESC research would be to amend or repeal the Dickey-Wicker Amendment. As Professor Davis writes, "Putting Dickey-Wicker back on the table will allow us to have an honest and robust national discussion about research with human embryos."[146] She suggests that the amendment be revised to exclude extracorporeal embryos, noting that polls show that a majority of Americans support embryonic stem cell research, just as they accept IVF, which creates the nearly half a million embryos now frozen in clinics across the country. Representative Diana DeGette (D-Colorado) agrees. Reacting to the Lamberth decision, she said, "This court opinion hit everybody by surprise. It calls all of these policies of the last 10 years into question. I think what it really underscores is the extreme urgency for Congress to act to codify ethical embryonic

142. Laura Meckler and Janet Adamy. 2010. "Stem-Cell Plaintiffs Cite Ethical Motivation," September 2. WSJ.com. http://online.wsj.com/article/SB10001424052748704791004575466081896678078.html. Accessed October 31, 2010.

143. Gardiner Harris. 2010. "U.S. Judge Rules Against Obama's Stem Cell Policy," August 23. *New York Times.* http://www.nytimes.com/2010/08/24/health/policy/24stem.html. Accessed September 8, 2010.

144. Laura Meckler. 2010. "Judge Is Asked to Lift Stem-Cell Funds Ban," September 1. WSJ.com. http://online.wsj.com/article/SB10001424052748703467004575463872413480384.html. Accessed September 8, 2010.

145. Gardiner Harris. 2010. "Stem Cell Financing Ban Ends, for Now," *New York Times,* September 10, A14.

146. Davis, "Restoring Human Embryonic Stem Cell Research" (see note 134).

stem cell research."[147] She has introduced a bill that would not repeal Dickey-Wicker but instead would clarify Congress's intention to exempt hESC research from the amendment.[148]

Is a political solution possible? While some doubt that legislators will have the political nerve to take on a controversial issue before midterm elections, others think that, given the popularity of embryonic stem cell research with the public, "a legislative fight on the issue could prove a tonic for Democrats battling a tough political environment."[149] In addition to Ms. DeGette's bill, both Senator Arlen Specter (D-Pennsylvania) and Senator Tom Harkin (D-Iowa) have introduced legislation to allow federal funding of hESC research. Conceivably, such legislation could receive bipartisan support, as it is supported by some who oppose abortion. For example, Senator Orrin Hatch (R-Utah), who is strongly pro-life, is nevertheless an enthusiastic supporter of hESC research because of its medical potential and because, in his view, "a frozen embryo stored in a refrigerator in a clinic" just isn't the same as "a fetus developing in a mother's womb."[150] Moreover, as Hatch said at a congressional hearing, "The reality today is that each year thousands of embryos are routinely destroyed [in fertility clinics]. Why shouldn't embryos slated for destruction be used for the benefit of mankind?"[151]

Cloning Policy

In 2002, the President's Council on Bioethics, appointed by President George W. Bush, revisited the question of human cloning.[152] It agreed with NBAC that cloning should not be used to create a child, but it was unable to reach consensus on the question of cloning for biomedical research. Seven members of the Council wanted to see the research go forward, but under strict regulation. Ten members were opposed to cloning for biomedical research, largely because it would be used primarily for stem cell research that involved destroying human embryos. Some members also were concerned that if cloning is permitted, it would be impossible to restrict it to biomedical research. They maintained that cloning-for-biomedical research will lead—intentionally or not—to cloning to produce children.[153] Still other Council

147. Sheryl Gaye Stolberg and Gardiner Harris. 2010. "Stem Cell Ruling Will Be Appealed," *New York Times,* August 24. http://www.nytimes.com/2010/08/25/health/policy/25stem.html. Accessed September 17, 2010.

148. Richard E. Cohen. 2010. "Stem Cell Bill Could See Vote," Politico.com, September 3. http://www.politico.com/news/stories/0910/41731.html. Accessed September 10, 2010.

149. Harris, "Stem Cell Financing Ban Ends, for Now" (see note 145).

150. Sharon Begley. 2001. Cellular Divide. *Newsweek.* July 9. http://www.newsweek.com/2001/07/08/cellular-divide.html. Accessed September 10, 2010.

151. "Research Foes Decry Embryo Slaughter." 2001. CNN.com/Health. http://archives.cnn.com/2001/HEALTH/07/17/stem.cell.hearing/. Accessed September 10, 2010.

152. The President's Council on Bioethics. 2002. *Human Cloning and Human Dignity: An Ethical Inquiry.* Washington, D.C.: U.S. Government Printing Office.

153. Ibid., p. 163.

members focused on possible dangers to, and exploitation of, women who are egg donors.

Several bills that would ban cloning, reproductive or therapeutic, have been introduced into Congress, but, as of this writing, none of these bills has passed (most remain stuck in committee). As a result, there is no federal law in the United States banning hESC research at this time. (Neither is there any federal law banning reproductive cloning, but that is because bills attempting to ban reproductive cloning have been held hostage by those who oppose therapeutic cloning and hESC research generally.) However, as mentioned earlier, according to the 2009 NIH Guidelines, federal funding may not be used on research with cloned embryos. Some states ban research on cloned embryos, including Arkansas, Indiana, Michigan, North Dakota, and South Dakota. Louisiana is the only state that specifically prohibits research on IVF embryos. California, Connecticut, Illinois, Iowa, Massachusetts, New Jersey, New York, and Rhode Island have statutes that prohibit reproductive cloning but allow cloning for research.[154] However, it is worth repeating that, to date, no stem cell lines have been created from cloned human embryos.

LAW AND POLICY IN OTHER COUNTRIES

Thirty-four countries, including Australia, Brazil, Canada, China, Denmark, Iran, Israel, Japan, Norway, Spain, Sweden, and the United Kingdom, support or have policies that are viewed as permissive for embryonic stem cell research. Most countries that have laws or policies on stem cell research have fairly standard guidelines requiring informed consent from egg or embryo donors, prevention of coercion, the keeping detailed records, and allowance for conscientious objection on the part of center workers. The differences center around whether it is permitted to create embryos for research purposes, and whether therapeutic cloning is allowed. However, it is not always easy to tell precisely what is permitted or forbidden, because the guidelines may be poorly written, with undefined terms, or even internally contradictory.[155]

In April 2005, the European Commissioner for Science and Research announced that the European Union (EU) would continue to fund embryonic stem cell research from 2007 to 2013. To allow initial EU funding for stem cell research, the EU had to clarify its stem cell rules in November 2003. It allowed funding of embryonic stem cell research regardless of the date that stem cells were procured from embryos. The creation of human embryos for purposes of stem cell procurement was not allowed, but it was implied (though not directly stated) that it would allow funding for research using spare embryos.

154. National Conference of State Legislatures (NCSL). 2008. "Stem Cell Research." http://www.ncsl.org/default.aspx?tabid=14413 Accessed September 17, 2010.

155. Søren Holm. 2007. "The Status of the Extracorporeal Embryo in Denmark From a Comparative Legal Perspective." In A. Eser, H. G. Koch, and C. Seith, eds., *International Perspectives on the Status and Protection of the Extracorporeal Embryo*, pp. 37–57. Baden-Baden, Germany: Nomos.

Among the countries characterized as permissive, China has been described as "probably the most liberal environment for embryo research in the world."[156] There are no laws governing hESC research in China, although such research must be endorsed by the Ministry of Health. Singapore and South Korea also have research-friendly policies,[157] although South Korea bans payment to oocyte donors.[158] This usually means fewer egg donors and "without willing donors, there will be less research on human embryonic stem cells."[159]

Israel bans reproductive cloning, but it allows both therapeutic cloning and the production of new embryonic stem cell lines. As a Jewish state, Israel's laws follow Halacha, or Talmudic law. According to an article in the *Jerusalem Post*, this has led to no restrictions being placed on embryonic stem cell research:

> As Halacha does not regard day-old human embryos as living things and encourages medical research aimed at saving lives, no restrictions have been placed in Israel on researchers in this field except a ban on their use for human cloning.[160]

This statement of Halacha and Israeli law is perhaps a bit misleading. The rationale for the use of extracorporeal embryos in research is not that "day-old embryos" are not "living things." For one thing, stem cells are not derived from "day-old embryos," but rather 4- to 5-day-old embryos. More important, extracorporeal embryos are clearly "living things"; if they were not, they could not be killed, the justification of which is precisely the issue at hand. The question is whether they count as living *human beings*, or to put the point another way, whether they have full moral or legal standing in Jewish law. According to one interpretation of Halacha, they do not:

> From the Talmudic discussion of abortion, we might expect that pre-embryos are not covered by the prohibition of abortion, because they have never been implanted. The rationale for such a decision is based on the concept that a pre-embryo left in its petri dish will die. It is not even potential life until it is implanted in an environment in which it can mature.[161]

156. Judith A. Johnson and Erin D. Williams. 2006. "Stem Cell Research." [Report for Congress]. http://www.usembassy.it/pdf/other/RL31015.pdf. Accessed September 17, 2010.

157. Ibid., p. 34.

158. Radhika Rao. 2006. "Coercion, Commercialization, and Commodification: The Ethics of Compensation for Egg Donors in Stem Cell Research," *Berkeley Technology Law Journal* 21 (3): 1055–1066, p. 1056.

159. Robert Steinbrook. 2006. "Egg Donation and Human Embryonic Stem-Cell Research," *New England Journal of Medicine* 4: 324–326, p. 324.

160. Judy Siegel. 2006. "Israeli Human Embryonic Stem Cell Research is 2nd in World." *Jerusalem Post*. October 6, p. 9.

161. Daniel Eisenberg. 2001. "Stem Cell Research in Jewish Law," *Jewish Law Articles*. http://www.jlaw.com/Articles/stemcellres.html. Accessed September 17, 2010.

Moreover, where there is a risk of transmitting a serious genetic disease, such as Tay-Sachs, Jewish law permits preimplantation genetic diagnosis on extracorporeal embryos and the discarding of affected embryos. From this, Eisenberg draws the following conclusion:

> If the pre-embryo may be destroyed, it certainly may be used for research purpose [sic] and other life-saving work. In fact, Rabbi Moshe Dovid Tendler, in testimony for the National Bioethics Advisory Commission, argued strongly in favor of the use of pre-embryos for stem cell research. Nevertheless, it is important to realize that this conclusion is not unanimous and that all of these rulings are predicated upon the understanding that the pre-embryo is not included in the prohibition of *retzicha* (murder).[162]

Australia, Canada, and the United Kingdom are characterized as permissive in their approach to hESC research. However, Canada prohibits all forms of human cloning, while both the United Kingdom and Australia allow grant licenses for therapeutic cloning. All three prohibit payments or other inducements for the donation of gametes or embryos. The reimbursement of reasonable out-of-pocket expenses is acceptable in these countries, but not compensation for time or lost wages, which contrasts with the recommendation given by the National Academy of Sciences in the United States. Sweden and Denmark are both characterized as permissive, although Sweden seems more permissive than Denmark, because Sweden allows the destruction of embryos for the derivation of new cell lines and the creation of embryos by NT, for example, whereas Denmark allows only the use of spare embryos and does not allow the cloning of human embryos to derive stem cell lines.[163]

In contrast to the most permissive countries, relative newcomers to hESC research, such as Brazil, are fairly restrictive. For example, Brazil passed legislation in 2005 that permits the derivation of stem cell lines only from embryos frozen for at least 3 years and considered unsuitable for human reproduction. Research on healthy, viable spare embryos is prohibited, as is the creation of embryos for research. Among the most restrictive countries are Germany, Austria, Italy, and Ireland, all of which ban the destruction of human embryos to create stem cell lines. The biggest influence on German and Austrian policy is the Nazi legacy, and the postwar German commitment to respecting human dignity. In part, this concern extended to the human embryo. However, in part, German opposition to cloning and human embryonic stem cell research is based on opposition to future genetic manipulation, and a slippery slope to eugenics,[164] while prohibitions in Italy and Ireland come primarily from the influence of the Roman Catholic Church. At the same time, the German Stem Cell Act passed in July 2002, which forbids either importing or deriving new stem cell lines, does not prohibit all hESC research. Instead, its policy resembles the Bush policy of permitting researchers to work with cell lines already derived, in this case,

162. Ibid.

163. E-mail communication from Søren Holm.

164. See, for example, Jurgen Habermas. 2003. *The Future of Human Nature*. Malden, MA: Polity Press.

before January 2002.[165] Similarly, while the Italian IVF law of February 2004 bans the creation or destruction of an embryo for research purposes, it does not specify any regulations regarding human stem cells, thus leaving researchers free to work on cell lines that are already established.[166]

In addition to the laws and policies of individual countries, the United Nations (UN) is a body that seeks to achieve "international co-operation in solving international problems of an economic, social, cultural, or humanitarian character,"[167] and thus it could be a forum for discussing the ethics of human embryonic stem cell research. To date, it has not done so, but the UN has adopted a nonbinding declaration urging the prohibition of all forms of human cloning.

United Nations Declaration on Human Cloning

In November 2004, the UN considered two international conventions against human cloning. One, introduced by Costa Rica, and backed by the United States, aimed to ban all human embryonic cloning. The other, introduced by Belgium, sought to proscribe only reproductive cloning. To avert a divisive vote, the General Assembly adopted Italy's proposal to take up the issue again in February as a declaration, rather than a convention, as declarations are nonbinding. On March 8, 2005, the General Assembly of the United Nations adopted a Declaration on Human Cloning, urging Member States to adopt "all measures necessary to prohibit all forms of human cloning inasmuch as they are incompatible with human dignity and the protection of human life."[168] The vote was 84 in favor to 34 against, with 37 abstentions. Several delegations voted against the declaration because the reference to "human life" could be interpreted as a call for a total ban on all forms of human cloning, including therapeutic cloning. The UK representative regretted the UN's having missed an opportunity for a global ban on reproductive cloning, "because of the intransigence of those who were not prepared to recognize that other sovereign States might decide to permit strictly controlled applications of therapeutic cloning."[169] Noting that it was a nonbinding resolution, he said that the vote would not affect UK policy. Similar statements were made by representatives of other countries favorable to hESC research. By contrast, those in favor of the Declaration said that it constituted an important step in the protection of human dignity and the promotion of human rights, as well as a first step toward a complete ban on human cloning.

165. Sarah Webb and Elisabeth Pain. 2006. "Navigating the Stem-Cell Research Maze," *Science Careers*. http://sciencecareers.sciencemag.org/career_development/previous_issues/articles/2006_12_01/navigating_the_stem_cell_research_maze. Accessed September 17, 2010.

166. Ibid.

167. Charter of the United Nations. Chapter 1, Article 1. http://www.un.org/en/documents/charter/chapter1.shtml. Accessed October 31, 2010.

168. Press Release. 2008. "General Assembly Adopts United Nations Declaration on Human Cloning by Vote of 84-34-37." http://www.un.org/News/Press/docs/2005/ga10333.doc.htm. Accessed September 17, 2010.

169. Ibid.

In my view, such appeals to human dignity and human rights are misplaced. Neither the cloning of embryos, nor their destruction in research, threatens human dignity or human rights. Indeed, exactly the opposite will be true, if hESC proves successful in curing disease and preventing premature death. Of course, at this point, no one knows whether the research will succeed—whether it will revolutionize medicine or prove to be a dead end. However, if uncertainty about success were a reason not to do research, there could never be any medical progress at all. Given its potential to cure such a wide range of diseases, it seems worth a serious effort.

Discarded-created distinction, 278–282.
  See also Embryo
Dresser, Rebecca, 276, 282
Dawson, Karen, 61
Dead people, 15
  as antemortem people, 16–17
  dead bodies, 15, 30, 274, 275 *n.* 80
  interests of, 16–17
  possibility of harming, 17
Decent minimum standard, 86–87, 90,
    91–92, 152, 213, 214, 225. *See also*
    Nonexistence condition
DES (diethylstilbestrol), 113–115.
    See also Preconception torts
Dietrich v. Northampton, 110, 128
Different People Choices, 34. *See also*
    Same People Choices
Disability critique, 143–144, 219–224
Discarded-created distinction. *See*
    Embryo
Double effect, principle of, 279–280
Down syndrome, 142–143, 152, 219,
    222
Drug use during pregnancy
  as child abuse, 169–172
  as criminal offense, 168
  and criminal prosecution for
    homicide, 172–174
  as dangerous to fetal health, 165–168
  difficulty in getting treatment for, 169
  incarceration to protect fetus from,
    176–179
  public health approach to, 175–176
  and termination of parental rights,
    155, 179–182
Dworkin, Ronald, 97 *n.* 167, 107

Egg donation, 243–254, 283–284.
    See also Gametes
Eisenstadt v. Baird, 97
Elective single embryo transfer (eSET),
    225–226, 228, 229
Elshtain, Jean, 54
Emanuel, Ezekiel, 228–229
Emanuel, Linda. *See* Emanuel, Ezekiel
Embodied mind account, 71–74
Embryo
  and autonomous goodness, 35
  and beginning of human
    organism, 269

and brain function, 45
and discarded-created distinction,
    278–282
dispositional problems with,
    230–239
implantation of, 50
impossibility of sentience in, 268, 271
moral standing of, 40, 268–270;
    contrasted with moral status of
    babies, 269–270
as potential person, 81
preimplantation, 232
respect for, 270–278
as source of embryonic stem
    cells, 268
spare, 259
symbolic value of, 35, 233
Empire State Stem Cell Board, 283
Engelhardt, H. Tristram, Jr., 54–55
Enright v. Lilly & Co., 113–114
Environmental ethic
  as consistent with interest view,
    11–12
Equal protection argument
  as basis for right to abortion, 97
  and fetal protection, 116, 188
Ethics Advisory Board (EAB),
    295 *n.* 139

Feinberg, Joel, 2, 5, 8–9, 11–12, 16–17,
    34 *n.* 95, 54 *n.* 56, 55, 63, 82,
    146–148, 151–152
Fertility Clinic Success Rate and
    Certification Act. *See* Wyden Act
Fetal alcohol syndrome (FAS). *See* Fetal
    health, dangers to
Fetal health, dangers to
  fetal alcohol syndrome (FAS),
    158, 163
  from moderate alcohol consumption,
    163–164
  from cocaine, 165–166
  from heroin, 166
  from marijuana, 167
  from methamphetamines, 166
  from poverty, 168
  from tobacco, 162–163
Fetal rights, 107, 109 *n.* 3, 115,
    116 *n.* 50, 118, 125 *n.* 75, 161.
    See also Fetus

CPSIA information can be obtained at www.ICGtesting.com
Printed in the USA
BVOW09s0511191214

379959BV00001B/4/P

9 780195 341621